Major Depressive Disorder

Major Depressive Disorder

Editor-in-Chief

ROGER S. MCINTYRE, M.D., FRCPC

Professor of Psychiatry and Pharmacology, University of Toronto, Toronto, Canada

Chairman and Executive Director, Brain and Cognition Discovery Foundation (BCDF), Toronto, Canada

Director, Depression and Bipolar Support Alliance (DBSA), Chicago, USA

Head, Mood Disorders Psychopharmacology Unit
Professor and Nanshan Scholar, Guangzhou Medical University, Guangzhou, China

Adjunct Professor College of Medicine, Korea University, Seoul, Republic of Korea

Clinical Professor State University of New York (SUNY) Upstate Medical University, Syracuse, New York, USA

Associate Editors

CAROLA RONG, MD
Department of Psychiatry and Behavioral Sciences
University of Texas Health Science Center at Houston
Houston, TX, United States

MEHALA SUBRAMANIAPILLAI, MSC
Mood Disorders Psychopharmacology Unit
Toronto Western Hospital
United Health Network
Toronto, ON, Canada

YENA LEE, HBSC
Mood Disorders Psychopharmacology Unit
Toronto Western Hospital
United Health Network
Toronto, ON, Canada

ELSEVIER

Major Depressive Disorder   ISBN: 978-0-323-58131-8

Publisher: Patrick Manley
Acquisition Editor: Lauren Boyle
Editorial Project Manager: Megan Ashdown
Production Project Manager: Poulouse Joseph
Cover Designer: Alan Studholme

3251 Riverport Lane
St. Louis, Missouri 63043

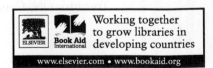

Working together
to grow libraries in
developing countries

www.elsevier.com • www.bookaid.org

List of Contributors

Fariya Ali, BS, MD
Resident Physician
Psychiatry
University of Miami Miller School of Medicine
Department of Psychiatry
Miami, FL, United States

Ali Bani-Fatemi, PhD
Centre for Addiction and Mental Health (CAMH)
Toronto, ON, Canada

Isabelle E. Bauer, PhD
Assistant Professor
University of Texas Health Science Center at Houston
McGovern Medical School
Department of Psychiatry and Behavioral Sciences
Houston, TX, United States

Bernhard T. Baune, PhD, MD, MPH, FRANZCP
Florey Institute of Neuroscience and Mental Health
Melbourne Brain Centre
University of Melbourne
Melbourne, VIC, Australia

Department of Psychiatry
Melbourne Medical School
University of Melbourne
Melbourne, VIC, Australia

Department of Psychiatry
University of Münster
Münster, Germany

Venkat Bhat, MD, MSc, FRCPC, DABPN
Department of Psychiatry
Sunnybrook Health Sciences Centre
Toronto, ON, Canada

Justin N. Chee, PhD(c), MSc, HonBSc
Research Staff
Psychiatry
Sunnybrook Health Sciences Centre
Toronto, ON, Canada

Amy Cheung, MD, MSc, FRCP(C)
Associate Professor
Psychiatry
University of Toronto
Sunnybrook Health Sciences Centre
Toronto, ON, Canada

Alexandria S. Coles, BA
Research Assistant
Mood Disorders Psychopharmacology Unit
Toronto Western Hospital
United Health Network
Toronto, ON, Canada

Timothy M. Cooper, MD
Resident Physician
Psychiatry, NYU School of Medicine
New York, NY, United States

Oluwagbenga O. Dada, BSc
Centre for Addiction and Mental Health (CAMH)
Toronto, ON, Canada

Vincenzo De Luca, MD, PhD
Centre for Addiction and Mental Health (CAMH)
Toronto, ON, Canada

Doctor
Psychiatry
University of Toronto
Toronto, ON, Canada

Erin C. Dunn, ScD, MPH
Assistant in Research
Psychiatric and Neurodevelopmental Genetics Unit
Center for Genomic Medicine
Massachusetts General Hospital
Boston, MA, United States

Assistant Professor
Department of Psychiatry
Harvard Medical School
Boston, MA, United States

Peter Giacobbe, MD, MSc, FRCPC
Department of Psychiatry
University of Toronto
Toronto, ON, Canada

Department of Psychiatry
Sunnybrook Health Sciences Centre
Toronto, ON, Canada

Faculty of Medicine
University of Toronto
Toronto, ON, Canada

Ariel Graff, MD, PhD
Centre for Addiction and Mental Health (CAMH)
Toronto, ON, Canada

Tracy L. Greer, BA, MS, PhD, MSCS
Associate Professor
Department of Psychiatry
UT Southwestern Medical Center
Center for Depression Research and Clinical Care
Dallas, TX, United States

Dan V. Iosifescu, MD, MSc
Associate Professor of Psychiatry
Psychiatry
NYU School of Medicine
New York, NY, United States

Director of Clinical Research
Nathan S. Kline Institute for Psychiatric Research
Orangeburg, NY, United States

Jeethu K. Joseph, BS
Clinical Data Specialist
Department of Psychiatry
UT Southwestern Medical Center
Center for Depression Research and Clinical Care
Dallas, TX, United States

Jungjin Kim, MD
Addiction Psychiatry Fellow
Harvard Medical School
Boston, MA, United States

Yena Lee, HBSc
Mood Disorders Psychopharmacology Unit
Toronto Western Hospital
United Health Network
Toronto, ON, Canada

Roger Chun Man Ho, MD, MRCPsych, FRCPC
Associate Professor and Senior Consultant
Department of Psychological Medicine
National University of Singapore
Singapore, Singapore

Roger S. McIntyre, MD, FRCP(C)
Head
Mood Disorders Psychopharmacology Unit
Toronto Western Hospital
United Health Network
Toronto, ON, Canada

Professor
Department of Psychiatry
University of Toronto
Toronto, ON, Canada

Department of Pharmacology
University of Toronto
Toronto, ON, Canada

Tomas Melicher, MD
Resident
Psychiatry
University of Texas Health Science Center at Houston
McGovern Medical School
Department of Psychiatry and Behavioral Sciences
Houston, TX, United States

Ying Meng, MD
Department of Psychiatry
Sunnybrook Health Sciences Centre
Toronto, ON, Canada

Department of Neurosurgery
University of Toronto
Toronto, ON, Canada

Karim Mithani, M.Eng
Department of Psychiatry
Sunnybrook Health Sciences Centre
Toronto, ON, Canada

Marcellino Monda, MD
University of Campania Vanvitelli
Naples, Italy

Charles B. Nemeroff, MD, PhD
Department of Psychiatry
University of Texas at Austin
Dell Medical School
Austin, TX, United States

Roy H. Perlis, MD, MSc
Center for Quantitative Health
Massachusetts General Hospital and Harvard
  Medical School
Boston, MA, United States

Arvind Rajagopalan, MBBS
Institute of Mental Health
Singapore, Singapore

Joshua D. Rosenblat, BSc, MD
Resident of Psychiatry
University of Toronto
Toronto, ON, Canada

Marsal Sanches, MD, PhD
Associate Professor
Department of Psychiatry and Behavioral Sciences
University of Texas Health Science Center at Houston
McGovern Medical School
Houston, TX, United States

Thomas L. Schwartz, MD
Professor
Department of Psychiatry
SUNY Upstate Medical University
Syracuse, NY, United States

Gaurav Singhal, M.Trop.V.Sc., B.V.Sc. & A.H.
Psychiatric Neuroscience Lab
Discipline of Psychiatry
University of Adelaide
Adelaide, SA, Australia

Jair C. Soares, MD, PhD
Professor and Chairman
University of Texas Health Science Center at Houston
McGovern Medical School
Department of Psychiatry and Behavioral Sciences
Houston, TX, United States

Mehala Subramaniapillai, MSc
Mood Disorders Psychopharmacology Unit
Toronto Western Hospital
United Health Network
Toronto, ON, Canada

Samia Tasmim, MSc
Centre for Addiction and Mental Health (CAMH)
Toronto, ON, Canada

Karen Wang, MD, MEd, FRCP(C)
Assistant Professor
Psychiatry
University of Toronto
Sunnybrook Health Sciences Centre
Toronto, ON, Canada

Kevin Z. Wang, BSc
Centre for Addiction and Mental Health (CAMH)
Toronto, ON, Canada

Min-Jung Wang, ScD
Graduate Student
Psychiatric and Neurodevelopmental Genetics Unit
Center for Genomic Medicine
Massachusetts General Hospital
Boston, MA, United States

Hanjing Wu, MD, PhD
Assistant Professor
University of Texas Health Science Center at Houston
McGovern Medical School
Department of Psychiatry and Behavioral Sciences
Houston, TX, United States

Preface

Globally, major depressive disorder (MDD) debases brain capital more than any other medical disorder. The high incidence and prevalence rate, as well as the early age of onset, low rates of recovery, and high rates of comorbidity account for the extraordinary loss of role function, and associated economic costs. There is no race, ethnic or demographic group, country, and/or culture that is immune from the hazards of MDD.

The foregoing portrait of MDD that I have sketched earlier is a very different portrait than was sketched as recently as 2 decades ago, wherein at that time, MDD was thought to be a relatively mild condition with most individuals recovering and returning to normal life "trajectory." The epidemiologic transition has shifted policy, public health, and clinical/research attention and resources toward noncommunicable disorders (NCD). Major depressive disorder is the most common NCD of young people and is associated with premature aging and shorter life span. Neurobiologic research indicates that the underlying pathogenesis of NCDs is overlapping providing a conceptual framework for why individuals with MDD are differentially affected by many other NCDs (e.g., obesity, cardiovascular disease, diabetes).

The future of MDD research will be guided by the principle of "disaggregation." What I mean by this is that the syndrome of MDD comprises agglutinated dimensions that are both overlapping and discrete in pathoetiology. For example, new treatments are required for general cognitive dysfunction in MDD. There is also an urgent need for novel treatments for disturbances in either motivation and/or reward dysfunction in MDD; critical unmet needs in most individuals affected by this disorder. An additional viable and valuable treatment for adults with MDD would be treatments that robustly and meaningfully improve the chronobiological alterations. This incomplete set of disaggregated targets comports with the biobehavioral matrix proffered by the US NIH the Research Domain Criteria (RDoC). Psychiatry will not develop genuinely novel disease modifying and/or curative therapies that are impactful and scalable by looking for "biomarkers" that correlate with treatment response to conventional antidepressants (e.g., selective serotonin reuptake inhibitors SSRIs) diagnosed with MDD according to DSM-5.0. Clearly, a more sophisticated and biologically informed disease model is required.

There are many metaphors that are suggested as a guiding lesson for psychiatry, including but not limited to metabolic syndrome. For example, it is well known that obesity, dyslipidemia, dysglycemia, and hypertension co-occur at a rate much higher than chance because of shared pathogenesis. Notwithstanding, parsing each phenotype separately has resulted in some major breakthroughs in pharmacologic treatment for several of these dimensions that can be used in combination in persons presenting with multicomponent metabolic syndrome. For MDD, there is a need to fully characterize the neurobiology that subserves the discrete dimensions with an aim to move away from exclusive symptom suppression approaches toward disease modification and cure.

Computational neuroscience, as well as advances in informatics, has given us a capability that is limited only by our knowledge of which variables should be interrogated. It seems very reasonable that using artificial intelligence machine learning, we should be able to fully characterize much of the operating characteristics of neural networks and critical intracellular cascades within neurons and glia that are altered in individuals with MDD. The monoaminergic hypothesis has provided us a rather surprising number of success stories given its serendipitous background. Future treatment discovery and development will be guided by disease models that focus on key targets including, but not limited to, amino acids (e.g., glutamate, GABA), immunoinflammatory systems, mitochondrial biogenesis, oxidative stress, neurotrophic systems, and opioidergics.

Psychosocial modalities of treatment for MDD will be further refined and subject to more rigorous study (e.g., exercise and computer-based manualized psychotherapy), as well as neurostimulatory approaches.

From a population health perspective, greater emphasis on the prevention and "immunization" from MDD is warranted (and already exists in some modalities!) (e.g., population-based exercise). It is concerning that many social determinants of MDD continue to be enduring problems for the global population (e.g., income inequality, wage stagnation, housing dislocation, obesity, exposure to infectious agents).

Taken together what the foregoing implies is that the neuroscientific advances regarding the causes and cures of MDD need to be yoked to public policy changes that target key social determinants. The digital economy has provided tremendous opportunity with respect to the provision of mental health care, as well as to guide treatment discovery and development. A negative externality of the digital economy however has been felt in both the public square (e.g., automation and workplace dislocation), as well as moderating to some extent social support and/or social networks (which may be protective and/or a vulnerability factor to MDD). We need to make the digital economy a "bull" market for our patients beginning with appreciating the negative externalities and mitigating them as much as possible, and exploiting the positive externalities.

In this textbook, I have invited input from global experts who have made independent and substantive contributions to the area of MDD. I purposely sought out individuals who I have identified as scholars who bring prescience, perspicacity, academic scholarship, and pragmatism to the research. The aim is to provide readers with a State of the Union on MDD from mechanisms to management with a view to provide a line of sight for the future. It is obvious that both the research and clinical community in MDD needs to supplant incrementalism with saltatory leaps forward. I thank all of the authors for their contribution. I particularly want to thank all of the patients and families that I have met throughout my career that have given me incredible privilege, incredible purpose, and calling in my life, and have inspired me to find cures (which we will) for MDD.

Roger S. McIntyre

Contents

CHAPTER 1

A Summary of Recent Updates on the Genetic Determinants of Depression*

ERIN C. DUNN, SCD, MPH • MIN-JUNG WANG, SCD • ROY H. PERLIS, MD, MSC

INTRODUCTION

With lifetime prevalence estimates of 6.2% among adolescents[1] and up to 19%[2] among adults, major depressive disorder (MDD) is one of the most common, costly, and disabling mental health conditions worldwide.[3] Its onset is typically early in life, with most individuals first experiencing depression during adolescence.[4] It is also a highly recurrent disorder, with nearly three quarters of people with MDD experiencing a second episode at some point in their lives.[5] Depression contributes substantially to excess mortality, either directly through suicide or indirectly through comorbid chronic conditions,[6] increasing mortality risk by 60%–80%.[7,8] The associated loss in productivity and years of life lived with disability due to MDD also impacts society as a whole.[9,10] For these reasons, depression is projected to be *the* leading cause of disease burden worldwide by 2030.[11]

Efforts to understand the ways in which genes and experience work in concert to shape risk for depression across the lifetime will be key to increasing knowledge about the etiology of this disorder and informing efforts to prevent and treat it. There are now numerous environmental risk factors for depression that are well established, including poverty,[12,13] negative family relationships and parental divorce,[14,15] child maltreatment,[16,17] and other stressful life events more generally.[18,19] Although the risk of depression is elevated in the immediate aftermath of experiencing these environmental adversities, the effects of adversity can persist over the life course.[20,21] Indeed, these environmental risk factors have been found to at least double the risk of youth- and adult-onset mental disorders.[22–24] Evidence is also beginning to suggest that there may be "sensitive periods," particularly during the first 5 years of life, when exposure to these adversities has more detrimental influences on the risk of depression. For example, prior studies have shown that individuals exposed to child maltreatment, financial instability, or acts of interpersonal violence during early childhood had depressive or other psychiatric symptoms that were up to twice as high as those who were first exposed to these adversities during middle childhood, adolescence, or adulthood.[21,25,26]

It is also clear that genetic variation confers risk for depression and other psychiatric disorders. MDD is known to run in families; people with this diagnosis are three times more likely than those without the disorder to have a first-degree relative who also has depression.[27] (Notably, they are also more likely to have family members with other neuropsychiatric disorders, including bipolar disorder.) Twin studies, which allow for the simultaneous quantification of genetic and environmental influences, suggest that depression is moderately heritable. Specifically, twin studies comparing monozygotic (identical) and dizygotic (fraternal) twins have estimated that approximately 40% of the variation in the population risk of MDD is attributable to genetic variation.[28]

For over a decade, the combination of advances in our understanding of human genomic variation (e.g., Human Genome Project,[29] HapMap Project,[30] 1000 Genomes Project[31]) and cost-effective genotyping techniques have led to unprecedented growth in molecular genetic studies of depression and other "complex" psychiatric phenotypes. These studies typically examine whether specific *alleles*, meaning alternative forms of DNA sequence at a specific locus, or *genotypes*, meaning the combination of alleles at a given locus, are associated with the phenotype of interest. As a starting point,

*Supported, in part, by the Harvard University Center on the Developing Child (Dr. Dunn) and by National Institute of Mental Health grant numbers: K01MH102403 (Dr. Dunn), R01MH113930 (Dr. Dunn), R56MH115187 (Dr. Perlis), and R01MH116270 (Dr. Perlis). The content is solely the responsibility of the authors and does not necessarily represent the official views of the National Institutes of Health.

Major Depressive Disorder. https://doi.org/10.1016/B978-0-323-58131-8.00001-X

molecular genetic studies of depression focused largely on candidate genes—that is, genes that are hypothesized to be implicated in the neurobiology of depression. Some of the most commonly studied candidate genes were those regulating serotonin (5-HT) and dopamine neurotransmission, given the suspected involvement of these neurotransmitters in the pathophysiology of depression and their role as targets of antidepressant drugs.[32–34] However, the lack of reproducibility of these studies led the field to instead focus on genome-wide association studies (GWAS), which adopt an *unbiased* approach that allows for a hypothesis-free analysis of a million or more common variants (known as single nucleotide polymorphisms (SNPs)) across the entire genome. The ultimate goal of GWAS is to increase understanding of the genetic basis of depression, including the mechanisms that give rise to the disorder, recognizing that at present there are no strong hypotheses about such mechanisms to guide focused genetic study. With greater insights into the genetic etiology of MDD, it may be possible to identify individuals at greatest risk for depression, develop novel treatment targets for the disorder (for both prevention as well as treatment), and tailor those targets in ways that maximize individual benefit; such efforts to improve diagnosis, prevention, and treatment are consistent with the goals of precision medicine.[35]

In this chapter, we review recent findings from genetic association studies and G×E studies related to depression, and outline some of the challenges for future research. Since a prior summary of this research published in 2015,[37] several key discoveries warrant a reconsideration of this expanding literature. As we describe later, such developments include ever larger collaborative consortia, which have enabled identification of novel variants associated with depression; aggregation of individual variants to account for the polygenicity of depression; and integration of systems biology via network and pathway analyses.[38,39] This summary is intended to be interpretable by nonspecialists who may be unfamiliar with genetic concepts and methods. In the first section, we provide updates from the past 3 years emerging from GWAS of depression and other work to identify the genetic basis of depression. In the second section, we summarize recent findings from G×E studies, which aim to simultaneously examine the respective roles of genetic variants and environmental exposures in the etiology of depression. As described later, G×E studies have the potential to help identify genetic variants associated with both the risk of, and resilience against, depression—which are revealed only in specific subgroups of the population that have experienced a given environment. In the third section, we address the challenges that face genetic studies of depression and describe emerging strategies that may be useful for overcoming these challenges.

FINDINGS FROM GENETIC ASSOCIATION STUDIES
Results From Genome-Wide Association Studies

As noted previously, GWAS have been one of the most widely used methods to identify genetic risk loci in the past decade.[40–42] An overview of GWAS is provided in Table 1.1.

One of the most important lessons emerging from GWAS performed starting in the early and mid 2000s—whether for depression and other complex diseases—was that the effect of most variants—and SNPs in particular—was small in magnitude, with results suggesting allelic odd ratios of around 1.3 or less. These findings meant that very large samples—on the order of tens of thousands, if not hundreds of thousands—would be needed to identify genetic risk

---

TABLE 1.1
What are Genome-Wide Association Studies (GWAS)?

- In a typical genome-wide association study, one million or more common variants known as single nucleotide polymorphisms (SNPs) are examined for their association to disease.
- Common risk variants are generally defined as those alleles carried by at least 5% of the population.
- GWAS are typically conducted using a case-control design in which allele frequencies are compared between cases with depression, for example, to controls without the disease.
- To account for the large number of statistical tests conducted in a GWAS, the threshold for declaring genome-wide significance is a P-value of less than 5×10^{-8}, which is equivalent to a P-value of 0.05 that has been corrected for a million independent tests ($P < 0.00000005$).[a]
- Because common variant effects are typically modest, large samples (in the order of 10,000 or more cases and controls) are usually needed to have sufficient power to detect such effects at this statistical threshold.

[a] Adapted from Pearson TA, Manolio TA. How to interpret a genome-wide association study. Journal of the American Medical Association 2008; 299:1335–44.

loci associated with depression. To achieve such large samples, individual groups were required to work together to form large collaborative consortia, rather than working solely on their own.

In one of the most well-known examples of such collaboration efforts, the Psychiatric Genomics Consortium (PGC) was established in 2007 as an international collaborative effort to define the spectrum of risk variants across psychiatric disorders (http://www.med.unc.edu/pgc/). One of the consortium's major goals has been to conduct mega-analyses for MDD as well as autism, attention-deficit/hyperactivity disorder, bipolar disorder, schizophrenia and other disorders.[43–45] In a mega-analysis, researchers pool individual-level phenotype and genotype data from across many studies; this approach differs from a meta-analysis, where the summary statistics produced by each study are analyzed. In 2012, the Consortium published the results of a GWAS mega-analysis of MDD comprising 9240 cases and 9519 controls across nine primary samples, all of European ancestry.[46] Although this sample was the largest to date, no SNP reached genome-wide significance. Around the same time, large-scale efforts to examine depressive symptoms were also not identifying genetic variants linked to depression. For example, even in the largest study conducted at that time, which was a meta-analysis comprising 17 population-based studies ($n = 34{,}549$ individuals) as the discovery sample—no SNP reached genome-wide significance.[47]

After many years of effort, GWAS of depression have begun making progress, as summarized in the review of results shown in Table 1.2. In 2015, researchers reported the first two genetic variants associated with depression. These two loci were detected in a sample of Chinese women with recurrent MDD.[48] One SNP (rs12415800) was near a gene involved in mitochondrial biogenesis (*SIRT1*), while the other (rs35936514) was near the *LHPP* gene, which has been found to influence regional brain activity.[49]

During 2015 and 2016, another 22 variants were identified within samples of European American adults. In the first such study, an additional 17 loci across 15 regions were identified using "crowd-sourced" data collected by consumer genomics platforms.[50] In this joint analysis of the 23andme cohort (75,607 individuals with self-reported depression and 231,747 individuals without self-reported history of depression) and PGC cohorts, the top loci (rs10514299) detected was in *TMEM161B-MEF2C*, which is expressed in the brain (*TMEM161B*)[51] and has been implicated in synaptic function regulation (*MEF2C*).[52] In a meta-analysis and proxy-phenotype analysis across three large

cohorts, including the PGC, UK Biobank, and the Resource for Genetic Epidemiology Research on Aging, four new loci were detected.[53] In this study, the two lead SNPs were rs7973260 in the *KSR2* (kinase suppressor of ras 2) gene, and rs62100776 in the *DCC* gene, which encodes a transmembrane receptor involved in axon guidance and helps establish synaptic connectivity.[54,55] Finally, one new locus was identified through efforts to examine a broad depression phenotype comprising lifetime MDD and depressive symptoms.[56]

In 2019, Howard and colleagues[57] presented results from the largest genome-wide meta-analysis of depression to date ($n = 807{,}~553$), which included participants from the three largest GWAS of depression published between 2016 and 2018: 23andme,[50] UK Biobank,[58] and PGC cohorts.[59] The study yielded several important findings. First, 102 independent genetic variants, of which 87 were significant in an independent replication sample, were associated with depression. Results from the gene-based analyses suggested that putative genes associated with depression may influence biological pathways related to synaptic functioning and stimuli response. Furthermore, partitioned heritability analysis revealed the importance of prefrontal brain regions in the pathophysiology of depression. Notably, there was significant genetic overlap between depression and other psychiatric disorders (e.g., schizophrenia, bipolar disorder), providing additional evidence that the current psychiatric classification system does not adequately distinguish between distinct pathological mechanisms, thus illustrating the need to refine psychiatric diagnoses. Overall, the results of this genome-wide association study provide novel insights into the neurobiological basis of depression and hint at potential new opportunities for pharmacological interventions.

On the other hand, several challenges in interpreting these studies should be noted. First, arguably the conclusion of a decade of genetic investigation is that MDD is a brain disease. That is, while identification of risk variants in brain-expressed genes is reassuring, it is perhaps not surprising. Second, the appropriate phenotype for investigation merits consideration. Initial publications using broad depression phenotypes, as with the 23andme results, were criticized for a lack of diagnostic precision (i.e., use of traditional multihour clinician assessments); however, the magnitude of effects identified in these cohorts appears to have been no different from studies using more traditional methods.

As has been the case for psychiatric genetics[60] and genetics research[61] more broadly, there has been a general

TABLE 1.2
Results for the Significant Loci (

Publication	rsid	CHR	Gene context[a]	Effect	P-value	Trait associations[b]
CONVERGE consortium, 2015	rs35936514	10	LHPP	OR = 0.84	6.43E-12	—
CONVERGE consortium, 2015	rs12415800	10	—	OR = 1.15	2.37E-10	—
Ware et al., 2015	rs1127233	3	MUC13	β = 0.2382	3.85E-08	—
Direk et al., 2016	rs9825823	3	FHIT	—	8.20E-09	Alcohol dependence (rs9825823, 2.3E-05)
Hyde et al., 2016	rs10514299	5	TMEM161B-AS1	—	9.99E-16	—
Hyde et al., 2016	rs1518395	2	VRK2	—	4.32E-12	Schizophrenia (rs2312147, <3E-07); Epilepsy (generalized) (rs2717068, <4E-07)
Hyde et al., 2016	rs2179744	22	CHADL; L3MBTL2	—	6.03E-11	—
Hyde et al., 2016	rs11209948	1	LOC105378797	—	8.38E-11	BMI (rs2815752, <2.0E-22); obesity (rs2568958, <4.0E-16); obesity—early onset (rs3101336, <2.0E-08); Subcutaneous adipose tissue (rs990871, <4.0E-06); weight (rs2568958, <2.0E-08); menarche (age-at-onset) (rs3101336, <5.0E-13)
Hyde et al., 2016	rs454214	5	—	—	1.09E-09	—
Hyde et al., 2016	rs301806	1	RERE	—	1.90E-09	Pelargonate (rs3795310, 2.03E-5); 3-methoxytyrosine (rs301816, 2.06E-05)
Hyde et al., 2016	rs1475120	6	LIN28B-AS1; LIN28B	—	4.17E-09	Menarche (age-at-onset) (rs314280, <2.0E-14); pubertal anthropometrics (rs11156429, <2.00E-07); waist circumference (rs4946651, 4.17E-08)
Hyde et al., 2016	rs10786831	10	SORCS3	—	8.11E-09	—
Hyde et al., 2016	rs12552	13	OLFM4	—	8.16E-09	Myo-inositol (rs12552, 1.5E-05)
Hyde et al., 2016	rs6476606	9	PAX5	—	1.20E-08	—
Hyde et al., 2016	rs8025231	15	—	—	1.23E-08	—
Hyde et al., 2016	rs12065553	1	—	—	1.32E-08	—
Hyde et al., 2016	rs1656369	3	LOC100996447	—	1.34E-08	—
Hyde et al., 2016	rs4543289	5	—	—	1.36E-08	—
Hyde et al., 2016	rs2125716	12	—	—	3.05E-08	Systemic lupus erythematosus (rs2125716, 1.13E-05)
Hyde et al., 2016	rs2422321	1	—	—	3.18E-08	—
Hyde et al., 2016	rs7044150	9	CARM1P1	—	4.31E-08	—

Study	rsID	Chr	Gene	Effect	P-value	Associated traits
Okbay et al., 2016	rs7973260	12	KSR2	β = 0.031	1.80E-09	Neuroticism (rs7973260, 2.40E-07)
Okbay et al., 2016	rs62100776	18	DCC	β = -0.025	8.50E-09	Neuroticism (rs62100776, 5.43E-05); educational attainment (rs62100776, 1.27E-05)
Howard et al., 2018	rs6699744	1	—	β = 0.0061	1.64E-13	—
Howard et al., 2018	rs3094054	6	—	β = -0.0061	1.79E-13	Myasthenia gravis (3.00E-71); idiopathic membranous nephropathy (9.47E-28); schizophrenia (2.35E-19); lung cancer (7.70E-14); type 1 diabetes (3.18E-09); triglycerides (1.43E-08); total cholesterol (4.80E-06); triglycerides (6.59E-06)
Howard et al., 2018	rs3807865	7	TMEM106B	β = 0.0057	7.28E-12	—
Howard et al., 2018	rs10501696	11	GRM5	β = 0.0008	6.73E-11	—
Howard et al., 2018	rs40465	5	RP11-6N13.1	β = 0.0052	4.45E-10	Educational attainment (1.26E-05); triglycerides (6.18E-05)
Howard et al., 2018	rs2402273	7	—	β = 0.0008	1.95E-09	—
Howard et al., 2018	rs9530139	13	B3GLCT	β = 0.0008	2.63E-09	—
Howard et al., 2018	rs1554505	7	MAD1L1	β = 0.0025	2.74E-09	—
Howard et al., 2018	rs7548151	1	ASTN1	β = 0.0051	3.87E-09	—
Howard et al., 2018	rs10929355	2	NBAS	β = -0.0053	5.84E-09	—
Howard et al., 2018	rs1021363	10	SORCS3	β = 0.0008	1.04E-08	Schizophrenia (1.76E-05)
Howard et al., 2018	rs5011432	7	TMEM106B	β = 0.0009	2.23E-08	—
Howard et al., 2018	rs263575	9	—	β = 0.0008	2.31E-08	—
Howard et al., 2018	rs28541419	15	—	β = 0.0008	2.78E-08	—
Howard et al., 2018	rs11018449	11	GRM5	β = 0.0008	4.52E-08	—
Wray et al., 2018	rs12552	13	[OLFM4]; LINC01065,80099	OR = 1.04	6.10E-19	Educational attainment (4.59E-05)
Wray et al., 2018	rs1432639	1	NEGR1,-64941	OR = 1.04	4.60E-15	Educational attainment (1.31E-06)
Wray et al., 2018	rs8025231	15	—	OR = 0.97	2.40E-12	—
Wray et al., 2018	rs12129573	1	LINC01360,-3486	OR = 1.04	4.00E-12	Schizophrenia (2.0E-12)
Wray et al., 2018	chr5_103942055_D	5	—	OR = 1.03	7.50E-12	—
Wray et al., 2018	rs115507122	6	Extended MHC	OR = 0.96	3.30E-11	Total cholesterol (1.71E-05)
Wray et al., 2018	rs12958048	18	[TCF4]; MIR4529,-44853	OR = 1.03	3.60E-11	Inflammatory bowel disease (2.02E-05)
Wray et al., 2018	chr5_87992715_I	5	LINC00461,-12095; MEF2C,21342	OR = 0.97	7.90E-11	—
Wray et al., 2018	rs61867293	10	[SORCS3]	OR = 0.96	7.00E-10	Schizophrenia (4.97E-06)

Continued

TABLE 1.2
Results for the Significant Loci (

Publication	rsid	CHR	Gene context[a]	Effect	P-value	Trait associations[b]
Wray et al., 2018	rs915057	14	[SYNE2]; MIR548H1,-124364; ESR2,7222	OR = 0.97	7.60E-10	Educational attainment (2.68E-05)
Wray et al., 2018	rs11135349	5	–	OR = 0.97	1.10E-09	–
Wray et al., 2018	rs1806153	11	[DKFZp686K1684]; [PAUPAR]; ELP4,44032	OR = 1.04	1.20E-09	–
Wray et al., 2018	rs4904738	14	[LRFN5]	OR = 0.97	2.60E-09	–
Wray et al., 2018	rs7430565	3	[RSRC1]; LOC100996447,155828; MLF1,-181772	OR = 0.97	2.90E-09	Height (4.70E-10)
Wray et al., 2018	rs34215985	4	[SLC30A9]; LINC00682,-163150; DCAF4L1,59294	OR = 0.96	3.10E-09	–
Wray et al., 2018	rs10149470	14	BAG5,4927; APOPT1,-11340	OR = 0.97	3.10E-09	Height (8.00E-09)
Wray et al., 2018	chr14_75356855_I	14	[DLST]; PROX2,-26318; RPS6KL1,13801	OR = 1.03	3.80E-09	–
Wray et al., 2018	rs11682175	2	RK2,-147192	OR = 0.97	4.70E-09	Schizophrenia (2.54E-12); genetic generalized epilepsy (1.00E-11); epilepsy (5.21E-05); BMI (8.98E-05)
Wray et al., 2018	rs10959913	9	–	OR = 1.03	5.10E-09	Neuroticism (9.52E-08)
Wray et al., 2018	rs4869056	5	[TENM2]	OR = 0.97	6.80E-09	–
Wray et al., 2018	rs8063603	16	[RBFOX1]	OR = 0.97	6.90E-09	–
Wray et al., 2018	rs116755193	5	LOC101927421,-120640	OR = 0.97	7.00E-09	–
Wray et al., 2018	rs5758265	22	[L3MBTL2]; EP300-AS1,-24392; CHADL,7616	OR = 1.03	7.60E-09	Schizophrenia (5.26E-09); neuroticism (3.40E-06)
Wray et al., 2018	rs7856424	9	[ASTN2]	OR = 0.97	8.50E-09	–
Wray et al., 2018	rs17727765	17	[CRYBA1]; MYO18A,-69555; NUFIP2,5891	OR = 0.95	8.50E-09	–
Wray et al., 2018	rs2389016	1	–	OR = 1.03	1.00E-08	Serum ratio of 1 palmitoylglycerol 1 monopalmitinerythronate (2.90E-06)
Wray et al., 2018	rs4261101	1	–	OR = 0.97	1.00E-08	–
Wray et al., 2018	rs7198928	16	[RBFOX1]	OR = 1.03	1.00E-08	–
Wray et al., 2018	rs62099069	18	[MIR924HG]	OR = 0.97	1.30E-08	–
Wray et al., 2018	rs12666117	7	–	OR = 1.03	1.40E-08	–
Wray et al., 2018	rs11663393	18	[DCC]; MIR4528,-148738	OR = 1.03	1.60E-08	Educational attainment (3.33E-05); neuroticism (5.64E-05)

Continued

Study		rs	Gene	OR	p-value	Associated traits
Wray et al., 2018	2	rs1226412	[LINC01876]; NR4A2,69630; GPD2,-180651	OR = 1.03	2.40E-08	—
Wray et al., 2018	9	rs1354115	PUM3,-139644; LINC01231,-197814	OR = 1.03	2.40E-08	—
Wray et al., 2018	16	rs7200826	[SHISA9]; CPPED1,-169089	OR = 1.03	2.40E-08	—
Wray et al., 2018	13	rs4143229	[ENOX1]; LACC1,-125620; CCDC122,82689	OR = 0.95	2.50E-08	—
Wray et al., 2018	7	rs10950398	[TMEM106B]; VWDE,105637	OR = 1.03	2.60E-08	—
Wray et al., 2018	18	rs1833288	[RAB27B]; CCDC68,50833	OR = 1.03	2.60E-08	—
Wray et al., 2018	9	rs7029033	[DENND1A]; LHX2,-91820	OR = 1.05	2.70E-08	—
Wray et al., 2018	6	rs9402472	FBXL4,-170672; C6orf168,154271	OR = 1.03	2.80E-08	—
Wray et al., 2018	1	rs9427672	DENND1B,-10118	OR = 0.97	3.10E-08	Neuroticism (4.01E-06)
Wray et al., 2018	12	rs4074723	PAX6,-1	OR = 0.97	3.10E-08	—
Wray et al., 2018	1	rs159963	[RERE]; SLC45A1,100194	OR = 0.97	3.20E-08	Schizophrenia (2.03E-06)
Wray et al., 2018	16	rs11643192	PMFBP1,-7927; DHX38,67465	OR = 1.03	3.40E-08	Educational attainment in females (6.72E-08); circulating haptoglobin levels (2.41E-06); height (7.40E-05)
Wray et al., 2018	3	chr3_44287760_I	[TOPAZ1]; TCAIM,-91850; ZNF445,193501	OR = 1.03	4.60E-08	—
Howard et al., 2019	1	rs2568958	—	OR = 1.038	8.47E-25	BMI (2.79E-19 - 1.50E-37); hip circumference (6.27E-19 - 1.20E-08); overweight/obese (4.00E-16 - 1.10E-11); waist circumference (1.23E-15 - 6.50E-13); weight (4.52E-14); gene expression (1.30E-27); NEGR1 expression, blood (4.20E-13); age at menarche (3.80E-12 - 8.10E-13); arm fat/fat-free mass left (2.92E-18 - 1.37E-11); basal metabolic rate (5.60E-12); body fat percentage (1.02E-15); impedance of arm/whole body (5.67E-10 - 1.19E-08); leg fat/fat-free mass (2.39E-22 - 3.51E-11); number of self-reported noncancer illnesses (1.29E-08); qualifications (6.08E-16); seen doctor for nerves, anxiety, tension or depression (8.52E-14); sodium in urine (3.87E-08); trunk fat mass (3.10E-16 - 2.96E-12); whole body fat mass (3.95E-19 - 8.94E-10)

TABLE 1.2
Results for the Significant Loci (

Publication	rsid	CHR	Gene context[a]	Effect	P-value	Trait associations[b]
Howard et al., 2019	rs200949	6	–	OR = 1.049	2.53E-19	Eosinophil count/percentage (3.79E-22 - 2.70E-09); granulocyte count (2.58E-13); hematocrit (4.07E-19); hemoglobin concentration (2.73E-27); high light scatter reticulocyte count (4.07E-08); lymphocyte count (7.68E-34); mean corpuscular hemoglobin concentration (3.76E-10); monocyte count (1.46E-25); myeloid white cell count (8.93E-16); neutrophil count/percentage (2.44E-10 - 7.54E-10); red blood cell count (2.76E-09); reticulocyte count (5.75E-18); white blood cell count (6.58E-31); IgA deficiency (2.42E-29); primary sclerosing cholangitis (1.39E-71); diastolic blood pressure (3.18E-08); doctor diagnosed sarcoidosis (1.18E-13); forced expiratory volume (1.83E-17); forced vital capacity (6.14E-12); guilty feelings (9.16E-09); hearing difficulty or problems with background noise (7.84E-09); intestinal malabsorption (2.47E-40); medication for pain relief, constipation, heartburn (4.23E-09 - 6.43E-10); mouth or teeth dental problems: dentures (4.20E-14); number of days or week of moderate physical activity 10 + min (1.06E-08); peak expiratory flow (1.78E-16); potassium in urine (1.56E-08); seen a doctor/psychiatrist for nerves, anxiety, tension or depression (1.25E-11 - 3.64E-10); self-reported hyperthyroidism or thyrotoxicosis (6.26E-22); self-reported hypothyroidism or myxoedema (2.95E-12); self-reported malabsorption or celiac disease (2.62E-134); self-reported sarcoidosis (1.18E-11); treatment with insulin (6.01E-14 - 9.97E-09); treatment with levothyroxine sodium (1.71E-14); schizophrenia (1.51E-16)
Howard et al., 2019	rs1343605	13	–	OR = 1.032	6.23E-18	Sleeplessness or insomnia (4.42E-10)
Howard et al., 2019	rs11135349	5	AC109466.1	OR = 0.971	6.04E-17	Hip circumference (4.69E-08)

Study	SNP	Chr	Gene	OR	p-value	Associated traits
Howard et al., 2019	rs30266	5	AC099520.1	OR = 1.031	1.45E-16	Ever depressed for a whole week (3.52E-08); leg fat percentage (2.40E-09 - 3.08E-08); long-standing illness, disability or infirmity (2.49E-08); seen doctor for nerves, anxiety, tension or depression (1.08E-12); sleeplessness or insomnia (3.19E-08)
Howard et al., 2019	rs12967143	18	TCF4	OR = 0.969	3.70E-16	Irritability (1.74E-10); neuroticism (6.87E-10); seen doctor for nerves, anxiety, tension or depression (1.04E-09)
Howard et al., 2019	rs1021363	10	SORCS3	OR = 1.031	4.41E-16	Seen doctor for nerves, anxiety, tension or depression (2.13E-08)
Howard et al., 2019	rs7932640	11	GRM5	OR = 1.028	1.62E-15	Seen doctor for nerves, anxiety, tension or depression (6.61E-09)
Howard et al., 2019	rs10890020	1	—	OR = 0.973	4.03E-15	—
Howard et al., 2019	rs3099439	5	TMEM161B	OR = 0.973	5.05E-15	Alcohol intake frequency (1.63E-08)
Howard et al., 2019	rs2043539	7	TMEM106B	OR = 1.028	9.89E-15	Miserableness (1.83E-08); mood swings (5.09E-09); neuroticism score (9.23E-09); seen doctor for nerves, anxiety, tension, or depression (6.89E-12)
Howard et al., 2019	rs10149470	14	—	OR = 0.974	3.72E-14	Monocyte count (1.01E-13); height (8.00E-09); cognitive ability (3.00E-09); intelligence (5.00E-11); trunk fat-free mass (2.84E-08); trunk predicted mass (3.11E-08)
Howard et al., 2019	rs1095626	3	RSRC1	OR = 0.974	7.13E-14	BMI (1.86E-08); force vital capacity (1.80E-12); height (2.18E-18)
Howard et al., 2019	rs17641524	1	DENND1B	OR = 0.969	1.52E-13	Lymphocyte percentage of white cells (2.45E-09); primary biliary cirrhosis (1.00E-11); worrier or anxious feelings (2.33E-10)
Howard et al., 2019	rs61990288	14	—	OR = 0.974	1.68E-13	—
Howard et al., 2019	rs10913112	1	—	OR = 0.974	3.40E-13	—
Howard et al., 2019	rs1045430	14	AREL1	OR = 0.975	7.31E-13	Nervous feelings (1.31E-08); neuroticism (1.68E-10); worrier/anxious feelings (1.72E-09)
Howard et al., 2019	rs12967855	18	CELF4	OR = 1.027	1.18E-12	Fed-up feelings (2.52E-12); guilty feelings (3.48E-08); mood swings (9.11E-09); neuroticism (3.24E-16); overall health rating (4.11E-13); qualifications (6.83E-23-4.90E-15); seen doctor for nerves, anxiety, tension or depression (3.09E-09); sensitivity or hurt feelings (9.33E-15); time spent watching television (1.25E-09); worrier or anxious feelings (9.45E-09); years of educational attainment (1.41E-10); neuroticism (1.45E-09)

Continued

TABLE 1.2
Results for the Significant Loci (

Publication	rsid	CHR	Gene context[a]	Effect	P-value	Trait associations[b]
Howard et al., 2019	rs301799	1	RERE, AL096855.1	OR = 0.975	1.36E-12	Eosinophil count/percentage (5.49E-19 - 2.49E-12); lymphocyte count (6.08E-11); nneutrophil percentage of granulocytes (1.36E-15); sum eosinophil basophil counts (4.54E-11); allergic disease (3.62E-16); aarm fat percentage (2.73E-09 - 3.99E-08); asthma (1.86E-08); body fat percentage (3.88E-10); diastolic blood pressure (1.13E-12); hay fever, allergic rhinitis or eczema (3.07E-11); heel bone mineral density (5.53E-14 - 9.84E-11); leg fat mass left (2.17E-11 - 4.27E-09); no blood clot, bronchitis, emphysema, asthma, rhinitis, eczema, or allergy diagnosed by doctor (2.18E-11); self-reported asthma (1.97E-08); self-reported hypertension (3.74E-08); systolic blood pressure (1.16E-08); trunk fat percentage (7.50E-09); vascular or heart problems diagnosed by doctor (4.22E-08)
Howard et al., 2019	rs61902811	11	–	OR = 0.975	1.40E-12	Guilty feelings (4.99E-08); miserableness (1.85E-11); mood swings (1.23E-10); neuroticism score (6.65E-15); seen doctor for nerves, anxiety, tension or depression (1.51E-08); schizophrenia (8.30E-09); neuroticism (2.30E-09)
Howard et al., 2019	rs56887639	16	–	OR = 0.973	1.51E-12	Depressive symptoms (4.00E-09 - 5.00E-8)
Howard et al., 2019	rs7030813	9	PAX5	OR = 1.026	3.07E-12	–
Howard et al., 2019	rs1002656	1	–	OR = 0.974	3.74E-12	Neuroticism (5.51E-11)
Howard et al., 2019	rs7200826	16	SHISA9	OR = 1.028	3.74E-12	–
Howard et al., 2019	rs1568452	2	–	OR = 1.025	8.12E-12	Impedance of leg (9.81E-10 - 1.64E-09)
Howard et al., 2019	rs12966052	18	–	OR = 0.969	1.25E-11	Mood swings (4.83E-08)
Howard et al., 2019	rs5995992	22	–	OR = 0.974	1.30E-11	Neutrophil percentage of granulocytes (1.46E-08); irritability (2.97E-08); mood swings (1.39E-11); neuroticism score (1.46E-08)
Howard et al., 2019	rs1982277	9	–	OR = 1.028	1.45E-11	Neuroticism (2.02E-08)

Reference	SNP	Chr	Gene	OR	p-value	Associated phenotypes
Howard et al., 2019	rs7227069	18	DCC	OR = 1.024	1.50E-11	Fed-up feelings (1.61E-10); frequency of depressed mood in last 2 weeks (4.55E-13); frequency of tiredness or lethargy in last 2 weeks (2.25E-09; frequency of unenthusiasm or disinterest in last 2 weeks (6.70E-15); miserableness (1.14E-08); mood swings (4.97E-10); neuroticism score (5.14E-09); sitting height (1.39E-12); tense or highly strung (4.77E-08)
Howard et al., 2019	rs58104186	7	—	OR = 1.024	1.82E-11	Frequency of tiredness or lethargy (2.65E-08)
Howard et al., 2019	rs7807677	7	CTTNBP2	OR = 1.024	1.82E-11	Ever smoked (5.34E-11)
Howard et al., 2019	rs1890946	1	NRDC	OR = 0.977	2.68E-11	—
Howard et al., 2019	rs10817969	9	ASTN2	OR = 1.026	3.11E-11	—
Howard et al., 2019	rs8037355	15	—	OR = 0.977	3.94E-11	—
Howard et al., 2019	rs7198928	16	RBFOX1	OR = 1.024	4.45E-11	Neuroticism score (4.09E-08); worrier or anxious feelings (5.18E-10)
Howard et al., 2019	rs72710803	1	AL122019.1	OR = 0.960	5.29E-11	—
Howard et al., 2019	rs9363467	6	—	OR = 1.024	6.44E-11	—
Howard et al., 2019	rs10061069	5	FAM172A, POU5F2	OR = 0.973	8.15E-11	—
Howard et al., 2019	rs3793577	9	ELAVL2	OR = 0.977	8.41E-11	Frequency of depressed mood in last 2 weeks (1.20E-08); guilty feelings (8.67E-09); neuroticism score (5.57E-09)
Howard et al., 2019	rs2670139	9	DENND1A	OR = 0.974	1.21E-10	Waist circumference (1.44E-08)
Howard et al., 2019	rs2876520	6	—	OR = 0.977	2.29E-10	Height (6.30E-14)
Howard et al., 2019	rs1933802	6	LIN28B-AS1	OR = 0.978	2.57E-10	Age at menarche (7.81E-88); forced expiratory volume (1.32E-11); hand grip strength right (1.58E-08); height (1.01E-60); impedance of arm/whole body (3.28E-19 - 1.49E-14)
Howard et al., 2019	rs7241572	18	—	OR = 1.028	2.70E-10	Wheeze or whistling in the chest in last year (1.57E-08)
Howard et al., 2019	rs56314503	12	—	OR = 0.975	2.95E-10	—

Continued

TABLE 1.2
Results for the Significant Loci (

Publication	rsid	CHR	Gene context[a]	Effect	P-value	Trait associations[b]
Howard et al., 2019	rs198457	11	DAGLA	OR = 0.971	2.99E-10	Granulocyte percentage of myeloid white cells (1.89E-08); monocyte percentage of white cells (4.38E-08)
Howard et al., 2019	rs263645	9	–	OR = 1.022	3.70E-10	Seen doctor for nerves, anxiety, tension or depression (1.18E-09)
Howard et al., 2019	rs4772087	13	STK24	OR = 1.023	3.91E-10	–
Howard et al., 2019	rs7193263	16	RBFOX1	OR = 0.976	4.33E-10	Depressive symptoms multi trait analysis 4.00E-11
Howard et al., 2019	rs12052908	2	LINC01830	OR = 0.978	4.44E-10	Walking for pleasure (1.21E-08)
Howard et al., 2019	rs7758630	6	–	OR = 0.978	5.56E-10	–
Howard et al., 2019	rs11579246	1	ELAVL4	OR = 1.039	5.71E-10	–
Howard et al., 2019	rs1152578	14	ESR2	OR = 0.978	6.36E-10	–
Howard et al., 2019	rs4346585	3	–	OR = 0.977	7.13E-10	–
Howard et al., 2019	rs62188629	2	AC007879.1	OR = 1.024	7.13E-10	Medication for pain relief, constipation, heartburn (2.63E-08)
Howard et al., 2019	rs3213572	12	SPPL3	OR = 1.022	7.61E-10	Allergic disease (1.65E-11); height (9.96E-09)
Howard et al., 2019	rs141954845	3	FHIT	OR = 1.023	8.15E-10	–
Howard et al., 2019	rs9592461	13	PCDH9	OR = 1.022	9.10E-10	–
Howard et al., 2019	rs67436663	8	–	OR = 0.974	9.37E-10	–
Howard et al., 2019	rs12923444	16	METTL9	OR = 0.979	1.30E-09	Seen doctor for nerves, anxiety, tension or depression (1.36E-08)
Howard et al., 2019	rs1448938	11	DCDC1	OR = 1.022	1.30E-09	Red blood cell count (1.72E-08); impedance of arm/whole body (8.90E-09, 2.62E-09)
Howard et al., 2019	rs35553410	4	–	OR = 0.976	1.42E-09	–
Howard et al., 2019	rs1409379	13	–	OR = 1.025	1.67E-09	–
Howard et al., 2019	rs62091461	18	RAB27B	OR = 0.975	1.95E-09	Arm fat-free/overall mass (2.14E-09 - 3.07E-08); basal metabolic rate (3.61E-09); BMI (1.73E-08); hip circumference (3.22E-11); leg fat/fat-free/overall mass (6.83E-09 - 1.37-08); weight (2.66E-10); whole body fat/fat-free/water mass (2.00E-08 - 3.27E-08)

Howard et al., 2019	7	MAD1L1	rs3823624	OR = 1.028	1.99E-09	Age at first live birth (4.64E-08); arm fat mass/percentage (1.58E-12 - 8.14E-11); body fat percentage/mass (2.54E-13 - 2.72E-09); hip circumference (4.13E-09); impedance of leg (1.37E-09 - 3.23E-08); irritability (3.75E-08); leg fat mass/percentage (1.79E-08 - 3.66E-08); miserableness (4.21E-09); number of self-reported noncancer illnesses (1.44E-11); overall health rating (2.43E-10); qualifications (6.90E-12); taking other prescription medications (1.69E-08); trunk fat mass/percentage (2.27E-08 - 2.38E-08); types of physical activity in last 4 weeks: Other exercises (5.36E-10); whole body fat mass (4.45E-09)
Howard et al., 2019	9	—	rs34653192	OR = 0.977	2.23E-09	—
Howard et al., 2019	20	—	rs143186028	OR = 1.028	2.29E-09	—
Howard et al., 2019	8	CYP7B1	rs7837935	OR = 0.971	3.34E-09	—
Howard et al., 2019	2	LINC01876	rs1226412	OR = 1.026	3.46E-09	Neuroticism (3.50E-08)
Howard et al., 2019	7	PCLO	rs2247523	OR = 0.980	4.38E-09	—
Howard et al., 2019	13	—	rs9545360	OR = 0.973	5.02E-09	—
Howard et al., 2019	15	SEMA6D, AC023905.1	rs34488670	OR = 0.975	6.03E-09	Current tobacco smoking (4.08E-08); years of educational attainment (4.28E-08)
Howard et al., 2019	3	—	rs13084037	OR = 0.976	7.08E-09	Mean corpuscular hemoglobin (4.64E-09); mean corpuscular volume (3.97E-08); age at menarche (8.32E-10); frequency of tiredness or lethargy (1.28E-10); impedance of arm/whole body (8.17E-14 - 3.48E-12); miserableness (6.91E-10); overall health rating (3.18E-08); pulse rate (3.01E-10); qualifications (4.48E-09); age at menarche (2.00E-14)
Howard et al., 2019	9	CARM1P1	rs1354115	OR = 1.021	7.08E-09	—

Continued

TABLE 1.2
Results for the Significant Loci (

Publication	rsid	CHR	Gene context[a]	Effect	P-value	Trait associations[b]
Howard et al., 2019	rs7117514	11	SHANK2	OR = 0.980	7.29E–09	–
Howard et al., 2019	rs12624433	20	SLC12A5	OR = 1.024	7.44E–09	Rheumatoid arthritis (4.10E–10)
Howard et al., 2019	rs16887442	7	–	OR = 1.021	8.62E–09	–
Howard et al., 2019	rs2509805	11	–	OR = 1.022	9.17E–09	Average weekly red wine intake (4.80E–08); duration walking for pleasure (3.34E–09); neuroticism score (1.72E–10); types of physical activity in last 4 weeks: heavy DIY (2.05E–09); worry too long after embarrassment (3.82E–09)
Howard et al., 2019	rs59283172	9	–	OR = 0.968	1.02E–08	–
Howard et al., 2019	rs2029865	6	–	OR = 0.980	1.20E–08	–
Howard et al., 2019	rs7655414	4	–	OR = 0.980	1.20E–08	Impedance of leg (2.84E–13 – 1.28E–11)
Howard et al., 2019	rs60157091	5	–	OR = 1.020	1.42E–08	Mean platelet volume (1.51E–09)
Howard et al., 2019	rs58621819	11	LTBP3	OR = 0.976	1.57E–08	Platelet count (1.00E–08); plateletcrit (1.88E–09); red cell distribution width (2.45E–10); arm fat/fat-free mass (5.19E–11 – 1.76E–08); basal metabolic rate (9.53E–09); body fat percentage (3.02E–08); BMI (2.79E–09); heel bone mineral density (9.82E–12); impedance of right arm (2.50E–08); leg fat mass/percentage (2.42E–11 – 2.58E–10); pulse rate (9.50E–09); trunk fat mass (6.24E–09); waist circumference (3.66E–10); weight (6.97E–11); whole body fat mass (7.71E–10)
Howard et al., 2019	rs57344483	11	–	OR = 0.963	1.82E–08	–
Howard et al., 2019	rs45510091	4	KIAA1109	OR = 1.046	1.83E–08	Depressive symptoms (3.00E–09 - 3.97E–09); fed-up feelings (2.11E–10); miserableness (2.31E–09)

Source	SNP	CHR	Gene context	OR	P	Trait associations
Howard et al., 2019	rs113188507	1	—	OR = 1.022	1.87E-08	Body fat percentage (2.54E-08); leg fat (4.03E-08-1.36E-08); waist circumference (3.01E-08)
Howard et al., 2019	rs725616	6	SAMD5	OR = 1.021	1.87E-08	—
Howard et al., 2019	rs1956373	14	RTN1	OR = 0.978	2.06E-08	—
Howard et al., 2019	rs913930	9	—	OR = 0.979	2.42E-08	—
Howard et al., 2019	rs7685686	4	HTT	OR = 1.020	2.57E-08	Alcohol intake frequency (2.29E-08); frequency of tiredness or lethary in last 2 weeks (4.04E-08)
Howard et al., 2019	rs7585722	2	RNF103-CHMP3, AC015971.1	OR = 0.973	2.68E-08	—
Howard et al., 2019	rs6783233	3	AC092691.1, AC092691.3	OR = 1.022	2.90E-08	Age at menarche (8.39E-11); seen doctor for nerves, anxiety, tension or depression (1.44E-08); age at menarche (9.40E-13)
Howard et al., 2019	rs169235	1	CACNA1E	OR = 0.977	2.98E-08	Neuroticism (5.00E-13)
Howard et al., 2019	rs75581564	17	PIPOX	OR = 1.031	3.17E-08	—
Howard et al., 2019	rs78337797	12	SOX5	OR = 1.031	3.37E-08	Height (4.84E-08)
Howard et al., 2019	rs10774600	12	ATP2A2	OR = 0.974	3.39E-08	Red blood cell count (4.94E-08); eosinophil/basophil counts (1.66E-08)
Howard et al., 2019	rs2187490	11	—	OR = 0.967	3.82E-08	—
Howard et al., 2019	rs7624336	3	—	OR = 1.024	3.96E-08	—
Howard et al., 2019	rs1466887	1	—	OR = 0.980	4.12E-08	—
Howard et al., 2019	rs34937911	4	—	OR = 1.031	4.13E-08	—
Howard et al., 2019	rs10789214	1	SGIP1	OR = 1.019	4.44E-08	—
Howard et al., 2019	rs33431	19	ZNF536	OR = 1.020	4.81E-08	—
Howard et al., 2019	rs997934	10	—	OR = 1.020	4.81E-08	—

CHR, chromosome.

[a] The gene context column indicates the closest gene or gene in which the SNP is found. Parentheses (|I|) indicates that the SNP was within that gene.

[b] Trait associations ($P < 1 \times 10^{-5}$) were obtained from the following sources: Ware et al., 2016; Okbay et al., 2016; Howard et al., 2018; Wray et al., 2018 and Howard et al., 2019: PhenoScanner; Hyde et al., 2016: SNiPA and include publicly available GWAS (made available through the GWAS catalog).

underrepresentation of non-European populations in research into the genetic underpinnings of depression.[62,63] To increase the diversity of genetic association studies, several groups have performed GWAS within racial/ethnic minority samples of African Americans and Hispanics.[64,65] For example, Dunn and colleagues[36] conducted the largest genome-wide association study of depressive symptoms using data from 12,310 adults in the Hispanic Community Health Study/Study of Latinos. The authors did not identify any genome-wide significant loci in the overall analysis of the entire sample, though they did find seven genome-wide significant associations in sex-stratified analyses. Importantly, neither these loci nor any others with suggestive evidence were replicated in subsequent analyses across three independent cohorts. However, through a transethnic generalization analysis, they did find some evidence of overlap in genetic vulnerability to depression across ancestry; these findings suggest that the genetic contributors to depression are likely both unique to specific populations and common across ancestral populations.

Results From Structural and Rare-Variant Association Studies

In one of the largest GWAS of MDD described earlier, common genetic variants (meaning SNPs) explained more than 8% of SNP heritability in depression,[59] suggesting the important influence of other genetic factors, such as structural and rare variants, that are not captured by GWAS.[66] Structural variations are variations in the DNA sequence that involve the duplication or deletion of thousands or more than a million base pairs. Rare variants can include genetic single-nucleotide variances (SNVs; present in < 1% of the population) and copy number variants (CNVs). Such variants have been shown to play a role in autism,[67,68] schizophrenia,[69,70] and bipolar disorder,[71] and there is now limited but emerging evidence for the role of these variations in depression.

Structural variation including CNVs, which can be inherited or spontaneous (de novo), is a potential source of depression risk loci, as suggested by six studies[72–77]. In a large study with more than 6000 participants published almost a decade ago, Glessner and colleagues[77] found 12 CNV regions that were exclusive to cases with MDD. The region with the highest frequency in cases was a locus on chromosome 5 (5q35.1) that overlapped the genes SLIT3, CCDC99, and DOCK2. The finding of a CNV overlapping the gene SLIT3 is interesting, since SLIT3 is known to play a role in axon development and neurodevelopmental

disorders. A subsequent study examining ~1200 individuals with treatment-resistant MDD, as a putative extreme phenotype, found enrichment in duplications among individuals with TRD, with a greater than expected number of CNV's intersecting genes related to actin cytoskeleton.[72] In the largest of these studies, which included over 450,000 individuals, Kendall and colleagues[73] found that four CNVs that had previously been implicated in neurodevelopmental disorders were associated with an increased risk of depression, although these CNV loci did not overlap with the top hits in the PGC GWAS of MDD.

In contrast to traditional Sanger sequencing, which sequences a single DNA fragment at a time, high-throughput sequencing allows for massive parallel sequencing of millions of DNA fragments in a single run.[78] Such advancements in sequencing technology have dramatically reduced the cost of direct DNA sequencing and provided greater discovery power and more opportunities to explore the role of rare SNVs.[79,80] There appear to be five studies that have identified rare variants associated with depression using these newer genomic technologies.[81–85] In the most recent study, Amin and colleagues[85] sequenced the exomes of over 1300 individuals in the Erasmus Rucphen Family study to examine exonic variants influencing depression. A rare variant in the RCL1 gene on chromosome 9 (rs115482041) segregated with depression across multiple generations and explained more than half of the variation of depression in an extended family. Although RCL1 protein is known to be present in human neurons and astrocytes, the mechanism through which it influences depression pathophysiology needs clarification. In the largest study to date, Peterson and colleagues[83] used high-throughput sequencing to sequence more than 250,000 exons across almost 22,000 genes, in ~10,000 Han Chinese women. The study revealed that compared to controls, MDD cases had significantly more deleterious exonic SNPs and that rare deleterious variants were overrepresented in nuclear-encoded mitochondrial genes affected the risk of depression. The latter finding is consistent with prior clinical reports of MDD comorbidity in some human mitochondrial disease and clinical symptoms of MDD that imply disruption of mitochondrial processes.

Substantial progress has been made in unraveling the "missing heritability" of MDD, meaning that gap between the expected heritability in the disorder based on twin studies (37%) and the amount of variation identified through SNP-based studies (8%). However, rare-variant association methods are still in early stages of development and further work is needed to match the comprehensiveness and specificity of CNV catalogs to that of SNP catalogs.

FINDINGS FROM GENE–ENVIRONMENT INTERACTION STUDIES

Interest in statistical gene–environment interactions (GxE) in depression has been motivated by the recognition that depression likely results from a complex interplay between genes and life experience. GxE studies assess the degree to which genetic variants modify the association between environmental factors and depression (or similarly, the extent to which environmental factors modify the gene–depression relationship).[86–88] Conventionally GxE studies have assumed a *diathesis-stress* model, where a genetic liability or diathesis interacts with an adverse environmental experience to give rise to depression. In this model, genes either exacerbate or buffer the effects of stress.[89] More recently, theoretical GxE models have also sought to account for different relationships between genes and experience, such as incorporating positive aspects of the environment, including social support, psychosocial interventions, and other protective factors that reduce the risk of depression.[90,91] The *differential susceptibility* model,[92,93] for instance, suggests that genetic variation makes individuals more likely to respond differentially to all environments, meaning more adversely to negative environments, but also more positively to salutary environments. The *vantage sensitivity* model[94] on the other hand proposes that genetic differences in response to environmental experiences are only evident when studying positive experiences or environmental advantages. That is, some people might be more likely to benefit only from positive experiences or environments, while other people would have diminished or completely eliminated positive responses to the same positive conditions; this model suggests that genetic differences are only apparent when studying the effects of positive, but makes no claims regarding genetic differences that would be observed among people exposed to negative, environments. Regardless of the specific GxE model studied, GxE research can ultimately help identify high-risk populations most at risk for depression who would benefit most from interventions. Ultimately, such insights could guide intervention strategies and inform efforts to allocate resources to those most in need.

Historically, GxE studies have focused primarily on a limited set of candidate genes, which with recent exceptions (see for example Van der Auwera and colleagues work[95]) have typically been underpowered, creating a risk of both false-positive and false-negative results. As a result, we still know little about whether experience plays a role in shaping genetic effects and, if so, which genetic variants may be involved.

One approach to address this gap has been to perform genome-wide environment interaction studies (GWEIS).[96,97] In a GWEIS, investigators test for GxE, where *G* is defined as the genetic loci (e.g., SNPs) included in a GWAS and the *E* is defined as a known environmental exposure. Different from candidate gene GxE, GWEIS are genetically unbiased searches in which prior genetic or biologic hypotheses are not required. In one type of GWEIS, investigators could focus on loci that have already shown a genetic main effect in a prior GWAS. In this scenario, loci that have been identified by GWAS become candidates for GxE analysis, but with the advantage over traditional candidate gene studies that the locus is already known to influence the phenotype of interest.

Several studies have identified significant genome-wide G×E interactions in cancer,[98,99] diabetes[100] and insulin resistance,[101] Parkinson's disease,[102] pulmonary function,[103] and nonsyndromic cleft palate.[104] In a large GWEIS study of esophageal squamous cell carcinoma (ESCC), totaling over 10,000 cases and 10,000 controls, Wu and colleagues[98] identified three genomic regions, involved in alcohol-metabolizing pathways, that significantly interacted with alcohol consumption to increase the risk of ESCC. The results indicated the importance of reducing alcohol consumption among carriers of these high-risk alleles for ESCC.

To our knowledge, only two GWEIS of depression has been published to date.[64,105] In the largest of these analyses, Dunn and colleagues[64] performed a GWAS and GWEIS of depressive symptoms among African American and Hispanic/Latino populations. While no significant associations were identified in the GWAS, a locus (rs4652467) near the *CEP350* gene showed significant interaction with stressful life events (SLEs). Specifically, individuals who had more exposure to SLEs and had more copies of the major allele had the highest depressive symptoms. However, this GxE was not observed in a smaller independent replication cohort, suggesting the need for larger samples to confirm these findings.

Although interest in GWEIS is growing, several challenges exist with respect to conducting this type of study.[96] The first is identifying the best methods to test for genome-wide GxE. Several methodological approaches have been developed (see reviews by Winham & Biernacka[106] and Gauderman et al.[107]), though there remains no consensus as to which approach is the best.

Selection of a specific analytic method depends largely on whether the goal is to leverage GxE to discover novel loci, or to characterize the joint effect of genetic variants and environmental factors.[108] Second, achieving sufficient sample size and statistical power is a major challenge; it has been reported that the sample size for a GWEIS should be at least 3–4 times that of a GWAS.[96] Unsuccessful replication efforts for GxE have also been attributed to underpowered studies. Methods such as the two-stage testing procedures can potentially reduce the multiple testing burden and improve power to detect smaller interaction effects.[109]

Recognizing that depression is a polygenic disorder, meaning a condition influenced by multiple genes of individually small effect, many studies have also tested for GxE in the context of polygenic risk scores (PRS), which capture the aggregate effect of risk loci across the genome.[110,111] PRS are constructed in a target sample, typically by summing the count of the risk alleles weighted by the corresponding effect size from the discovery GWAS.[110] By aggregating across multiple loci, each of small effect,[111] PRS can be statistically more powerful than single variant approaches without requiring large sample sizes.[110,112] PRS using genome-wide data are particularly advantageous as they can explain more phenotypic variance than scores confined to certain genes, such as candidate genes.[113,114] Indeed, a large GWAS of MDD study found that PRS explain 1.9% of variance in MDD.[59,115]

Of the handful of published GxE studies of depression, most have focused on the interaction between PRS and childhood maltreatment, as child maltreatment is common worldwide[116] and has been associated with adverse psychological consequences that often persist into adulthood.[116–121] To date, four studies in adult populations have tested for GxE of depression using MDD PRS derived from genome-wide data[36,122–124] and some indicator of childhood maltreatment assessed retrospectively, whether through a single type of childhood maltreatment (e.g., sexual abuse) or multiple types considered simultaneously. These studies have generally yielded mixed results. In the earliest GxE study comprised of approximately 2000 individuals, Peyrot and colleagues found a significant GxE with childhood abuse, such that the PRS for depression was positively associated with risk for depression among individuals with high exposure to childhood maltreatment, but not among those with no or low exposure to childhood maltreatment.[123] In a larger sample of ~1600 MDD cases and ~1000 controls, Mullins and colleagues[124] found a significant interaction for childhood maltreatment in the opposite

direction, such that among individuals who had experienced moderate/severe childhood maltreatment, the PRS was inversely associated with MDD.[125] The authors of this study speculated that these opposing results may reflect differences in study design, including the measures of depression, the nature and timing of stressful life events, as well as differences in the sample populations studied.

In the latest GxE study of MDD-PRS and childhood maltreatment, researchers reanalyzed the NESDA (Netherlands Study of Depression and Anxiety) and RADIANT-UK samples in an effort to better understand the sources of the discrepant results. Using a more accurate PRS, obtained from a larger discovery sample (~110,000 individuals vs. ~15,000 in prior studies), Peyrot and colleagues meta-analyzed the results from NESDA and RADIANT-UK with additional PGC cohorts,[36] yielding the largest sample size yet for a PRS GxE study of child maltreatment on depression ($n = 5765$). The authors did not find evidence for an interaction between MDD-PRS and childhood maltreatment, suggesting that prior reports of interaction effects may be chance findings and that further studies are required to determine the true source of genetic heterogeneity in MDD.

CURRENT AND FUTURE DIRECTIONS FOR RESEARCH

There are a number of areas of active inquiry that may help to extend these findings. We highlight three of these here.

Understanding the Biological Function of Loci Identified through GWAS

Since the advent of GWAS, over 1000 novel loci have been identified as associated with human diseases and traits.[126] However, most significant GWAS loci fall in noncoding intergenic or intronic regions, which are regions of the genome unlikely to have direct functional consequences on gene expression.[127] Nonetheless, these associational loci provide important clues that can be leveraged to ultimately identify the true causal variant and biological mechanisms through which they act. In the past decade, a range of methods have been developed and employed to elucidate the biological pathways through which genome-wide association study loci exert effects on a phenotype.[128–130]

Genetic fine mapping is a typical first step in the functional evaluation of genome-wide association study signals. This approach aims to identify the true causal variants and characterize the biological mechanisms through which the GWAS loci influence disease risk. These efforts have been mainly facilitated by large publicly available SNP catalogs, such as the 1000 Genomes Project, which sequenced the genomes of more than 1000 people.[131] In recent years, custom genotyping chips have also been developed for fine-mapping loci in specific disease groups, including the Immunochip,[132] Metabochip,[133] and iCOGs,[134] with an increasing emphasis on targeted sequencing when a smaller number of genes are of interest. These chips have been designed to perform deep replication of specific diseases (e.g., major autoimmune and inflammatory disease for Immunochip, and metabolic diseases for Metabochip), enabling identification of true disease-associated SNPs among GWAS hits.[135]

Expression quantitative trait locus (eQTL) analysis is also an increasingly common approach used to elucidate the molecular mechanisms of GWAS hits, given strong evidence for the enrichment of eQTLs in GWAS hits.[136,137] eQTLs are loci that explain all or a fraction of variation in gene expression levels.[138] eQTL data are particularly important for understanding the risk loci of complex psychiatric traits, since these loci appear to have more important roles in genetic regulation.[139] There are a number of eQTL databases with rich transcriptomics data; the major brain eQTL databases include the NIH funded Genotype-Tissue Expression (GTEx) (https://www.gtexportal.org/home/), the CommonMind consortium (https://www.synapse.org/#!Synapse:syn2759792/wiki/69613), and the UK Brain Expression Consortium (UKBEC) (http://www.braineac.org). A major goal of eQTL analyses is to identify the underlying mechanisms in the transcriptome that drive associations between genetic variants and outcomes of interest. Such insights can, in turn, inform subsequent experimental in vivo *or* in vitro testing, such as perturbing or knocking up/down expression of the eQTL target genes in culture cell lines and/or primary tissues, and examining the effects on relevant phenotypes.[140] Although these databases are important resources for uncovering disease mechanisms, they are not without technical limitations.[141] Current databases contain samples from a small number of participants due to challenges and costs associated with obtaining human tissues. Most tissue samples are also collected from adult populations, limiting their utility in understanding neurodevelopmental processes, which have long thought to be involved in shaping risk neuropsychiatric disorders.[142]

Application of these functional genomics methods to findings from GWAS has led to new discoveries about the molecular pathways that may be regulating risk for disease.[143,144] One area in psychiatry where such work has been most fruitful is through functional follow-up of schizophrenia GWAS results, where major new insights have been made in the past few years. For example, in 2016, prompted by findings from the PGC genome-wide association study of schizophrenia,[127] Stevens, McCarroll, and colleagues[145] characterized complement component 4 (C4), an immune molecule regulated by the *CSMD1* gene that was found to be associated with schizophrenia risk. The authors found that C4 variants were associated with greater C4A expression in postmortem human brain, and suggested an effect on pruning in rodent models. A subsequent study[146] demonstrated that synaptic pruning is abnormal in models derived from people with schizophrenia, and that this effect is moderated but not fully explained by C4A. Importantly, these two studies illustrate that genomics may be most useful in hypothesis generation, while actual hypothesis testing may require experiments rather than purely in silico analysis.

Similarly, using genome-wide gene expression data from postmortem human brain samples, a study by Hertzberg and colleagues[147] analyzed functional changes in GWAS-identified genes shown to predict risk for schizophrenia. The integration of GWAS and expression data improved the statistical power and biological reliability of their findings and their results provided evidence for a central role of calcium ion transport and calcium signaling in the pathogenesis of schizophrenia. Once again, such hypotheses still require experimental confirmation. Similar studies are underway for MDD[148] and may be accelerated by an expanding pool of candidate loci for investigation, but have thus far not yielded novel findings.

Identifying Best Practices to Study Gene–Environment Interaction

There is considerable interest in understanding how genes and life experience work together to shape risk for depression. Yet, as noted earlier, a number of major challenges remain with respect to how to design GxE studies and select analytic models for such analyses.

Arguably the biggest challenge relates to obtaining high quality and accurate measures of environmental exposures. As noted in our previous review,[37] the "environment" is unspecified, being unbounded in a way the genome is not. Such broadness produces challenges in deciding not just what is studied, but when and how such exposures are ascertained. One approach to test for GxE may be to focus on well-defined measures of specific environmental exposures, where robust and consistent evidence has been found to support a relationship between a given exposure and risk for depression. Examples of the kinds of exposures that could be studied with this criteria include in utero exposures to adverse biological or other substances (e.g., viruses, toxins, alcohol, and drugs), experiences of social deprivation during childhood or adolescence (e.g., poverty, maltreatment), and experiences of environmental enrichment (e.g., exercise; psychosocial interventions and treatments). However, as reflected in our earlier comments regarding PRS studies of child maltreatment, even efforts to study the same single environmental exposure can still produce mixed results, owing to differences in when the exposure is assessed and how.

For example, although commonly used and upheld as the current gold standard, retrospective and prospective self-reports of child maltreatment and other early life adversities have been shown to be susceptible to serious biases in recall, or willingness to self-disclose,[149–151] with low levels of agreement observed across time,[152,153] even when the same reporter is used.[154] Although official reports, such as health or social services records, represent an alternative strategy for measuring maltreatment exposure, these records likely dramatically underestimate the prevalence of maltreatment.[155,156] Similar measurement issues have been documented for a range of other psychosocial stressors, including financial difficulties, that can occur during prenatal and postnatal life.[157,158] Methods have been developed in the hopes of yielding more accurate self-reported information, such as the experience sampling method that involves daily reports of events, behavior, and feelings,[159] but new tools to objectively capture stressful life experiences in particular are needed. Recent research by Dr. Dunn's suggests that children's shed primary or "baby" could represent one such objective biomarker of past stress exposures and subsequent mental health risk.[160]

A second major challenge relates to the analytic models used to test for statistical interaction or GxE. GxE studies are generally more susceptible to potential biases than standard main effects models and could result in biased interaction estimates when underlying model assumptions, such as linearity, are violated.[161–163] One of the issues that has been raised in the past few years relates to adjustment for confounding. In 2015, Keller and colleagues argued that few studies completely adjust for potential covariates in statistical analyses in the GxE literature, leading them to encourage complete control for confounding by adjusting for all covariate-by-environment and covariate-by-gene interactions in the GxE analytic models.[164] Although such covariate adjustment could reduce

confounding bias and improve statistical power by removing residual variance, some have also raised concerns that controlling for certain covariates could also induce bias in genetic association studies. For instance, Aschard and colleagues[165] showed that adjusting for heritable covariates, or covariates with a strong genetic component, could introduce collider/selection bias and induce spurious associations. Recently, two methods have been proposed to concurrently avoid this bias and improve statistical power. The Covariates for Multiphenotype Studies (CMS) algorithm, developed by Aschard and colleagues,[166] selects covariates correlated with the exposure of interest, but not genotype. The other covariate adjustment approach, adjustment analysis using meta-statistic of covariates (AAMC), removes potential correlation between the covariate and exposure of interest due to shared genetics.[167] This method involves two steps: (1) adjusting for the residuals obtained from regressing the covariate on the genetic variant in the regression and (2) incorporating GWAS summary data of the covariate to reduce variance. However, both methods are limited in that they can currently only be applied to continuous outcomes, and further developments are needed for binary or categorical outcomes.

Finally, balancing the trade-off between large sample sizes and reliable environmental exposure data is a significant challenge. Study cohorts with detailed and repeated measures usually have small sample sizes and are largely underpowered to detect robust interaction effects. With the formation of international collaborations and consortia, studies have increasing statistical power for detecting G×E, but face issues with the lack of the depth and breadth of environmental or phenotype measures. Furthermore, harmonizing different measures of the environment across data sets is not a trivial task; environmental exposures can be highly heterogeneous and are prone to varying degrees of measurement error depending on the data collection modality. To address this problem, environmental phenotypes are often simplified or "watered-down," removing important variability within the study population (e.g., classifying respondents as either "exposed" or "nonexposed"). A selective sampling approach, known as recall-by-genotype or genotype-based recall, offers one potential solution for future GxE research.[168,169] In this study design, participants in a cohort are recalled for extensive phenotyping based on their genotypes. This sampling method provides adequate power even in smaller samples, as well as more precise environmental measures. A promising avenue for conducting GWEIS is through longitudinal birth cohort studies, which can include prospective and repeated measures of environmental exposures along with detailed phenotype data and genome-wide data. Such data will enable the assessment of GxE from a developmental and life-course perspective to determine whether GxE effects are particularly prominent in certain stages of life.[170]

Leveraging Genetics to Strengthen Causal Inference

Observational studies have traditionally been used to investigate environmental risk factors for depression. However, these types of studies are limited in their ability to infer causation given the potential influences of confounding, selection bias, and/or reverse causation on observed associations.[171] Although randomized controlled trials (RCTs) can confirm findings from observational studies and are considered the gold standard for determining causal effects, they are costly and cannot always be feasibly implemented.[172] For instance, psychiatric disorders tend to have risk factors that cannot be randomized, such as childhood maltreatment and life stressors, rendering RCTs an impractical and unethical approach to evaluate the causal role of many possible risk and protective factors linked to depression. This challenge has prompted the innovation of powerful genetic tools that exploit genotype or GWAS data to strengthen causal inference.

In the past few years, Mendelian randomization (MR) has rapidly gained popularity as a cost-effective method to test putative causal relationships.[173] MR is an instrumental variable approach that uses genetic instruments, typically SNPs identified through prior GWAS as associated with an exposure, to estimate the causal effect of the exposure on the outcome.[174,175] The premise of MR is that genes are randomly assorted at conception, and are therefore unlikely to be associated with potential confounders (of the exposure–disease relationship) in the population. As such, MR can be conceptualized as a natural randomized controlled trial, where the unconfounded gene–exposure and gene–outcome associations are used to estimate the causal effect of the exposure on the outcome. Three major assumptions must be met to conduct a valid MR analysis: (1) The genetic instrument must be strongly associated with the exposure; (2) the gene–exposure or gene–outcome associations must not be confounded by other factors; and (3) the genetic instrument must not be associated with the outcome of interest either directly or via other pathways (i.e., horizontal pleiotropy).

MR has been successfully applied across a range of diseases and traits.[176] In psychiatry, MR studies of risk factors for schizophrenia have identified a causal link between cannabis use,[177] lower C-reactive protein levels,[178] and higher interleukin-6 receptor levels[178] and an increased risk for schizophrenia. The same level of success, however, has not yet been achieved by MDD studies. A recent review by Kohler and colleagues[179] reported that the eight known MR studies of depression provided no consistent evidence supporting the causal effects of obesity, smoking, and alcohol consumption. Although these findings suggest that previously identified associations were likely spurious, the null results could also be attributed to weak instrument effects, meaning genetic instruments that have weak associations with the exposure, leading to low statistical power or violations of the MR assumptions due to pleiotropic effects.[172] Indeed, one recent MR analysis using genetic instruments with strong associations with the exposure, derived from a GWAS of over 370,000 individuals in the UK Biobank, yielded promising results. In their cross-sectional study, Choi and colleagues[180] found that physical activity was a protective factor associated with MDD.

Progress in genetic methods to produce more robust causal estimates is expected to continue in the coming years. With increasingly larger genome-wide data sets, stronger genetic instruments, such as polygenic scores, can be constructed to achieve higher statistical power in MR analyses.[181] Researchers have also proposed refining genetic instruments by incorporating information on their biological functions, as well as strategies to integrate genetic instruments with family-based designs to better understand the underlying causal mechanisms,[182] although these methods have not yet been developed. However, major challenges will need to be tackled along the way. For complex disorders such as MDD, the phenotypic variance explained by genetic instruments remains small, despite the size of the latest GWAS. Therefore, there may be insufficient power to detect weaker causal associations in the MR framework. In addition, while aggregating genetic instruments can improve statistical power, it simultaneously increases the likelihood that the genetic instrument affects the outcome of interest through pathways that are independent of the exposure; such associations violate the MR assumption that the selected genetic instrument does not have pleiotropic effects.[173] Finally, there are certain risk factors for psychiatric disorders, such as parental attitudes/behavior and neighborhood characteristics, for which strong genetic instruments may never be available due to small genetic effects. Alternative causal inference methods will have to be explored in these cases.

CONCLUSIONS

A decade of GWAS studies in MDD has yielded more than 100 regions within the genome associated with risk, complimented by a growing body of evidence supporting environmental risk, particularly linked to early adversity. Methods for making more efficient use of common variant data—for example, via polygenic risk scores—and for investigating GxE interactions are among areas of active work. In aggregate, genomic studies of MDD have begun to generate testable hypotheses about the pathophysiology of this common, costly, and complex disorder. Pursuit of these hypotheses may finally enable development of more effective strategies for diagnosis and treatment, and ultimately for prevention.

ACKNOWLEDGMENTS

The authors thank Kathryn Davis for her assistance in conducting the literature review for this article. The content is solely the responsibility of the authors and does not necessarily represent the official views of the National Institute of Mental Health or the National Institutes of Health.

REFERENCES

1. Erskine HE, Baxter AJ, Patton G, et al. The global coverage of prevalence data for mental disorders in children and adolescents. *Epidemiol Psychiatr Sci.* 2016; 26:395–402.
2. Kessler RC, Bromet EJ. The epidemiology of depression across cultures. *Annu Rev Public Health.* 2013;34: 119–138.
3. World Health Organization. *Depression and Other Common Mental Disorders: Global Health Estimates.* Geneva: World Health Organization; 2017.
4. Hankin BL. Adolescent depression: description, causes, and interventions. *Epilepsy Behav.* 2006;8:102–114.
5. Kessler RC, Zhao S, Blazer DG. Prevalence, course, and correlates of minor and MDD in the national comorbidity survey. *J Affect Disord.* 1997;45:19–30.
6. Jia H, Zack MM, Thompson WW, Crosby AE, Gottesman II . Impact of depression on quality-adjusted life expectancy (QALE) directly as well as indirectly through suicide. *Soc Psychiatr Psychiatr Epidemiol.* 2015;50:939–949.
7. Dembling BP, Chen DT, Vachon L. Life expectancy and causes of death in a population treated for serious mental illness. *Psychiatr Serv.* 1999;50:1036–1042.
8. Simon GE, Rutter CM, Peterson D, et al. Does response on the PHQ-9 depression questionnaire predict subsequent suicide attempt or suicide death? *Psychiatr Serv.* 2013;64:1195–1202.
9. Vos T, Abajobir AA, Abate KH, et al. Global, regional, and national incidence, prevalence, and years lived with disability for 328 diseases and injuries for 195 countries, 1990–2016: a systematic analysis for the Global Burden of Disease Study 2016. *Lancet.* 2017;390:1211–1259.
10. Lokkerbol J, Adema D, de Graaf R, et al. Non-fatal burden of disease due to mental disorders in The Netherlands. *Soc Psychiatr Psychiatr Epidemiol.* 2013;48:1591–1599.
11. Mathers C, Ma Fat D, Boerma JT. *The Global Burden of Disease: 2004 Update.* Geneva, Switzerland: World Health Organization; 2008.
12. Brooks-Gunn J, Duncan GJ, Aber JL, eds. *Neighborhood Poverty: Context and Consequences for Children.* New York, NY: Russell Sage Foundation; 1997.
13. McLeod JD, Shanahan MJ. Trajectories of poverty and children's mental health. *J Health Soc Behav.* 1996;37: 207–220.
14. Repetti RL, Taylor SE, Seeman TE. Risky families: family social environments and the mental and physical health of offspring. *Psychol Bull.* 2002;128:330–366.
15. Gilman SE, Kawachi I, Fitzmaurice GM, Buka SL. Family disruption in childhood and risk of adult depression. *Am J Psychiatry.* 2003;160:939–946.
16. Slopen N, Koenen KC, Kubzansky LD. Cumulative adversity in childhood and emergent risk factors for long-term health. *J Pediatr.* 2014;164:631–638.
17. Widom CS, DuMont K, Czaja SJ. A prospective investigation of major depressive disorder and comorbidity in abused and neglected children grown up. *Arch Gen Psychiatr.* 2007;64:49–56.
18. Kessler RC. The effects of stressful life events on depression. *Annu Rev Psychol.* 1997;48:191–214.
19. Hammen C. Stress and depression. *Annu Rev Clin Psychol.* 2005;1:293–319.
20. Dunn EC, Gilman SE, Slopen N, Willett JB, Molnar BE. The impact of exposure to interpersonal violence on gender differences in adolescent-onset major depression: results from the National Comorbidity Survey Replication (NCS-R). *Depress Anxiety.* 2012;29:392–399.
21. Dunn EC, McLaughlin KA, Slopen N, Rosand J, Smoller JW. Developmental timing of child maltreatment and symptoms of depression and suicidality in young adulthood: results from the National Longitudinal Study of Adolescent Health. *Depress Anxiety.* 2013;30: 955–964.
22. McLaughlin KA, Green JG, Gruber MJ, Sampson NA, Zaslavsky AM, Kessler RC. Childhood adversities and adult psychiatric disorders in the National Comorbidity Survey Replication II: associations with persistence of DSM-IV disorders. *Arch Gen Psychiatr.* 2010;67:124–132.
23. McLaughlin KA, Green JG, Gruber MJ, Sampson NA, Zaslavsky AM, Kessler RC. Childhood adversities and first onset of psychiatric disorders in a national sample of US adolescents. *Arch Gen Psychiatr.* 2012;69:1151–1160.

24. Gilman SE, Ni MY, Dunn EC, et al. Contributions of the social environment to first-onset and recurrent mania. *Mol Psychiatr.* 2015;20:329–336.

25. Dunn EC, Nishimi K, Powers A, Bradley B. Is developmental timing of trauma exposure associated with depressive and post-traumatic stress disorder symptoms in adulthood? *J Psychiatr Res.* 2017;84: 119–127.

26. Dunn EC, Soare TW, Raffeld MR, et al. What life course theoretical models best explain the relationship between exposure to childhood adversity and psychopathology symptoms: recency, accumulation, or sensitive periods? *Psychol Med.* 2018;48:2562–2572.

27. Sullivan PF, Neale MC, Kendler KS. Genetic epidemiology of major depression: review and meta analysis. *Am J Psychiatry.* 2000;157:1552–1562.

28. Rice F, Harold G, Thapar A. The genetic aetiology of childhood depression: a review. *J Child Psychol Psychiatry.* 2002;43:65–79.

29. International Human Genome Sequencing C, Lander ES, Linton LM, et al. Initial sequencing and analysis of the human genome. *Nature.* 2001;409:860.

30. The International HapMap Consortium, Gibbs RA, Belmont JW, et al. The international HapMap Project. *Nature.* 2003;426:789.

31. The 1000 Genomes Project Consortium, Auton A, Abecasis GR, et al. A global reference for human genetic variation. *Nature.* 2015;526:68.

32. Dunlop BW, Nemeroff CB. The role of dopamine in the pathophysiology of depression. *Arch Gen Psychiatr.* 2007;64:327–337.

33. Owens MJ, Nemeroff CB. Role of serotonin in the pathophysiology of depression: focus on the serotonin transporter. *Clin Chem.* 1994;40:288–295.

34. Thase ME, ed. *Neurobiological Aspects of Depression.* 2nd ed. New York, NY: The Guilford Press; 2009.

35. Smoller JW. Psychiatric genetics and the future of personalized treatment. *Depress Anxiety.* 2014;31:893–898.

36. Peyrot WJ, Van der Auwera S, Milaneschi Y, et al. Does childhood trauma moderate polygenic risk for depression? A meta-analysis of 5765 subjects from the psychiatric genomics consortium. *Biol Psychiatry.* 2018;84: 138–147.

37. Dunn EC, Brown RC, Dai Y, et al. Genetic determinants of depression: recent findings and future directions. *Harv Rev Psychiatry.* 2015;23:1–18.

38. Demkow U, Wolańczyk T. Genetic tests in major psychiatric disorders—integrating molecular medicine with clinical psychiatry—why is it so difficult? *Transl Psychiatry.* 2017;7:e1151.

39. Smoller JW. A quarter century of progress in psychiatric genetics. *Harv Rev Psychiatry.* 2017;25.

40. Manolio TA. Genomewide association studies and assessment of the risk of disease. *N Engl J Med.* 2010;36: 166–176.

41. Corvin A, Craddock N, Sullivan PF. Genome-wide association studies: a primer. *Psychol Med.* 2010;40:1063–1077.

42. Balding DJ. A tutorial on statistical methods for population association studies. *Nat Rev Genet.* 2006;7:781–791.

43. Psychiatric GWAS Consortium Coordinating Committee. Genomewide association studies: history, rationale, and prospects for psychiatric disorders. *Am J Psychiatry.* 2009;166:540–556.

44. Sullivan PF. The Psychiatric GWAS Consortium: big sciences comes to psychiatry. *Neuron.* 2010;68:182–186.

45. The Psychiatric GWAS Consortium Steering Committee. A framework for interpreting genome-wide association studies of psychiatric disorders. *Mol Psychiatr.* 2009;14: 10–17.

46. Major Depressive Disorder Working Group of the Psychiatric GWAS Consortium, Ripke S, Wray NR, et al. A megaanalysis of genome-wide association studies for major depressive disorder. *Mol Psychiatr.* 2013;18:497–511.

47. Hek K, Demirkan A, Lahti J, et al. A genome-wide association study of depressive symptoms. *Biol Psychiatry.* 2013; 73:667–678.

48. Converge Consortium. Sparse whole-genome sequencing identifies two loci for major depressive disorder. *Nature.* 2015;523:588–591.

49. Cui L, Gong X, Tang Y, et al. Relationship between the LHPP gene polymorphism and resting-state brain activity in major depressive disorder. *Neural Plast.* 2016;2016: 9162590.

50. Hyde CL, Nagle MW, Tian C, et al. Identification of 15 genetic loci associated with risk of major depression in individuals of European descent. *Nat Genet.* 2016;48: 1031–1036.

51. Muench C, Schwandt M, Jung J, Cortes CR, Momenan R, Lohoff FW. The major depressive disorder GWAS-supported variant rs10514299 in TMEM161B-MEF2C predicts putamen activation during reward processing in alcohol dependence. *Transl Psychiatry.* 2018;8:131.

52. Barbosa AC, Kim M-S, Ertunc M, et al. MEF2C, a transcription factor that facilitates learning and memory by negative regulation of synapse numbers and function. *Proc Natl Acad Sci U S A.* 2008;105:9391.

53. Okbay A, Baselmans BM, De Neve JE, et al. Genetic variants associated with subjective well-being, depressive symptoms, and neuroticism identified through genome-wide analyses. *Nat Genet.* 2016;48:624–633.

54. Manitt C, Eng C, Pokinko M, et al. Dcc orchestrates the development of the prefrontal cortex during adolescence and is altered in psychiatric patients. *Transl Psychiatry.* 2013;3:e338.

55. Torres-Berrío A, Lopez JP, Bagot RC, et al. DCC confers susceptibility to depression-like behaviors in humans and mice and is regulated by mir-218. *Biol Psychiatry.* 2017;81:306–315.

56. Direk N, Williams S, Smith JA, et al. An analysis of two genome-wide association meta-analyses identifies a new locus for broad depression phenotype. *Biol Psychiatry.* 2017;82:322–329.

57. Howard DM, Adams MJ, Clarke TK, et al. Genome-wide meta-analysis of depression identifies 102 independent

variants and highlights the importance of the prefrontal brain regions. *Nat Neurosci.* 2019;22:343−352.

58. Howard D, Adams M, Shirali M, et al. Genome-wide association study of depression phenotypes in UK Biobank identifies variants in excitatory synaptic pathways. *Nat Commun.* 2018;9:1−10.

59. Wray NR, Ripke S, Mattheisen M, et al. Genome-wide association analyses identify 44 risk variants and refine the genetic architecture of major depression. *Nat Genet.* 2018; 50:668.

60. Dalvie S, Koen N, Duncan L, et al. Large scale genetic research on neuropsychiatric disorders in african populations is needed. *EBioMedicine.* 2015;2:1259−1261.

61. Bentley AR, Callier S, Rotimi CN. Diversity and inclusion in genomic research: why the uneven progress? *J Commun Genet.* 2017;8:255−266.

62. Quansah E, McGregor NW. Towards diversity in genomics: the emergence of neurogenomics in Africa? *Genomics.* 2018;110:1−9.

63. Dalvie S, Koen N, McGregor N, et al. Toward a global roadmap for precision medicine in psychiatry: challenges and opportunities. *OMICS A J Integr Biol.* 2016;20:557−564.

64. Dunn EC, Wiste A, Radmanesh F, et al. Genome-wide association study (GWAS) and genome-wide by environment interaction study (GWEIS) of depressive symptoms in African American and Hispanic/Latina women. *Depress Anxiety.* 2016;33:265−280.

65. Ware EB, Mukherjee B, Sun YV, Diez-Roux AV, Kardia SL, Smith JA. Comparative genome-wide association studies of a depressive symptom phenotype in a repeated measures setting by race/ethnicity in the Multi-Ethnic Study of Atherosclerosis. *BMC Genet.* 2015;16:118.

66. Wray NR, Maier R. Genetic basis of complex genetic disease: the contribution of disease heterogeneity to missing heritability. *Cur Epidemiol Rep.* 2014;1:220−227.

67. Sanders SJ, Ercan-Sencicek AG, Hus V, et al. Multiple recurrent de novo CNVs, including duplications of the 7q11.23 Williams syndrome region, are strongly associated with autism. *Neuron.* 2011;70:863−885.

68. Sebat J, Lakshmi B, Malhotra D, et al. Strong association of de novo copy number mutations with autism. *Science.* 2007;316:445−449.

69. Stefansson H, Rujescu D, Cichon S, et al. Large recurrent microdeletions associated with schizophrenia. *Nature.* 2008;455:232−236.

70. Purcell SM, Moran JL, Fromer M, et al. A polygenic burden of rare disruptive mutations in schizophrenia. *Nature.* 2014;506:185−190.

71. Malhotra D, McCarthy S, Michaelson JJ, et al. High frequencies of de novo CNVs in bipolar disorder and schizophrenia. *Neuron.* 2011;72:951−963.

72. O'Dushlaine C, Ripke S, Ruderfer DM, et al. Rare copy number variation in treatment-resistant major depressive disorder. *Biol Psychiatry.* 2014;76:536−541.

73. Kendall KM, Rees E, Bracher-Smith M, et al. The role of rare copy number variants in depression. *bioR.* 2018;xiv.

74. Yu C, Baune BT, Wong M-L, Licinio J. Investigation of copy number variation in subjects with major depression based on whole-genome sequencing data. *J Affect Disord.* 2017;220:38−42.

75. Degenhardt F, Priebe L, Herms S, et al. Association between copy number variants in 16p11.2 and major depressive disorder in a German case−control sample. *Am J Med Genet Part B.* 2012;159B:263−273.

76. Glessner JT, Li J, Wang D, et al. Copy number variation meta-analysis reveals a novel duplication at 9p24 associated with multiple neurodevelopmental disorders. *Genome Med.* 2017;9.

77. Glessner JT, Wang K, Sleiman PMA, et al. Duplication of the SLIT3 locus on 5q35.1 predisposes to major depressive disorder. *PLoS One.* 2010;5:e15463.

78. Reuter JA, Spacek DV, Snyder MP. High-throughput sequencing technologies. *Mol Cell.* 2015;58:586−597.

79. Bras J, Guerreiro R, Hardy J. Use of next-generation sequencing and other whole-genome strategies to dissect neurological disease. *Nat Rev Neurosci.* 2012;12:453−464.

80. Rizzo JM, Buck MJ. Key principles and clinical applications of "next-generation" DNA sequencing. *Cancer Prev Res.* 2012;5:887−900.

81. Amin N, Jovanova O, Adams HH, et al. Exome-sequencing in a large population-based study reveals a rare Asn396Ser variant in the LIPG gene associated with depressive symptoms. *Mol Psychiatry.* 2017;22:537−543.

82. Pirooznia M, Wang T, Avramopoulos D, Potash JB, Zandi PP, Goes FS. High-throughput sequencing of the synaptome in major depressive disorder. *Mol Psychiatr.* 2016;21:650−655.

83. Peterson RE, Cai N, Bigdeli TB, et al. The genetic architecture of major depressive disorder in han Chinese women. *JAMA Psychiatry.* 2017;74:162−168.

84. Yu C, Baune BT, Licinio J, Wong M-L. A novel strategy for clustering major depression individuals using whole-genome sequencing variant data. *Sci Rep.* 2017;7.

85. Amin N, De Vrij FMS, Baghdadi M, et al. A rare missense variant in RCL1 segregates with depression in extended families. *Mol Psychiatr.* 2017;23.

86. Moffitt TE, Caspi A, Rutter M. Strategy for investigating interactions between measured genes and measured enviornments. *Arch Gen Psychiatr.* 2005;62:473−481.

87. Dick. Gene-environment interaction in psychological traits and disorders. *Annual Review of Clinical Psychology.* 2011;7:383−409.

88. Dunn EC, Uddin M, Subramanian SV, Smoller JW, Galea S, Koenen KC. Gene-environment interaction (GxE) research in youth depression: a systematic review with recommendations for future research. *J Child Psychol Psychiatry.* 2011;52:1223−1238.

89. Monroe SM, Simons AD. Diathesis-stress theories in the context of life stress research: implications for the depressive disorders. *Psychol Bull.* 1991;110:406−425.

90. Bakermans-Kranenburg MJ, Van Ijzendoorn MH, Pijlman FTA, Mesman J, Juffer F. Experimental evidence for differential susceptibility: dopamine D4 receptor polymorphism (DRD4 VNTR) moderates intervention effects on toddlers' externalizing behavior in a randomized controlled trial. *Dev Psychol.* 2008;44:293−300.

91. Brody GH, Beach SRH, Philibert RA, Chen Y-F, Murry VM. Prevention effects moderate the association of 5-HTTLPR and youth risk behavior initiation: gene × environment hypotheses tested via a randomized prevention design. *Child Dev.* 2009;80:645–661.

92. Belsky J, Pleuss M. Beyond diathesis stress: differential susceptibility to environmental influences. *Psychol Bull.* 2009;135:885–908.

93. Ellis BJ, Boyce WT. Biological sensitivity to context. *Curr Dir Psychol Sci.* 2008;17:183–187.

94. Pluess M, Belsky J. Vantage sensitivity: individual differences in response to positive experiences. *Psychol Bull.* 2013;139:901–916.

95. Van der Auwera S, Peyrot WJ, Milaneschi Y, et al. Genome-wide gene-environment interaction in depression: a systematic evaluation of candidate genes: the childhood trauma working-group of PGC-MDD. *Am J Med Genet B Neuropsychiatr Genet.* 2018;177:40–49.

96. Thomas D. Gene-environment-wide association studies: emerging approaches. *Nat Rev Genet.* 2010;11.

97. Thomas D. Methods for investigating gene-environment interactions in candidate pathway and genome-wide association studies. *Annu Rev Public Health.* 2010;31:21–36.

98. Wu C, Kraft P, Zhai K, et al. Genome-wide association analyses of esophageal squamous cell carcinoma in Chinese identify multiple susceptibility loci and gene-environment interactions. *Nat Genet.* 2012;44:1090–1097.

99. Seigert S, Hampe J, Schafmayer C, et al. Genome-wide investigation of gene-environment interactions in colorectal cancer. *Hum Genet.* 2013;132:219–231.

100. Cornelis MC, Tchetgen EJ, Liang L, et al. Gene-environment interactions in genome-wide association studies: a comparative study of tests applied to empirical studies of type 2 diabetes. *Am J Epidemiol.* 2012;175:191–202.

101. Manning AK, Hivert M-F, Scott RA, et al. A genome-wide approach accounting for body mass index identifies genetic variants influencing fasting glycemic traits and insulin resistance. *Nat Genet.* 2012;44.

102. Hamza TH, Chen H, Hill-Burns EM, et al. Genome-wide gene-environment study identifies glutamate receptor gene GRIN2A as a Parkinson's disease modifier gene via interaction with coffee. *PLoS Genet.* 2011;7:e1002237.

103. Hancock DB, Artigas MS, Gharib SA, et al. Genome-wide joint meta analysis of SNP and SNP-by-smoking interaction identifies novel loci for pulmonary function. *PLoS Genet.* 2012;8:e1003098.

104. Beaty TH, Ruczinski I, Murray JC, et al. Evidence for gene-environment interaction in a genome wide study of nonsyndromic cleft palate. *Genet Epidemiol.* 2011;35:469–478.

105. Ikeda M, Shimasaki A, Takahashi A, et al. Genome-wide environment interaction between depressive state and stressful life events. *J Clin Psychiatry.* 2016;77:e29–30.

106. Winham SJ, Biernacka JM. Gene-environment interactions in genome-wide association studies: current

approaches and new directions. *J Child Psychol Psychiatry.* 2013;54:1120–1134.

107. Gauderman WJ, Zhang P, Morrison JL, Lewinger JP. Finding novel genes by testing GxE interactions in a genome-wide association study. *Genet Epidemiol.* 2013;37:603–613.

108. Hutter CM, Mechanic LE, Chatterjee N, Kraft P, Gillanders EM, NCI Gene-Environment Think Tank. Gene-environment interactions in cancer epidemiology: a national cancer institute think tank report. Genet Epidemiol in press.

109. Dai JY, Kooperberg C, Leblanc M, Prentice RL. Two-stage testing procedures with independent filtering for genome-wide gene-environment interaction. *Biometrika.* 2012;99:929–944.

110. Wray NR, Lee SH, Mehta D, Vinkhuyzen AA, Dudbridge F, Middeldorp CM. Research review: polygenic methods and their application to psychiatric traits. *J Child Psychol Psychiatry.* 2014;55:1068–1087.

111. Khera AV, Emdin CA, Drake I, et al. Genetic risk, adherence to a healthy lifestyle, and coronary disease. *N Engl J Med.* 2016;375:2349–2358.

112. Chang SC, Glymour MM, Walter S, et al. Genome-wide polygenic scoring for a 14-year long-term average depression phenotype. *Brain Behav.* 2014;4:298–311.

113. Evans DM, Visscher PM, Wray NR. Harnessing the information contained within genome-wide association studies to improve individual prediction of complex disease risk. *Hum Mol Genet.* 2009;18:3525–3531.

114. International Schizophrenia C, Purcell SM, Wray NR, et al. Common polygenic variation contributes to risk of schizophrenia and bipolar disorder. *Nature.* 2009;460:748–752.

115. Demirkan A, Penninx BW, Hek K, et al. Genetic risk profiles for depression and anxiety in adult and elderly cohorts. *Mol Psychiatr.* 2011;16:773–783.

116. Akmatov MK. Child abuse in 28 developing and transitional countries—results from the Multiple Indicator Cluster Surveys. *Int J Epidemiol.* 2011;40:219–227.

117. Jud A, Fegert JM, Finkelhor D. On the incidence and prevalence of child maltreatment: a research agenda. *Child Adolesc Psychiatr Ment Health.* 2016;10:17.

118. Kaplow JB, Widom CS. Age of onset of child maltreatment predicts long-term mental health outcomes. *J Abnorm Psychol.* 2007;116:176–187.

119. Scott KM, McLaughlin KA, Smith DAR, Ellis PM. Childhood maltreatment and DSM-IV adult mental disorders: comparison of prospective and retrospective findings. *Br J Psychiatry.* 2012;200:469–475.

120. Khan A, McCormack HC, Bolger EA, et al. Childhood maltreatment, depression, and suicidal ideation: critical importance of parental and peer emotional abuse during developmental sensitive periods in males and females. *Front Psychiatry.* 2015;6:42.

121. Briere J, Elliott DM. Prevalence and psychological sequelae of self-reported childhood physical and sexual abuse in a general population sample of men and women. *Child Abuse Negl.* 2003;27:1205–1222.

122. Musliner KL, Seifuddin F, Judy JA, Pirooznia M, Goes FS, Zandi PP. Polygenic risk, stressful life events and depressive symptoms in older adults: a polygenic score analysis. *Psychol Med.* 2015;45:1709–1720.

123. Peyrot WJ, Milaneschi Y, Abdellaoui A, et al. Effect of polygenic risk scores on depression in childhood trauma. *Br J Psychiatry.* 2014;205:113–119.

124. Mullins N, Power RA, Fisher HL, et al. Polygenic interactions with environmental adversity in the aetiology of major depressive disorder. *Psychol Med.* 2015:1–12.

125. Mullins N, Power RA, Fisher HL, et al. Polygenic interactions with environmental adversity in the aetiology of major depressive disorder. *Psychol Med.* 2016;46:759–770. https://doi.org/10.1017/S0033291715002172. Epub 2015 Nov 3.

126. Hindorff LA, MacArthur J, Morales J, et al. A catalog of published genome-wide association studies. www.genome.gov/gwastudies2013.

127. Schizophrenia Working Group of the Psychiatric Genomics C, Ripke S, Neale BM, et al. Biological insights from 108 schizophrenia-associated genetic loci. *Nature.* 2014;511:421–427.

128. Xiao X, Chang H, Li M. Molecular mechanisms underlying noncoding risk variations in psychiatric genetic studies. *Mol Psychiatr.* 2017;22:497–511.

129. Nurnberg ST, Zhang H, Hand NJ, et al. From loci to biology: functional genomics of genome-wide association for coronary disease. *Circ Res.* 2016;118:586–606.

130. Edwards Stacey L, Beesley J, French Juliet D, Dunning Alison M. Beyond GWASs: illuminating the dark road from association to function. *Am J Hum Genet.* 2013;93: 779–797.

131. The 1000 Genomes Project Consortium, McVean GA, Altshuler DM, et al. An integrated map of genetic variation from 1,092 human genomes. *Nature.* 2012;491:56.

132. Trynka G, Hunt KA, Bockett NA, et al. Dense genotyping identifies and localizes multiple common and rare variant association signals in celiac disease. *Nat Genet.* 2011;43:1193.

133. Voight BF, Kang HM, Ding J, et al. The Metabochip, a custom genotyping array for genetic studies of metabolic, cardiovascular, and anthropometric traits. *PLoS Genet.* 2012;8:e1002793.

134. Michailidou K, Hall P, Gonzalez-Neira A, et al. Large-scale genotyping identifies 41 new loci associated with breast cancer risk. *Nat Genet.* 2013;45:353.

135. Cortes A, Brown MA. Promise and pitfalls of the Immunochip. *Arthritis Res Ther.* 2011;13:101.

136. Nicolae DL, Gamazon E, Zhang W, Duan S, Dolan ME, Cox NJ. Trait-associated SNPs are more likely to Be eQTLs: annotation to enhance discovery from GWAS. *PLoS Genet.* 2010;6:e1000888.

137. Dimas AS, Deutsch S, Stranger BE, et al. Common regulatory variation impacts gene expression in a cell type–dependent manner. *Science.* 2009;325:1246.

138. Nica AC, Dermitzakis ET. Expression quantitative trait loci: present and future. *Phil Trans Biol Sci.* 2013:368.

139. Straub RE, Weinberger DR. Schizophrenia genes — famine to feast. *Biol Psychiatry.* 2006;60:81–83.

140. Lawrenson K, Li Q, Kar S, et al. Cis-eQTL analysis and functional validation of candidate susceptibility genes for high-grade serous ovarian cancer. *Nat Commun.* 2015;6.

141. Gupta RM, Musunuru K. Mapping novel pathways in cardiovascular disease using eQTL data: the past, present, and future of gene expression analysis. *Front Genet.* 2012;3:232.

142. Hagan CC, Graham JME, Wilkinson PO, et al. Neurodevelopment and ages of onset in depressive disorders. *Lancet Psychiat.* 2015;2:1112–1116.

143. Ledo N, Ko Y-A, Park A-SD, et al. Functional genomic annotation of genetic risk loci highlights inflammation and epithelial biology networks in CKD. *J Am Soc Nephrol.* 2015;26:692–714.

144. Calabrese GM, Mesner LD, Stains JP, et al. Integrating GWAS and Co-expression network data identifies bone mineral density genes SPTBN1 and MARK3 and an osteoblast functional module. *Cell Sys.* 2017;4:46–59.e4.

145. Sekar A, Bialas AR, de Rivera H, et al. Schizophrenia risk from complex variation of complement component 4. *Nature.* 2016;530:177.

146. Sellgren CM, Gracias J, Watmuff B, et al. Increased synapse elimination by microglia in schizophrenia patient-derived models of synaptic pruning. *Nat Neurosci.* 2019;22:374–385.

147. Hertzberg L, Katsel P, Roussos P, Haroutunian V, Domany E. Integration of gene expression and GWAS results supports involvement of calcium signaling in Schizophrenia. *Schizophr Res.* 2015;164:92–99.

148. Hall LS, Adams MJ, Arnau-Soler A, et al. Genome-wide meta-analyses of stratified depression in generation Scotland and UK Biobank. *Transl Psychiatry.* 2018;8:9.

149. Hardt J, Rutter M. Validity of adult retrospective reports of adverse childhood experiences: review of the evidence. *J Child Psychol Psychiatry.* 2004;45:260–273.

150. Tajima EA, Herrenkohl TI, Huang B, Whitney SD. Measuring child maltreatment: a comparison of prospective parent reports and retrospective adolescent reports. *Am J Orthopsychiatry.* 2004;74:424–435.

151. Fisher HL, Bunn A, Jacobs C, Moran P, Bifulco A. Concordance between mother and offspring retrospective reports of childhood adversity. *Child Abuse Negl.* 2011;35: 117–122.

152. Newbury JB, Arseneault L, Moffitt TE, et al. Measuring childhood maltreatment to predict early-adult psychopathology: comparison of prospective informant-reports and retrospective self-reports. *J Psychiatr Res.* 2018;96: 57–64.

153. Reuben A, Moffitt TE, Caspi A, et al. Lest we forget: comparing retrospective and prospective assessments of adverse childhood experiences in the prediction of adult health. *J Child Psychol Psychiatry.* 2016;57:1103–1112.

154. Patten SB, Wilkes TCR, Williams JVA, et al. Retrospective and prospectively assessed childhood adversity in

association with major depression, alcohol consumption and painful conditions. *Epidemiol Psychiatr Sci.* 2015;24: 158.

155. Gilbert R, Widom CS, Browne K, Fergusson D, Webb E, Janson S. Burden and consequences of child maltreatment in high-income countries. *Lancet.* 2009;373:68–81.

156. MacMillan HL, Jamieson E, Walsh CA. Reported contact with child protection services among those reporting child physical and sexual abuse: results from a community survey. *Child Abuse Negl.* 2003;27:1397–1408.

157. Sheikh MA, Abelsen B, Olsen JA. Differential recall bias, intermediate confounding, and mediation analysis in life course epidemiology: an analytic framework with empirical example.(report)(author abstract). *Front Psychol.* 2016;7.

158. Kauhanen L, Lakka H-M, Lynch JW, Kauhanen J. Social disadvantages in childhood and risk of all-cause death and cardiovascular disease in later life: a comparison of historical and retrospective childhood information. *Int J Epidemiol.* 2006;35:962–968.

159. Menne-Lothmann C, Jacobs N, Derom C, Thiery E, Os J, Wichers M. Genetic and environmental causes of individual differences in daily life positive affect and reward experience and its overlap with stress-sensitivity. *Behav Genet.* 2012;42:778–786.

160. Dunn, E.C. (2019, February 15). Biomarkers in psychiatry: A review of possibilities spanning genes to teeth. Paper presented as part of the symposium "Teeth as a Biomarker for Environmental stress and risk of disease" at *The American Association for the Advancement of Science Annual Meeting*, Washington, D.C.

161. Dick DM, Agrawal A, Keller MC, et al. Candidate gene-environment interaction research: reflections and recommendations. *Perspect Psychol Sci.* 2015;10:37–59.

162. Moore SR, Thoemmes F. What is the biological reality of gene–environment interaction estimates? An assessment of bias in developmental models. *J Child Psychol Psychiatry.* 2016;57:1258–1267.

163. Gauderman WJ, Mukherjee B, Aschard H, et al. Update on the state of the science for analytical methods for gene-environment interactions. *Am J Epidemiol.* 2017; 186:762–770.

164. Keller MC. Gene × environment interaction studies have not properly controlled for potential confounders: the problem and the (simple) solution. *Biol Psychiatry.* 2014;75:18–24.

165. Aschard H, Vihjalmsson BJ, Joshi AD, Price AL, Kraft P. Adjusting for heritable covariates can bias effect estimates in genome-wide association studies. *Am J Hum Genet.* 2015;96:329–339.

166. Aschard H, Guillemot V, Vilhjalmsson B, et al. Covariate selection for association screening in multiphenotype genetic studies. *Nat Genet.* 2017;49:1789.

167. Wang T, Xue X, Xie X, Ye K, Zhu X, Elston RC. Adjustment for covariates using summary statistics of genome-wide association studies. *Genet Epidemiol.* 2018;42:812–825.

168. Corbin LJ, Tan VY, Hughes DA, et al. Formalising recall by genotype as an efficient approach to detailed phenotyping and causal inference. *Nat Commun.* 2018.

169. Franks PW, Timpson NJ. Genotype-based recall studies in complex cardiometabolic traits. *Circ Genom Precis Med.* 2018;11.

170. Assary E, Vincent JP, Keers R, Pluess M. Gene-environment interaction and psychiatric disorders: review and future directions. *Semin Cell Dev Biol.* 2018; 77:133–143.

171. Salanti G, Ioannidis JPA. Synthesis of observational studies should consider credibility ceilings. *J Clin Epidemiol.* 2009;62:115–122.

172. Pingault J-B, Cecil CAM, Murray J, Munafò MR, Viding E. Causal inference in psychopathology: a systematic review of mendelian randomisation studies aiming to identify environmental risk factors for psychopathology. *Psychopathol Rev.* 2016;a4:4–25.

173. Pingault J-B, O'Reilly PF, Schoeler T, Ploubidis GB, Rijsdijk F, Dudbridge F. Using genetic data to strengthen causal inference in observational research. *Nat Rev Genet.* 2018;19:566.

174. Smith GD, Ebrahim S. What can mendelian randomisation tell us about modifiable behavioural and environmental exposures? *BMJ.* 2005;330:1076.

175. Davey Smith G, Hemani G. Mendelian randomization: genetic anchors for causal inference in epidemiological studies. *Hum Mol Genet.* 2014;23:R89–R98.

176. Zheng J, Baird D, Borges M-C, et al. Recent developments in mendelian randomization studies. *Cur Epidemiol Rep.* 2017;4:330–345.

177. Vaucher J, Keating BJ, Lasserre AM, et al. Cannabis use and risk of schizophrenia: a Mendelian randomization study. *Mol Psychiatr.* 2017;23:1287.

178. Hartwig F, Borges M, Horta B, Bowden J, Davey Smith G. Inflammatory biomarkers and risk of schizophrenia: a 2-sample mendelian randomization study. *JAMA Psychiatry.* 2017;74:1226–1233.

179. Köhler CA, Evangelou E, Stubbs B, et al. Mapping risk factors for depression across the lifespan: an umbrella review of evidence from meta-analyses and Mendelian randomization studies. *J Psychiatr Res.* 2018;103: 189–207.

180. Choi KW, Chen CY, Stein MB, Klimentidis YC, Wang MJ, Koenen KC, Smoller JW. Major Depressive Disorder Working Group of the Psychiatric Genomics C. Assessment of Bidirectional Relationships Between Physical Activity and Depression Among Adults: A 2-Sample Mendelian Randomization Study. *JAMA Psychiatry.* 2019.

181. Burgess S, Thompson SG. Use of allele scores as instrumental variables for Mendelian randomization. *Int J Epidemiol.* 2013;42:1134–1144.

182. Pingault JB, O'Reilly PF, Schoeler T, Ploubidis GB, Rijsdijk F, Dudbridge F. Using genetic data to strengthen causal inference in observational research. *Nat Rev Genet.* 2018;19:566–580.

CHAPTER 2

Epigenetics of Major Depressive Disorder

KEVIN Z. WANG, BSC • OLUWAGBENGA O. DADA, BSC • ALI BANI-FATEMI, PHD •
SAMIA TASMIM, MSC • MARCELLINO MONDA, MD • ARIEL GRAFF, MD, PHD •
VINCENZO DE LUCA, MD, PHD

INTRODUCTION

Major depressive disorder (MDD) is a multifactorial disease involving complex interactions among social, psychological, and biological factors.[1] Genetic variations were initially believed to be responsible for the development of this disease, with twin studies estimating the heritability to be approximately 37%.[2,3] Recent findings, however, have shown that variations in the nucleotide sequence alone cannot adequately account for MDD susceptibility.[4]

In fact, genome-wide association studies (GWAS) indicate that the risk of MDD is unlikely to be increased by the effect of one or a few common genetic variants but instead is highly polygenic with only a small portion of the heritability explained by combining several variants.[5] As a result, in recent years, attention has shifted to epigenetic processes to help understand the potential links to depression.

Epigenetic modifications have been defined as changes "in addition to changes in genetic sequence."[6] Epigenetic mechanisms alter gene expression independently of DNA sequence changes and are reversible, and in some instances they are also heritable.[7,8,9]

Epigenetic modifications can account for a significant portion of the "missing heritability" discrepancy attributed to the low heritability of MDD.[10] Some of the major epigenetic mechanisms involve DNA methylation, histone modifications, and noncoding RNAs (ncRNAs).[1,11] Fundamentally, epigenetic regulation of gene expression is accomplished through altered chromatin structure and DNA accessibility, such as preventing the binding of transcription factors and other elements required for downstream events.[12,13] Epigenetic mechanisms are dynamic processes that can be modified by changes in the state of individuals and their respective environmental stressors.[2] In the context of transgenerational inheritance, the epigenetic

modifications that occur can be further passed on to future generations, potentially conferring additional risk for the development of MDD.[9]

In this chapter, we will first introduce the concept of DNA methylation. Furthermore, we will describe twin studies of depression that have suggested the involvement of DNA methylation in MDD, as well as the three most validated neurobiological models of depression. We will also review the implications of histone modifications and ncRNAs in MDD pathophysiology.

DNA METHYLATION

DNA methylation is the most widely studied epigenetic modification, and thus will be the primary focus of this chapter. Methylation involves the covalent addition of a methyl group (CH_3) to the fifth carbon of the aromatic pyrimidine ring of the cytosine DNA base.[14,15] This process results in the formation of 5-methyl-cytosine (5 mC), and is regulated by a family of DNA methyltransferases that transfer a methyl group from the universal methyl-donor S-adenosyl-L-methionine.[15] DNA methylation in somatic cells occurs mainly at cytosines in the context of cytosine—phosphate—guanine (CpG) dinucleotides (over 98% of all methylation sites).[14,15] CpG islands are short genomic regions, averaging 1000 base pairs in length, with increased numbers of CpG sites.[16] In these regions, the content of guanines and cytosines is greater than 50%, and the percentage ratio of observed to expected CpG sites is greater than 60%.[17] CpG islands are particularly important, in that approximately 40% of genes contain CpG islands in their promoter regions.[18] Thus, the methylation of cytosine nucleotides in the CpG islands of promoters plays an integral role in regulating gene expression levels, specifically by repressing transcription.[2,15] This is done by 5 mC's ability to prevent proper binding of

Major Depressive Disorder. https://doi.org/10.1016/B978-0-323-58131-8.00002-1

transcription factors to regulatory elements.[15] Additionally, aside from some exceptions, hypermethylation is often typically indicative of repressed transcription, whereas hypomethylation reflects a more active and regular gene transcriptional state.[15,19] DNA methylation is profoundly important, as it plays a role in many developmental processes including genomic imprinting, embryonic development, X-chromosome inactivation, chromosomal stability, and transposable element silencing.[20,14,15] At the same time, aberrant DNA methylation patterns have been recently associated with many human diseases, such as Beckwith–Wiedemann, Prader–Willi, Angelman syndrome, Albright hereditary osteodystrophy, transient neonatal diabetes, pseudohypoparathyroidism 1a (PHP-1a), and PHP-1b.[21]

TWIN STUDIES OF DEPRESSION

Twin studies are frequently used to determine the importance of heritable and environmental influences on particular traits, and are done by comparing the phenotypic similarity of monozygotic and dizygotic twins.[22] Dizygotic twins, also known as fraternal twins, are derived from two separate zygotes; whereas, monozygotic twins, or identical twins, are derived from a single zygote resulting in almost identical genetic profiles.[22] In this section, we will focus on studies involving monozygotic twins, as these twin pairs share almost identical genetic profiles and environmental influences both before and after birth. However, it is well known that even between monozygotic twin pairs, there are often still phenotypic discordances of many complex traits.[23,24] In epigenetic studies, monozygotic twins can help to rule out genetic variations as confounding factors.[4]

Despite sharing common genetic and environmental backgrounds, it has been shown that methylation profiles in monozygotic twins slightly differ.[25,26] To offer insight into monozygotic twins in the context of MDD, we outline several key findings of an influential manuscript published by Córdova-Palomera et al.[27] To investigate differences in DNA methylation, their group utilized analytical strategies to identify sites of differentially methylated probes (DMPs) and variably methylated probes (VMPs).[27,28] They hypothesized that DMPs can account for environmental influences that affect only one of the twins, whereas VMPs cover stochastic factors that may arise by chance.[27,28] Utilizing a study sample of 17 monozygotic twin pairs comprising a total of 34 participants, the group found several DMPs of interest only in the discordant twin

pairs for depression, but not in diagnostic-concordant or healthy twin pairs.[27] In terms of VMPs, they found that each classification of twin pairs had a unique set of variably methylated CpG sites.

From this study, several notable DMPs were found to be located in WDR26 (WD repeat domain 26), VCAN (versican), CBR3 (carbonyl reductase 3), and RPL3 (ribosomal protein L3), genes that are known to be associated with depressive phenotypes. The most discussion-worthy CpG site was cg01122889, located in WDR26, where hypomethylation was associated with reduced gene expression and a lifetime diagnosis of depression. This finding is consistent with previous studies implicating single-nucleotide polymorphisms in WDR26 predisposing for MDD,[29,30] as well as animal studies suggesting that lower blood transcript levels of WDR26, attributed to hypomethylation in areas of the gene body, are associated with depression.[31] Furthermore, cg01122889 was found to be differentially methylated only in diagnostic-discordant twin pairs, and not in diagnostic-concordant or healthy twin pairs.[27] This site could then potentially serve as a marker of environmental influences that increase the risk for MDD.[27] For VCAN, CBR3, and RPL3, it was found that CpG sites within the gene bodies were also hypomethylated, resulting in lower gene expression in patients with depression.[27,32,33]

As previously mentioned, VMPs were examined to investigate stochastic factors, such as nonsystematic epigenetic instability.[27,28] Feinberg et al.[28] suggested that epigenetic variations could mediate genetic variability of a given phenotype, and accordingly, the model of inherited stochastic variation attempts to elucidate heritable variations of complex diseases.[28] Córdova-Palomera et al. identified unique VMP sites within each of the groups studied that are concordant, discordant, and healthy twin pairs.[27] Particularly interesting for depression studies were the VMP sites associated with depression-discordant twin pairs. The significantly variable VMPs found in the discordant twin pairs were located in CACNA1C (calcium voltage-gated channel subunit alpha1 C), IGF2 (insulin like growth factor 2), and MAPK11 (mitogen-activated protein kinase 11), genes that have also been previously associated with depression.[27] In support of these findings, previous studies have found that VMP sites tend to be located within genes that play critical roles in the context of the phenotype being studied.[28] Córdova-Palomera et al. detailed the links of these genes with depression. For instance, CACNA1C methylation variability has previously been associated with early-life adversities such as stress, one of the major risks for depression and other psychiatric disorders.[27] Other studies have also linked the *IGF2* and *MAPK11* genes to depression.[34−37] In summary, this study suggested that differentially and variably methylated sites may contribute to certain clinical aspects of MDD.

THEORIES OF DEPRESSION

Traditionally, there have been several theories regarding the etiology of MDD, of which, we will focus on three: 1) the stress model of depression, 2) neurotrophic hypothesis of depression, and 3) the monoamine hypothesis of depression. In this section, we will discuss the epigenetic mechanism of DNA methylation in candidate genes that have been identified relating to each of these three theories of depression.

Stress Model of Depression

Numerous studies have suggested that methylation patterns can be influenced by environmental factors, particularly early-life adversities, stress, and trauma.[38,39,40] Furthermore, these events have been recognized as risk factors for the development of psychiatric disorders, with epidemiological studies showing that they greatly increase susceptibility to MDD.[41−43] Here, we will briefly introduce the hypothalamic−pituitary−adrenal (HPA) axis, and subsequently, its relationship with stress and MDD by the means of DNA methylation. The HPA axis is a neuroendocrine system involved in maintaining homeostasis in an adaptive response to stress.[44] This system mediates the release of glucocorticoids, a class of steroid hormones that help the body to respond to stressful physical or emotional events.[44] The glucocorticoid receptor (GR), encoded by the *NR3C1* gene, is one of the key regulators of the stress response. This is accomplished through the binding of glucocorticoids to the GR at times when there are excessively high levels of circulating glucocorticoids, as is the case during stressful events.[45] Following binding, GR signals for glucocorticoid inhibition through various mechanisms include those involving the hypothalamic paraventricular nucleus, limbic system, and neuropeptide drivers of the HPA axis.[45] These means of action can occur often within minutes, and it is imperative in the negative feedback regulation of the HPA axis once a stressor has been resolved.[46] However, dysregulation of the negative feedback mechanism involving the GR has been shown to be associated with depression.[47]

To clinically assess the functioning of the HPA axis in patients with MDD, neuroendocrine challenge tests are frequently utilized. The most common test is the dexamethasone suppression test (DST), in which patients are given a synthetic corticosteroid dexamethasone (DEX) in the evening, and cortisol levels are assessed in the following morning.[48] Inhibition of cortisol release due to the GR negative feedback regulation in response to DEX would be observed under normal HPA axis functioning, whereas measurement of cortisol levels in excess of a clinically determined threshold would be indicative of a patient with "DST nonsuppression."[49] To effectively show a link between dysregulation of the GR negative feedback loop and MDD, studies have determined the sensitivity of the suppression test as the rate of "DST nonsuppression" in patients with MDD. The sensitivity was found to be approximately 43%, though an updated neuroendocrine challenge test involving both DEX and corticotrophin-releasing hormone, secreted by the hypothalamus in the HPA axis, has a sensitivity of up to 90%.[50,51] Dysregulation of the HPA axis in the negative feedback mechanisms has been found to be due to the reduced *NR3C1* gene expression and subsequent reduced GR protein levels.[52]

Based on these findings, the specific mechanism leading to the reduced *NR3C1* gene expression has been of particular interest. There has been strong evidence demonstrating that this decreased expression is correlated with hypermethylation of the *NR3C1* promoter region.[53−55] Several notable studies have focused on GR gene hypermethylation and early-life adversities. In postmortem hippocampal samples from suicide victims, McGowan et al.[56] found decreased levels of GR 1F splice variant expression and hypermethylation of the promoter region of the *NR3C1* gene in subjects with histories of childhood abuse, compared to those without histories of such abuse.[56] Efstathopoulos et al.[57] also found hypermethylation in the exon 1F region of *NR3C1* in adolescents who reported social and environmental stressors, such as bullying and social isolation.[57] A study by Shields et al.[58] found that women reporting a history of being victims of childhood abuse had increased methylation levels in a CpG site located within a CpG island shore region of the *NR3C1* promoter. Furthermore, they reported a dose-response relationship in methylation levels in subjects receiving childhood emotional support.[58]

Recent studies have also found important associations between prenatal stress and increased GR gene methylation in infants. For instance, a landmark paper by Oberlander et al.[59] documented that maternal depression and anxiety during the third trimester of pregnancy was associated with hypermethylation of CpG sites in the promoter and exon 1F regions of the *NR3C1* gene in fetus.[59] At birth, infants showed increased salivary cortisol stress responses when tested at 3 months of age. This study effectively demonstrated a critical link where *NR3C1* gene methylation status can be sensitive to maternal stresses, in addition to early-life adversities. Considering the findings from the previous papers, there appears to be compelling evidence suggesting that both prenatal stress and early-life adversities have the ability to make lasting impacts on the regulation of HPA axis functioning, thus leading to future adult psychopathologies, including MDD.[60]

Neurotrophic Hypothesis of Depression

According to the neurotrophic hypothesis of depression, depressive symptoms arise from decreased neurotrophic support involved in the development, maintenance, and survival of neurons, as well as in synaptic plasticity.[61,,4] Neurotrophic factors are proteins that are responsible for neurotropic support; the brain-derived neurotrophic factor (BDNF) is the most well examined.[62] Studies from multiple avenues have shown that decreased expression of BDNF in both the brain and blood is associated with patients with MDD, and conversely, that the use of antidepressants alleviates depression by upregulating BDNF expression.[63–65] It has been further suggested that decreased BDNF expression is due to epigenetic modifications of the *BDNF* gene, specifically through DNA methylation.[63] Here, we will briefly discuss the impact of *BDNF* methylation on clinical depression.

In one of the largest epigenetic studies of depression, Januar et al.[66] found that patients with depression had increased methylation in *BDNF* promoters I and IV, resulting in decreased gene expression.[66] As patients with MDD frequently exhibit altered brain structures, including decreased neuron numbers, neuronal atrophy, and reduced cortical thickness, it can prove useful to identify the functional relevance of methylation status in MDD.[4,63] Na et al.[67] found that increased methylation of the *BDNF* promoter was associated with reduced cortical thickness in patients with MDD.[67] They suggested that because the prefrontal cortex regulates emotion and executive functions, prefrontal dysfunction could then account for some symptoms of MDD, including those relating to "cognitive," "executive," "emotional," and "affective" functions.[68,,67] Similarly, Choi et al.[69] found that increased methylation of the *BDNF* promoter was associated with reduced white matter integrity in the anterior corona radiata of patients with MDD, which can contribute to the emotional and cognitive pathophysiology of MDD.

Antidepressant treatment and clinical improvement have been closely related to BDNF expression,[70] with multiple studies reporting increased BDNF levels in patients taking antidepressants.[71,72] In cases where the serum BDNF levels do not increase early in response to antidepressant treatment, there is a high likelihood of treatment failure in MDD patients.[73] Furthermore, Lopez et al.[74] found that treatment-naïve MDD patients who responded to antidepressants after 8 weeks showed increases in BDNF expression and improvements in depressive symptoms. This increased BDNF expression was further found to be due to reductions of methylation levels in the *BDNF* promoter region.[74] Taken together with other studies, findings show substantial support for assessing *BDNF* methylation status and expression levels as potential diagnostic biomarkers for depression and predicting the efficacy of antidepressant treatment.[66,75,76]

Monoamine Hypothesis of Depression

Neurotransmitters, simply defined, are chemical messengers that act as signals among neurons in the central nervous system. One of the oldest theories regarding depression is the monoamine hypothesis of depression, which states that the pathophysiological basis of depression is dependent on decreased levels of neurotransmitters.[77] Studies have investigated the implications of the monoamine neurotransmitter 5-hydroxytryptamine (5-HT), more commonly known as serotonin, on mood regulation and depression.[78] With relation to MDD, a key candidate gene is *SLC6A4*, which encodes the serotonin transporter (5-HTT) that transports serotonin from synaptic spaces into presynaptic neurons.[78,,4] It has been widely suggested that decreased level of 5-HTT protein leads to increased susceptibility to MDD.[79] A case-control study by Shi et al.[80] found hypermethylation of several CpG sites within the *SLC6A4* promoter region to be significantly associated with MDD in the Han Chinese population.[80] Philibert et al.[81] found trends for association between overall methylation of *SLC6A4* and a lifetime history of MDD.[81] From these and other findings in the literature, it is plausible that DNA methylation may provide a significant link between the serotonin transporter and MDD, although further studies are required.[82,83]

In addition to serotonin, preclinical and clinical evidence also suggests that disturbances in norepinephrine (NE), also known as noradrenaline, are linked to the development of depression.[84] Patients with MDD show increased amounts of NE and its extraneuronal metabolite, normetanephrine.[85] These findings can be attributed to the reduced function of the norepinephrine transporter (NET), encoded by the *SLC6A2* gene.[86] Genetic studies have yielded inconclusive findings regarding *SLC6A2* sequence variations in contributing to MDD, thus interest has shifted to transcriptional silencing through DNA methylation. *SLC6A2* methylation status had been previously examined in the context of diseases such as hypertension and panic disorder.[87−89] Investigating MDD, Bayles et al. did not find differences in the methylation status of the *SLC6A2* promoter region, but found significant correlations in methylation levels at several CpG sites elsewhere within the gene.[86] As a result, further studies and analyses are recommended to elucidate the impact of DNA methylation on NE and NET dysregulation, in the context of MDD.

INFLUENCE OF OTHER EPIGENETIC MODIFICATIONS
Histone Modifications

DNA molecules can be over a meter in length, and to package the genetic material into a cell's nucleus, histones play a crucial role in organizing DNA into chromatin.[90] The basis for chromatin lies in the nucleosome core particle, which comprises an octamer of histones.[91] The structural state of the histone proteins can determine DNA replication status and downstream gene expression.[90] These histone proteins are subject to posttranscriptional modification at their tails, and such modifications include acetylation, methylation, phosphorylation, ubiquitination, SUMOylation, and ADP-ribosylation.[92] Although histone modifications serve many purposes, we will focus only on transcriptional regulation mechanisms such as histone acetylation.

Histone acetylation involves the transfer of an acetyl group to the histone tail by enzymes known as histone acetyltransferases, resulting in chromatin decondensation and promoting gene expression.[2] On the other hand, histone deacetylation involves the removal of the acetyl group from the histone tail by enzymes known as histone deacetylases (HDACs), thus resulting in chromatin condensation and a decrease in gene expression.

Several studies using psychotropic medications found that some antidepressants act on histone modifications.[2] For instance, monoamine oxidase inhibitors are a class of antidepressant drugs that act by inhibiting histone demethylase LSD1,[93] whereas the mood stabilizer valproate acts by inhibiting HDACs.[2,93] Furthermore, other studies revealed that certain HDACs were upregulated in patients with MDD. Hobara et al.[94] found that there was an increase in HDAC2 and

HDAC5 mRNA in peripheral white blood cells of patients with MDD compared to healthy controls.[94] Although we have some observations implicating HDACs in the pathophysiology of MDD, the overall understanding of histone modifications relating to depression is still largely unclear.

Noncoding RNAs (ncRNAs)

There are a variety of noncoding RNAs (ncRNAs), which are RNAs that are not translated into proteins, yet still have functional roles with regards to regulation of gene expression.[2] Although there are several different classes of ncRNAs, the most widely studied are the microRNAs (miRNAs), a family of small RNAs approximately 21−25 nucleotides in length that exert negative regulation of gene expression at the posttranscriptional level.[95,,2] The miRNAs have the ability to regulate gene expression through methods of posttranscriptionally regulating the cleavage of target mRNAs or through translational repression of mRNAs.[96] Furthermore, it has been shown that one miRNA has the ability to regulate the expression of more than one target, and conversely, a single mRNA target can be regulated by several miRNAs. Although miRNAs can play numerous roles, including cell proliferation and death, fat metabolism and immunity, we will focus on functions from a behavioral point of view.[97] Recent studies have found miRNAs to play important roles in MDD symptoms at the level of neurogenesis, synaptic plasticity, and regulation of components of various signaling pathways.[2]

The general observed trend is that upregulation of certain key miRNAs is associated with depressive symptoms. For instance, Uchida et al.[98] found that in a rat model, increased expression of miRNA 18a inhibited the translation of GR, as previously mentioned in the stress model of depression.[98] This key finding could further serve to explain some aspects of the dysregulation of the HPA axis negative feedback loop and elevated cortisol levels after a stressful event has passed. With regards to the neurotropic hypothesis of depression, Li et al.[99] found that miRNA 182 and 132 were upregulated in patients with MDD, and this resulted in decreased neurotropic support, specifically by a reduction in BDNF expression.[99] Finally, recent studies have shown that miRNAs can be detected in both blood and cerebrospinal fluid, and that the increased levels of miRNAs can be associated with several pathologies.[2] As a result, with further research, miRNAs can potentially serve as a biomarker for MDD in the clinical setting.

CONCLUSION

Although genetics may play a role in terms of heritability, studies have shown that despite sharing common genetic features, monozygotic twins still have diagnostic discordance with relation to MDD and other psychiatric disorders. As such, other methods should be carefully examined to account for the missing heritability. Epigenetic mechanisms should not be overlooked, as these modifications can address important roles of environmental factors such as stress and early-life adversities. These stressful events have been shown to explain several key features of clinical depression. As multiple studies have shown, epigenetic mechanisms can prove extremely useful as biomarkers to predict susceptibility, identify disease onset, and potentially even improve clinical outcomes in patients with MDD.

REFERENCES

1. Hoffmann A, Sportelli V, Ziller M, Spengler D. Epigenomics of major depressive disorders and schizophrenia: early life decides. *Int J Mol Sci.* 2017;18(1711).
2. Saavedra K, Molina-Marquez AM, Saavedra N, Zambrano T, Salazar LA. Epigenetic modifications of major depressive disorder. *Int J Mol Sci.* 2016;17(1279).
3. Sullivan PF, Neale MC, Kendler KS. Genetic epidemiology of major depression: review and meta-analysis. *Am J Psychiatry.* 2000;157(10):1552–1562.
4. Pishva E, Rutten BPF, van den Hove D. DNA methylation in major depressive disorder. In: Delgado-Morales R, ed. *Neuroepigenomics in Aging and Disease.* New York City, NY: Springer International Publishing; 2017:185–196.
5. Mullins N, Lewis CM. Genetics of depression: progress at last. *Curr Psychiatr Rep.* August 2017;19(8):43.
6. Weinhold B. Epigenetics: the science of change. *Environ Health Perspect.* 2006;114(3):A160–A167.
7. El-Sayed AM, Koenen KC, Galea S. Putting the 'epi' into epigenetics research in psychiatry. *J Epidemiol Community Health.* 2013;67(7):610–616.
8. Henikoff S, Matzke MA. Exploring and explaining epigenetic effects. *Trends Genet.* 1997;13(8):293–295.
9. Yung PYK, Elsasser SJ. Evolution of epigenetic chromatin states. *Curr Opin Chem Biol.* 2017;41:36–42.
10. Trerotola M, Relli V, Simeone P, Alberti S. Epigenetic inheritance and the missing heritability. *Hum Genom.* 2015;9:17.
11. Bani-Fatemi A, Howe AS, De Luca V. Epigenetic studies of suicidal behavior. *Neurocase.* 2015;21(2):134–143.
12. Bird A. Perceptions of epigenetics. *Nature.* 2007; 447(7143):396–398.
13. Handy DE, Castro R, Loscalzo J. Epigenetic modifications: basic mechanisms and role in cardiovascular disease. *Circulation.* 2011;123(19):2145–2156.
14. Jin B, Li Y, Robertson KD. DNA methylation: superior or subordinate in the epigenetic hierarchy? *Genes Cancer.* 2011;2(6):607–617.
15. Singhal SK, Usmani N, Michiels S, et al. Towards understanding the breast cancer epigenome: a comparison of genome-wide DNA methylation and gene expression data. *Oncotarget.* 2015;7(3):3002–3017.
16. Deaton AM, Bird A. CpG islands and the regulation of transcription. *Genes Dev.* 2011;25(10):1010–1022.
17. Jiang N, Wang L, Chen J, Wang L, Leach L, Luo Z. Conserved and divergent patterns of DNA methylation in higher vertebrates. *Genome Biol Evol.* 2014;6(11): 2998–3014.
18. Fatemi M, Pao MM, Jeong S, et al. Footprinting of mammalian promoters: use of a CpG DNA methyltransferase revealing nucleosome positions at a single molecule level. *Nucleic Acids Res.* 2005;33(20):e176.
19. Bock C, Walter J, Paulsen M, Lengauer T. CpG island mapping by epigenome prediction. *PLoS Comput Biol.* 2007; 3(6):e110.
20. Ikeda Y, Nishimura T. The role of DNA methylation in transposable element silencing and genomic imprinting. In: Pontes O, Jin H, eds. *Nuclear Functions in Plant Transcription, Signalling, and Development.* New York City, NY: Springer Science and Business Media; 2015:13–29.
21. Robertson KD. DNA methylation and human disease. *Nat Rev Genet.* 2005;6(8):597–610.
22. van Dongen J, Slagboom PE, Draisma HHM, Martin NG, Boomsma DI. The continuing value of twin studies in the omics era. *Nat Rev Genet.* 2012;13(9):640–653.
23. Castillo-Fernandez JE, Spector TD, Bell JT. Epigenetics of discordant monozygotic twins: implications for disease. *Genome Med.* 2014;6(7):60.
24. Johnson W, Turkheimer E, Gottesman II, Bouchard TJ. Beyond heritability: twin studies in behavioral research. *Curr Dir Psychol Sci.* 2010;18(4):217–220.
25. Kaminsky ZA, Tang T, Wang SC, et al. DNA methylation profiles in monozygotic and dizygotic twins. *Nat Genet.* 2009;41(2):240–245.
26. Li C, Zhang S, Que T, Li L, Zhao S. Identical but not the same: the value of DNA methylation profiling in forensic discrimination within monozygotic twins. *Forensic Sci Int- Gen.* 2011;3(1):e337–e338.
27. Córdova-Palomera A, Fatjo-Vilas M, Gasto C, Navarro V, Krebs MO, Fananas L. Genome-wide methylation study on depression: differential methylation and variable methylation in monozygotic twins. *Transl Psychiatry.* 2015; 5:e557.
28. Feinberg AP, Irizarry RA. Stochastic epigenetic variation as a driving force of development, evolutionary adaptation, and disease. *P Natl Acad Sci USA.* 2010; 107(suppl 1):1757.
29. Major Depressive Disorder Working Group of the Psychiatric GWAS Consortium [PGC-MDD], Ripke S, Wray NR, et al. A mega-analysis of genome-wide association studies for major depressive disorder. *Mol Psychiatr.* 2013;18(4): 497–511.
30. Wray NR, Pergadia ML, Blackwood DH, et al. Genome-wide association study of major depressive disorder: new results, meta-analysis, and lessons learned. *Mol Psychiatr.* 2012;17(1):36–48.

31. Pajer K, Andrus BM, Gardner W, et al. Discovery of blood transcriptomic markers for depression in animal models and pilot validation in subjects with early-onset major depression. *Transl Psychiatry*. 2012;2:e101.

32. Karanges EA, Kashem MA, Sarker R, et al. Hippocampal protein expression is differentially affected by chronic paroxetine treatment in adolescent and adult rats: a possible mechanism of "paradoxical" antidepressant responses in young persons. *Front Pharmacol*. 2013;4:86.

33. Lee HC, Chang DE, Yeom M, et al. Gene expression profiling in hypothalamus of immobilization-stressed mouse using cDNA microarray. *Brain Res Mol Brain Res*. 2005;135(1):293−300.

34. Bruchas MR, Schindler AG, Shankar H, et al. Selective p38α MAPK deletion in serotonergic neurons produces stress resilience in models of depression and addiction. *Neuron*. 2011;71(3):498−511.

35. Cline BH, Steinbusch HW, Malin D, et al. The neuronal insulin sensitizer dicholine succinate reduces stress-induced depressive traits and memory deficit: possible role of insulin-like growth factor 2. *BMC Neurosci*. 2012;13:10.

36. Luo YW, Xu Y, Cao WY, et al. Insulin-like growth factor 2 mitigates depressive behavior in rat model of chronic stress. *Neuropharmacology*. 2015;59:318−324.

37. Raison CL, Capuron L, Miller AH. Cytokines sing the blues: inflammation and the pathogenesis of depression. *Trends Immunol*. 2006;27(1):24−31.

38. Henn FA, Vollmayr B. Stress models of depression: forming genetically vulnerable strains. *Neurosci Biobehav Rev*. 2005;29(4−5):799−804.

39. Matosin N, Cruceanu C, Binder EB. Preclinical and clinical evidence of DNA methylation changes in response to trauma and chronic stress. *Chronic Stress*. 2017;1.

40. Weber M, Schubeler D. Genomic patterns of DNA methylation: targets and function of an epigenetic mark. *Curr Opin Cell Biol*. 2007;19(3):273−280.

41. Agid O, Kohn Y, Lerer B. Environmental stress and psychiatric illness. *Biomed Pharmacother*. 2000;54(3):135−141.

42. Chirita AL, Gheorman V, Bondari D, Rogoveanu I. Current understanding of the neurobiology of major depressive disorder. *Rom J Morphol Embryol*. 2015;56:651−658.

43. Zhou A, Han S, Yang H, Zhou ZJ. Major depressive disorder: understanding epigenetic basis for pharmacological care. *IOSR J Pharm*. 2016;6(11):36−41.

44. Juruena MF. Early-life stress and HPA axis trigger recurrent adulthood depression. *Epilepsy Behav*. 2014;38:148−159.

45. Herman JP, McKlveen JM, Solomon MB, Carvalho-Netto E, Myers B. Neural regulation of the stress response: glucocorticoid feedback mechanisms. *Braz J Med Biol Res*. 2012;45(4):292−298.

46. Tasker JG, Herman JP. Mechanisms of rapid glucocorticoid feedback inhibition of the hypothalamic-pituitary-adrenal axis. *Stress*. 2011;14(4):398−406.

47. Myers B, McKlveen JM, Herman JP. Neural regulation of the stress response: the many faces of feedback. *Cell Mol Neurobiol*. 2012;32(5):683−694.

48. Ness-Abramof R, Nabriski D, Apovian CM, et al. Overnight dexamethasone suppression test: a reliable screen for cushing's syndrome in the obese. *Obes Res*. 2002;10(12):1217−1221.

49. Varghese FP, Brown ES. The hypothalamic-pituitary-adrenal Axis in major deppressive disorder: a brief primer for primary care physicians. *Prim Care Companion J Clin Psychiatry*. 2001;3(4):151−155.

50. Arana GW, Baldessarini RJ, Ornsteen M. The dexamethasone suppression test for diagnosis and prognosis in psychiatry. Commentary and review. *Arch Gen Psychiatr*. 1985;42(12):1193−1204.

51. Heuser I, Yassouridis A, Holsboer F. The combined dexamethasone/CRH test: a refined laboratory test for psychiatric disorders. *J Psychiatr Res*. 1994;24(4):341−356.

52. Yin H, Galfalvy H, Pantazatos SP, et al. Glucocorticoid receptor-related genes: genotype and brain gene expression relationships to suicide and major depressive disorder. *Depress Anxiety*. 2016;33(6):531−540.

53. Mata-Greenwood E, Jackson PN, Pearce WJ, Zhang L. Endothelial glucocorticoid receptor promoter methylation according to dexamethasone sensitivity. *J Mol Endocrinol*. 2015;55(2):133−146.

54. Nesset KA, Perri AM, Mueller CR. Frequent promoter hypermethylation and expression reduction of the glucocorticoid receptor gene in breast tumors. *Epigenetics*. 2014;9(6):851−859.

55. Steiger H, Labonté B, Groleau P, Turecki G, Israel M. Methylation of the glucocorticoid receptor gene promoter in bulimic women: associations with borderline personality disorder, suicidality, and exposure to childhood abuse. *Int J Eat Disord*. 2013;46(3):246−255.

56. McGowan PO, Sasaki A, D'Alessio AC, et al. Epigenetic regulation of the glucocorticoid receptor in human brain associates with childhood abuse. *Nat Neurosci*. 2009;12(3):342−348.

57. Efstathopoulos P, Andersson F, Melas PA, et al. NR3C1 hypermethylation in depressed and bullied adolescents. *Transl Psychiatry*. 2018;8(1):121.

58. Shields AE, Wise LA, Ruiz-Narvaez EA, et al. Childhood abuse, promoter methylation of leukocyte NR3C1 and the potential modifying effect of emotional support. *Epigenomics*. 2016;8(11):1507−1517.

59. Oberlander TF, Weinberg J, Papsdorf M, Grunau R, Misri S, D'evlin AM. Prenatal exposure to maternal depression, neonatal methylation of human glucocorticoid receptor gene (NR3C1) and infant cortisol stress responses. *Epigenetics*. 2008;3(2):97−106.

60. Perroud N, Paoloni-Giacobino A, Prada P, et al. Increased methylation of glucocorticoid receptor gene (NR3C1) in adults with a history of childhood maltreatment: a link with the severity and type of trauma. *Transl Psychiatry*. 2011;1:e59.

61. Duman RS, Li N. A neurotrophic hypothesis of depression: role of synaptogenesis in the actions of NMDA receptor antagonists. *Philos Trans R Soc Lond B Biol Sci*. 2012;367(1601):2475−2484.

62. Skaper SD. The neurotrophin family of neurotrophic factors: an overview. In: Skaper SD, ed. *Neurotrophic Factors: Methods and Protocols*. Totowa, NJ: Humana Press; 2012:1−12.

63. Dwivedi Y. Brain-derived neurotrophic factor: role in depression and suicide. *Neuropsychiatric Dis Treat.* 2009;5: 433–449.

64. Kang HJ, Kim JM, Lee JY, et al. BDNF promoter methylation and suicidal behavior in depressive patients. *J Affect Disord.* 2013;151(2):679–685.

65. Keller S, Sarchiapone M, Zarrilli F, et al. Increased BDNF promoter methylation in the wernicke area of suicide subjects. *Arch Gen Psychiatr.* 2010;67(3):258–267.

66. Januar V, Ancelin ML, Ritchie K, Saffery R, Ryan J. BDNF promoter methylation and genetic variation in late-life depression. *Transl Psychiatry.* 2015;5:e619.

67. Na KS, Won E, Kang J, et al. Brain-derived neurotrophic factor promoter methylation and cortical thickness in recurrent major depressive disorder. *Sci Rep.* 2016;6: 21089.

68. Koenigs M, Grafman J. The functional neuroanatomy of depression: distinct roles for ventromedial and dorsolateral prefrontal cortex. *Behav Brain Res.* 2009;201(2):239–243.

69. Choi S, Han KM, Won E, Yoon BJ, Lee MS, Ham BJ. Association of brain-derived neurotrophic factor DNA methylation and reduced white matter integrity in the anterior corona radiata in major depression. *J Affect Disord.* 2015; 172:74–80.

70. Brunoni AR, Lopes M, Fregni F. A systematic review and meta-analysis of clinical studies on major depression and BDNF levels: implications for the role of neuroplasticity in depression. *Int J Neuropsychopharmacol.* 2008;11: 1169–1180.

71. Chen B, Dowlatshahi D, MacQueen GM, Wang JF, Young LT. Increased hippocampal bdnf immunoreactivity in subjects treated with antidepressant medication. *Biol Psychiatry.* 2001;50(4):260–265.

72. Duclot F, Kabbaj M. Epigenetic mechanisms underlying the role of brain-derived neurotrophic factor in depression and response to antidepressants. *J Exp Biol.* 2015;218(1): 21–31.

73. Tadić A, Wagner S, Schlicht KF, et al. The early non-increase of serum BDNF predicts failure of antidepressant treatment in patients with major depression: a pilot study. *Prog Neuro-Psychopharmacol Biol Psychiatry.* 2011;35: 415–420.

74. Lopez JP, Mamdani F, Labonte B, et al. Epigenetic regulation of BDNF expression according to antidepressant response. *Mol Psychiatr.* 2013;18(4):398–399.

75. Fuchikami M, Morinobu S, Segawa M, et al. DNA methylation profiles of the brain-derived neurotrophic factor (BDNF) gene as a potent diagnostic biomarker in major depression. *PLoS One.* 2011;6(8):e23881.

76. Zheleznyakova GY, Cao H, Schioth HB. BDNF DNA methylation changes as a biomarker of psychiatric disorders: literature review and open access database analysis. *Behav Brain Funct.* 2016;12(1):17.

77. Delgado PL. Depression: the case for a monoamine defiiency. *J Clin Psychiatry.* 2000;61:7–11.

78. Kuželová H, Ptáček R, Macek M. The serotonin transporter gene (5-HTT) variant and psychiatric disorders. *Neuroendocrinol Lett.* 2010;31(1):4–10.

79. Luddington NS, Mandadapu A, Husk M, El-Mallakh RS. Clinical implications of genetic variation in the serotonin transporter promoter region: a review. *Prim Care Companion J Clin Psychiatry.* 2009;11(3):93–102.

80. Shi M, Sun H, Xu Y, et al. Methylation status of the serotonin transporter promoter CpG island is associated with major depressive disorder in Chinese han population: a case-control study. *J Nerv Ment Dis.* 2017;205(8): 641–646.

81. Philibert RA, Sandhu H, Hollenbeck N, Gunter T, Adams W, Madan A. The relationship of 5HTT (SLC6A4) methylation and genotype on mRNA expression and liability to major depression and alcohol dependence in subjects from the Iowa Adoption Studies. *Am J Med Genet B Neuropsychiatr Genet.* 2008;147B(5):543–549.

82. Okada S, Morinobu S, Fuchikami M, et al. The potential of SLC6A4 gene methylation analysis for the diagnosis and treatment of major depression. *J Psychiatr Res.* 2014;53: 47–53.

83. Olsson CA, Foley DL, Parkinson-Bates M, et al. Prospects for epigenetic research within cohort studies of psychological disorder: a pilot investigation of a peripheral cell marker of epigenetic risk for depression. *Biol Psychol.* 2010;83(2):159–165.

84. Moret C, Briley M. The importance of norepinephrine in depression. *Neuropsychiatric Dis Treat.* 2011;7(suppl 1): 9–13.

85. Potter WZ, Manji HK. Catecholamines in depression: an update. *Clin Chem.* 1994;40(2):279–297.

86. Bayles R, Baker EK, Jowett JBM, et al. Methylation of the SLC6a2 promoter in major depression and panic disorder. *PLoS One.* 2013;8(12):e83223.

87. Esler M, Alvarenga M, Peir C, et al. The neuronal noradrenaline transporter, anxiety and cardiovascular disease. *J Psychopharmacol.* 2006;20:60–66.

88. Esler M, Eikelis N, Schlaich M, et al. Human sympathetic nerve biology: parallel influences of stress and epigenetics in essential hypertension and panic disorder. *Ann N Y Acad Sci.* 2008;1148:338–348.

89. Millis RM. Epigenetics and hypertension. *Curr Hypertens Rep.* 2011;13:21–28.

90. Mariño-Ramírez L, Kann MG, Shoemaker BA, Landsman D. Histone structure and nucleosome stability. *Expert Rev Proteomics.* 2005;2(5):719–729.

91. Thatcher TH, Gorovsky MA. Phylogenetic analysis of the core histones H2A, H2B, H3, and H4. *Nucleic Acids Res.* 1994;22(2):174–179.

92. Portela A, Esteller M. Epigenetic modifications and human disease. *Nat Biotechnol.* 2010;28(10):1057–1068.

93. Sun H, Kennedy PJ, Nestler EJ. Epigenetics of the depressed brain: role of histone acetylation and methylation. *Neuropsychopharmacology.* 2013;38(1):124–137.

94. Hobara T, Uchida S, Otsuki K, et al. Altered gene expression of histone deacetylases in mood disorder patients. *J Psychiatr Res.* 2010;44(5):263–270.

95. Lin H, Hannon GJ. MicroRNAs: small RNAs with a big role in gene regulation. *Nat Rev Genet.* 2004;5: 522–531.

96. Cai Y, Yu X, Hu S, Yu J. A brief review on the mechanisms of miRNA regulation. *Genom Proteom Bioinform*. 2009;7(4): 147—154.

97. Wahid F, Shehzad A, Khan T, Kim YY. MicroRNAs: synthesis, mechanism, function, and recent clinical trials. *Biochim Biophys Acta*. 2010;1803(11):1231—1243.

98. Uchida S, Nishida A, Hara K, et al. Characterization of the vulnerability to repeated stress in Fischer 344 rats: possible involvement of microRNA-mediated down-regulation of the glucocorticoid receptor. *Eur J Neurosci*. 2008;27(9): 2250—2261.

99. Li YJ, Xu M, Gao ZH, et al. Alterations of serum levels of BDNF-related miRNAs in patients with depression. *PLoS One*. 2013;8(5):e63648.

CHAPTER 3

Brain Structural Abnormalities of Major Depressive Disorder

HANJING WU, MD, PHD • TOMAS MELICHER, MD • ISABELLE E. BAUER, PHD • MARSAL SANCHES, MD, PHD • JAIR C. SOARES, MD, PHD

INTRODUCTION

Major depressive disorder (MDD) is one of the leading causes of morbidity, mortality, and disability. The worldwide lifetime prevalence of MDD approaches 12%[1] and the World Health Organization (WHO) ranks MDD as the 11th leading cause of disability and mortality.[2] In the United States, MDD is the second leading cause of disability, and therefore this condition poses a considerable burden, both in terms of prevalence and public health impact.

Despite the remarkable progress in psychiatry research over the last several decades, the pathophysiological mechanisms underlying MDD are still poorly understood. Current areas of investigation involve biological markers, postmortem studies, and neuroimaging techniques. For decades, the most prominent theory on the pathophysiology of depression focused on altered levels of monoamine neurotransmitters.[3,4] Other compelling theories argue for a role of inflammation,[5] stress sensitivity,[6] and gene—environment interactions[7,8] in the development and recurrence of MDD.

Neuroimaging studies converge in implicating brain networks related to emotional behavior and mood regulation in the pathophysiology of MDD.[9] Several lines of evidence suggest that regions in the limbic—cortical system mediate mood, affective processing, and stress responsiveness. Regions of specific relevance for MDD include the limbic regions, orbital and medial prefrontal cortex, thalamic nuclei, and ventral pallidum.[10] The orbital prefrontal network is of relevance for the affective evaluation of stimuli, for example, reward, aversion, and relative value.[11] A second frontal network called "medial prefrontal network" includes dorsomedial, dorsal, and anterolateral prefrontal regions, the mid- and posterior cingulate, the anterior superior temporal gyrus and sulcus, and the entorhinal and posterior parahippocampal cortex. These regions connect to limbic structures and visceral regions such as the entorhinal and posterior parahippocampal cortex, subgenual anterior cingulate cortex, amygdala, and ventral striatum.[12,13] Visceral regions are particularly important for emotional introspection and "physiological" reactions to emotions. They also appear to play a role in anxiety, which is often comorbid with MDD.[14]

In this chapter we specifically focus on recent neuroimaging literature examining neuroimaging findings in MDD based on structural magnetic resonance imaging (MRI), diffusion tensor imaging (DTI), and white matter structural connectivity data.

REGIONAL BRAIN ABNORMALITIES

Numerous structural MRI studies have been conducted to identify the key brain areas involved in the pathogenesis of MDD. Typical analytical MRI methods to quantify structural abnormalities include the traditional region of interest (ROI) approach and whole-brain morphometrics. The ROI method, with manual delineation of the different brain regions, is time consuming and vulnerable to ROI selection bias despite substantial anatomical validity. Whole-brain morphometrics include voxel-based morphometry (VBM) and vertex-based morphometry.

VBM is a fully automated method for analyzing neuromorphological MRI data that allow unbiased integration of differences in brain structure between groups.[15] VBM shows comparable accuracy to that of manual volumetry.[16,17] It does not require manually drawing regions of interests and overcomes the drawbacks of ROI-based methods. It is noted that disadvantages of VBM include lacking of precise localization of regional volumetric differences and sensitivity to artifacts with risk of false positives. It has been largely utilized to identify

Major Depressive Disorder. https://doi.org/10.1016/B978-0-323-58131-8.00003-3

neuroanatomical abnormalities in a number of psychiatric ailments including MDD. Vertex-based morphometry, on the other hand, is used to quantify cortical thickness. For example, Surface-based morphometry (SBM) is a non-ROI-based approach used to analyze structural deficits by measuring and comparing the cortical thickness according to vertex. SBM has been used to investigate regional cortical thinning.

CORTICAL REGIONS
Frontal Lobe
Some VBM studies reported volume reductions in the right superior frontal gyrus,[18] orbitofrontal cortex,[19] and the right middle and inferior frontal gyrus.[20] Nonremitted MDD patients showed an even greater volumetric reduction in the orbitofrontal cortex bilaterally compared with controls.[19] A recent meta-analysis of 2124 structural images[21] identified decreased gray matter in the right dorsolateral prefrontal cortex conjoining with functional abnormality in the same region.

Recent evidence suggests that medication status may contribute to the brain structural findings observed in MDD patients. Zhao et al.[22] found gray matter reductions in the bilateral orbital frontal cortex (OFC) in medication-naïve MDD patients. Another study reported significant gray matter volume deficits in bilateral superior frontal gyri, left middle frontal gyrus, and left medial frontal gyrus in first-episode medication-naïve MDD patients.[23] One meta-analysis of VBM studies consisting of 14 datasets comprising 400 medication-free MDD patients and 424 healthy controls found significantly reduced gray matter in the prefrontal and limbic regions.[24] There is also evidence of reduced gray matter volume in the frontal lobe in adolescent medication-naïve MDD patient compared to healthy controls (HCs).[130]

Besides the volumetric findings, cortical thickness was found to be decreased in subjects with familial risk for MDD.[25] Cortical thinning was found in the prefrontal cortex of MDD patients especially in the bilateral superior frontal gyrus.[26] This study also reported that the cortical thinning in the prefrontal cortex seems to be modulated by the numbers of past depressive episodes. Another study in untreated, first-episode midlife MDD patients showed a modest negative correlation between cortical thickness in the rostral middle frontal cortex and depression severity.[27] Zhao et al.[22] reported cortical thickening in the bilateral medial prefrontal cortex, posterior dorsolateral prefrontal cortex, and cortical thinning in the left lateral OFC and bilateral rostral middle frontal cortex among medication-naïve MDD patients.

Overall, there is evidence of cortical volume loss and cortical thinning/thickening in different areas of the frontal lobe in MDD patients on medications versus medication-naïve MDD patients. The frontal lobe appears to be a key region in regard to neuroanatomical findings implicated in MDD.

Temporal Lobe
MDD patients have been found to have volumetric reductions in the right middle temporal pole when compared to controls.[19] Similarly, Yuan et al.[18] found smaller right middle temporal gyrus in remitted first-episode elder MDD patients compared with HC, while Shad et al. (2012) reported smaller gray matter volume in right superior and middle temporal gyri in medication-naïve adolescent MDD patients. Furthermore, one meta-analysis revealed gray matter reductions in the right middle temporal gyrus in first-episode MDD patients compared with the HCs.[28] In another study, medication-naïve MDD patients were found to have significantly reduced cortical thickness in the left inferior temporal cortex[29] and temporal lobe.[26,30] Zhao et al.[22] detected cortical thickening in the left temporal pole among medication-naïve MDD patient, and Wang et al.[21] described decreased gray matter in the right inferior temporal and increased gray matter in the left temporal pole in medication-naïve MDD patients compared HCs in a meta-analysis of 2124 structural imagines.

In conclusion, volumetric reductions in the right middle temporal have been consistently replicated among MDD patients, including remitted patients, without apparent medication effects. However, findings on cortical thickness are controversial. Further studies with better designs, larger samples, and more precise analytic methods of structure should be applied to better localize the structural abnormalities in the left temporal lobe.

Parietal Lobe
In a study by Yuan et al.[18] the left postcentral cortex was significantly smaller in remitted first-episode elderly MDD patients compared with HCs. Another study reported cortical thinning in the bilateral inferior parietal cortex in MDD patients on medications.[26] Zhao et al.[22] concluded that there was cortical thickening in the right superior parietal cortex of medication-naïve MDD patient. Thus, structural findings on the parietal lobe appears restricted to certain areas. Due to the limited number of reports, findings of structural abnormalities in the parietal lobe among MDD patients appear to be nonspecific.

CINGULATE CORTEX

Robust VBM studies described bilateral volumetric reductions in the anterior cingulate cortex (ACC)[20,31–34] in patients with MDD. Two meta-analysis of ROI-based imaging studies also reported volumetric reductions in the ACC of MDD patients.[35,36] One study found reduction of gray matter volume in the ACC[37] in first-episode, drug-naïve MDD patients. In their meta-analysis of VBM studies consisting of 14 datasets comprising 400 medication-free MDD patients and 424 HCs medication-free MDD, Zhao et al.[24] suggested that increased ACC volumes may be an effect of medication. Thicker right ACC volumes at baseline in MDD patients on medications were shown in another study.[38] Last, a longitudinal study revealed that a thicker right caudal ACC at baseline is associated with greater symptoms improvements.[38]

Besides ACC area, Yang reported that, compared to HCs, medication-free patients with MDD showed significant increase in gray matter volume in the left posterior cingulate gyrus and gray matter volume decrease in the left lingual gyrus.[39] Furthermore, Yuan et al.[18] found larger left cingulate gyrus volume in remitted first-episode elder MDD patients compared with HCs.

Overall, volumetric reductions in the ACC of MDD patients have been shown by multiple studies. It is noteworthy that the increase in ACC volume and thickness of ACC may be associated with symptom improvement. However, more studies are required to proper elucidate the effect of medications on ACC volume.

OTHER CORTICAL REGIONS

There are two other cortical area abnormalities previously reported in structural MRI studies in MDD: the insula and the occipital lobe. Zhao et al.[22] observed gray matter reductions in insular cortex in medication-naïve MDD patients, and Stratmann et al.[40] found that MDD patients showed gray-matter reductions in the right anterior insula in MDD patients compared to HCs. Lai et al. reported significant gray matter volume deficits in the left insula in first-episode medication-naïve MDD patients.[23] Another meta-analysis revealed gray matter reductions in the left insula in first-episode MDD patients compared with HCs.[28] However, a recent meta-analysis of 2124 structural images[21] identified increased gray matter in right insula. Finally, one study described cortical thinning in the occipital lobes.[26] However, the above results have not been replicated in other studies.

SUBCORTICAL REGIONS

Hippocampus

The hippocampal gyrus and the parahippocampal region are extensively connected with other cortical and subcortical structures in the frontal and temporal lobes and seem to play an important role in the normal cognitive function in MDD patients.[41] Hippocampal volume reduction in MDD patients has been most extensively studied and widely replicated in the past.[40,42–50] Similarly, VBM studies found volumetric reductions in the parahippocampal gyrus and hippocampus of MDD patients.[20] Gray matter reduction in the hippocampal gyrus and the parahippocampal region in MDD were further identified in three ROI-based meta-analyses of MDD.[51–53] Furthermore, one study found reductions in the gray matter volume in the hippocampus[54] among first-episode drug-naïve MDD patients. Zhao et al.[24] pointed out that female medication-free MDD patients may have smaller right hippocampus than male medication-free MDD patients. It has also been shown that the factors affecting hippocampal volumes in MDD include recurrence of depressive episodes, age of onset, disease severity, antidepressant medication, illness duration, and child abuse.[52,55] Another study reported differences in the gray matter volumes (atrophic and hypertrophic) at the subiculum CA1 of the hippocampus among MDD patients compared to HCs, with negative correlation between number of days untreated and changes in gray matter.[56] Moreover, a mega-analysis of structural MRI findings in a very large sample of 1728 MDD patients identified significantly lower hippocampus volume compared to 7199 HCs.[57] It is noteworthy that the hippocampal volume reductions were mainly present in recurrent and/or early onset ($\leq$ 21 years) MDD, while were absent in first-episode patients and less pronounced in patients with later age of onset (> 21 years) MDD. It is consistent with the report from another recent study, which described smaller hippocampal volumes among MDD patients compared to healthy adolescents.[58] One longitudinal study also mentioned slower reductions of the right hippocampal volume in patients with early-onset depression than patients with late-onset depression.[59] Notably, the course of depression could be related to neuroanatomical brain changes in MDD. Previous findings reveal smaller hippocampal volume to be associated with multiple depressive episodes,[60,61] chronic depression,[62] a longer course of illness,[50] and an earlier age onset of depressive symptoms.[47]

In conclusion, reduction of hippocampal volume is one of the most replicated finding in MDD. Furthermore, evidence indicates that hippocampal volume reductions are typically present in recurrent and/or early-onset MDD, whereas hippocampal volume reductions are absent in first-episode patients and less pronounced in patients with later-onset MDD. It is possible that these decreases in the hippocampal volume are related to hypercortisolism, secondary to the hyperactivation of the hypothalamic–pituitary–adrenal axis in MDD.

Amygdala

A single episode of depression and antidepressant use has been found to be associated with enlarged amygdala volume in MDD patients.[63–65] A high number of episodes and a family history of MDD have been reported associated with smaller amygdala volume.[65,66] Decreased amygdala volume was observed in a meta-analysis of six VBM-MRI studies including a total of 176 depressed patients and 175 controls, which is in line with findings in postmortem brains of patients who had suffered from MDD[67,68] and another two studies.[37,66]

Thus, decreased amygdala volume appears to be related to recurrent MDD, while enlarged amygdala is linked to current first depressive episode and antidepressant use. The structural changes in the amygdala lend further support to the limbic–cortical–striatal–pallidal–thalamic model of mood regulation implicated in mood disorder.[131]

Thalamus

Zhao et al.[22] reported gray matter reductions in the thalamus among medication-naïve MDD patient. Another study also found significant volume reductions in the left thalamus among medication-naïve first-episode MDD patients.[69] The gray matter reductions in the thalamus are consistent with findings of a postmortem study that showed decreases in the total thalamus volume in depressed individuals.[70] Zhao et al.[24] also pointed out that female unmedicated MDD patients may have increased right thalamus volume compared to male patients. However, a recent meta-analysis of 2124 structural images[21] identified increased gray matter bilateral thalamus in medication-naïve MDD patient compared with HCs. Qiu et al.[27] also found increased cortical thickness in the thalamus among medication-naïve MDD patients compared to HCs.

Overall, MRI studies have given conflicting evidence with respect to thalamic abnormalities in MDD. Given that the thalamus is a major relay center in the brain for sensorial information, further studies examining the role of thalamus in mood regulation is warranted.

Basal Ganglia

A recent meta-analysis of 2124 structural images[21] identified increased gray matter in the right putamen. Another study observed caudate enlargement following long-term antipsychotics intake in MDD patients.[57] Three studies reported bilateral smaller gray matter volume in the caudate nucleus of depressed drug-naïve patients (Shad et al., 2012,[71] and.[34] Zhao et al.[22] showed gray matter reductions in the putamen among medication-naïve MDD patients. Lu et al. found that medication-naïve, first-episode MDD patients had significant volume reductions in the bilateral putamen.[69] There is consistent evidence of volumetric reductions in the basal ganglia region in MDDs. The basal ganglia are, therefore, a crucial area in the neuroanatomical model of MDD.

Cerebellum

It has been suggested that the cerebellar hemispheres may be involved in the pathophysiology of MDD. This is not surprising given its role in both motor and cognitive control and feedback loops. Two studies found significant gray matter reductions in the cerebellum among first-episode MDD patients compared to HCs[72,73]). One postmortem study reported decreased cerebellar volume in patients with MDD compared to patients with bipolar disorder, schizophrenia, and HCs.[74] The prefrontal-cerebellar circuit is assumed to be of critical importance to the regulation of emotional and cognitive functions. Therefore, a smaller cerebellum may be a consistent feature of the neuroanatomical profile of MDD.

BRAIN STEM

Few studies addressed structural abnormalities of the brainstem in MDD patients. Conflicting results have been reported due to small sample size, clinical characteristic of samples, and effect of medications. Becker suggested decreased echogenicity of the brainstem raphe in MDD,[75,76] which was not replicated in one recent study.[77] One longitudinal study found smaller medulla among MDD patients but the finding was no longer identified at the time of the follow-up 11 years later.[78] Another study showed increased midbrain volume in MDD patients compared to HCs,[79] while another study detected a reduction in gray matter concentration in the midbrain encompassing the dorsal raphe nucleus.[80] One recent study with a larger sample reported that drug-naïve patients with MDD had significantly greater midbrain volumes compared to HCs, while no significant differences between the antidepressant treatment group and HCs.[81] Thus, there are heterogeneous results regarding brain stem structural abnormalities in MDD. Further studies are needed to draw definite conclusions regarding this important brain region.

NEGATIVE FINDINGS

It is noteworthy to mention that two studies found no differences in regard to whole-brain volume and ROI between MDD and HCs.[82,83] This heterogeneity of findings may be partially explained by differences in the clinical characteristics of the sample such as illness duration, severity, comorbidity sample size, imaging protocols, and treatment status.

WHITE MATTER

Abnormalities in structural and functional connectivity have been implicated in the pathophysiology of MDD. In this chapter, we will address white matter structural findings, specifically white matter (WM) microstructure and tractography studies using diffusion weighted imaging, as well as WM volumetric studies, in addition to studies assessing macroscopic WM lesions.

It has been previously established that brain regions that are anatomically connected by white matter tracts show a high degree of functional connectivity.[84] WM microstructure underlies resting state regional functional networks,[85] and can therefore be used as a proxy measure. Although structural connectivity correlates positively with functional connectivity, some evidence suggests that even areas that are not directly anatomically connected exhibit functional connections.[86]

As discussed earlier in this chapter, structural neuroimaging studies have identified a number of cortical and subcortical structures that appear to be implicated, in the pathophysiology of depression.[87,88] Furthermore, it has been suggested that microstructural changes in the WM of cortico-subcortical circuits (including frontotemporal regions, amygdala, and hippocampus) may lead to a disconnection syndrome.[89] This profile could explain the poor emotional regulation and cognitive control characterizing MDD.

Neuroimaging studies of in vivo human white brain matter fall into three categories—macroscopic studies (typically using T2 or FLAIR MRI sequences), microstructural studies (using diffusion indices), and tractographic studies. In the next sections, we will review current literature on structural brain changes in MDD based on the previously mentioned methodology.

WHITE MATTER HYPERINTENSITIES

White matter hyperintensities (WMHs) are age-related changes in white matter integrity[90] that are more pronounced in late-life depression (LLD), and to an even greater extent late-onset depression.[91] Patients with late-onset depression (LOD) were found to be about 4.5 more likely to have WMHs than patients with early-onset depression (EOD). Similarly, the severity of WMHs was higher in LOD than EOD patients. These findings suggest likely different etiological mechanisms between early-onset and late-onset depression, in accordance with the theory of "cerebrovascular depression"[92] in late onset. Ischemic WMHs are usually larger in size than WMHs of other etiologies, such as dilated perivascular spaces.[93]

The lesions tend to be located primarily in frontal and temporal areas, and the disruption of the frontostriatal circuits involved in mood regulation may lead to a disconnection syndrome,[94] which corresponds with the clinical profile of LLD.

WMHs increase over time in patients with LLD, and this increase is more pronounced among those who do not achieve remission than among remitters.[95] The severity of WMHs was also found to be associated with poor response to electroconvulsive therapy.[96]

Moreover, the presence of WMHs in patients with LLD is associated with worse cognitive skills, predominantly poorer executive function,[97] and an increased risk for functional decline.[98]

VOLUMETRIC STUDIES

Most imaging studies assessing the volume of brain structures focus on the cortex or gray matter, and WM is typically excluded. We identified one study looking at WM volume in depressed adolescents.[99] The authors report significantly smaller frontal WM volumes and significantly larger frontal GM volumes in the patients, which suggest an abnormality in developmental myelination in depressed adolescents. An adult study[100] found no group difference in WM volume between depressed patients and HCs.

WM MICROSTRUCTURE

The following section reviews findings from diffusion weighted MRI studies, analyzing the microstructural integrity of WM. For the purposes of this chapter, we will first review the findings in adults with MDD, and then talk about special populations (late life, child, and adolescent).

Adults

In 2013, Liao et al. published the first systematic review and meta-analysis of diffusion tensor imaging (DTI) studies in MDD.[101,102] It included the results of 11 studies and found significantly reduced fractional anisotropy (FA) in MDD patients in the right and left frontal lobes, right temporal lobe, and right fusiform gyrus. The authors tracked the fibers passing through the areas of significantly decreased FA, and identified the following affected tracts: genu and body of the corpus callosum, right inferior longitudinal fasciculus, right inferior fronto-occipital fasciculus and right posterior thalamic radiation. A later meta-analysis of DTI studies in MDD and bipolar disorder (BD) found decreased FA in the genu of the corpus callosum in both conditions.[103] This meta-analysis included 23 studies of MDD patients, and 17 studies of patients with BD, and BD patients showed more marked reduction in left cingulum FA when comparing these two groups. All studies included in these meta-analyses employed either voxel-based approach or Tract-based spatial statistics (TBSS).[104]

A later review[105] carried newer tractography and found alterations in the cingulum bundle, uncinate fasciculus, and superolateral medial forebrain bundle. This review pointed to differences between the findings of meta-analyses of voxel-based and tractographic studies. This might have resulted from the fact that meta-analyses include data from heterogeneous populations that may differ anatomically, as well as different data acquisition schemes and analysis methods, that may lead to different results. Of note, the largest single DTI study to date, that set out to reconcile the inconsistencies in published data, found no differences in FA between MDD patients and Hs.[106] A recent meta-analysis studied medication-free patients with MDD, and identified decreased FA in the WM of right cerebellum hemispheric lobule, body of the CC, bilateral ventral component of the SLF, and the long segment of the arcuate network, as compared with HCs.[107]

The next sections will discuss findings specific to WM tracts and regions that are relevant to the symptomatology of MDD.

Areas

Corpus callosum. The corpus callosum (CC) is the largest fiber bundle in the human brain connecting the right and left hemispheres. It is divided into the anterior part (genu) consisting of fibers connecting the prefrontal and orbitofrontal regions, a central part (body) connecting precentral frontal regions and parietal lobes, and a posterior part connecting the occipital

(splenium) and temporal (tapetum) lobes.[108] Corpus callosum fibers in the left frontal lobe were found to have decreased FA in Liao's 2011[101,102] meta-analysis. This was the only left hemisphere region identified in the study, along with a number of contralateral areas, suggesting a role for functional impairment of information transfer between hemispheres in MDD.

Fusiform Gyrus

The fusiform gyrus is a part of the temporal and occipital lobe in Brodmann area (BA) 37. One study suggested that biased memory processing in the fusiform gyrus and prefrontal cortex may contribute to symptom maintenance and cognitive vulnerability in depression.[109] The right fusiform gyrus is responsible for facial recognition, and its activation is reduced in response to happy faces in comparison with HCs.[110] Modulation of activity in the facial processing area has been suggested to contribute to changes in the salience of such emotional stimuli.[111] The earlier cited meta-analysis[101,102] found evidence of impairment in the connectivity of the fusiform face recognition region.

Superior Longitudinal Fasciculus

The superior longitudinal fasciculus (SLF) is a bilateral associative tract that connects the frontal, occipital, parietal, and temporal lobes.[112] It comprises three subcomponents: SLF I is involved in regulating motor behavior; SLF II is the major component, connecting parietal lobes to the dorsolateral prefrontal cortex, and carries information about the perception of visual space and spatial attention; SLF III connects the parietal lobes to the ventral premotor and prefrontal cortex, and carries somatosensory information.[113]

Inferior Longitudinal Fasciculus

The inferior longitudinal fasciculus (ILF) is an associative fiber tract connecting the temporal and occipital lobes. The long fibers of the ILF connect visual areas to the amygdala and hippocampus,[114] which are limbic system components connected to emotional regulation. It is involved in face recognition,[115] visual perception,[116] reading,[117] visual memory,[118] and other functions involving in language processing.[119]

Inferior Fronto-Occipital Fasciculus

The inferior fronto-occipital (alternatively referred to as occipitofrontal) fasciculus is an associative bundle subdivided into a superficial and dorsal component connecting the ventral occipital lobe and the orbitofrontal cortex,[120] and a deep and ventral component connecting the frontal lobe with inferior occipital gyrus and the posterior temporobasal area, and is a functional part of the semantic system.[121] It plays an essential role in semantic processing,[122] and is likely involved in reading,[117,132] attention,[119] and visual processing.[115,123]

Thalamic Radiations

The thalamic radiations are two-way fiber connections originating in the thalamic nuclei that run through the internal capsule, and enter the corona radiata and terminal in the cortex of ipsilateral hemispheres. They are divided into four groups—anterior, superior, posterior, and inferior.[124] The posterior thalamic radiation includes fibers connecting the lateral geniculate nucleus with the primary visual cortex, as posterior thalamus with the association areas of the occipital cortex, and it is involved in visual processing. The involvement of thalamic radiations in the pathophysiology of MDD gives evidence for a role of the occipital lobe, possibly related to dysfunctional facial recognition in patients with MDD.[101,102]

In the following section, we will discuss the findings in children and adolescents, as well as elderly patients with MDD.

Several studies have investigated the WM microstructure in adolescents with MDD. The findings include decreased FA in the tract connecting anterior cingulate to the amygdala,[125] in the anterior cingulum and anterior corona radiata,[126] and bilateral uncinated fasciculi.[127] It is important to note that all of these studies analyzed relatively small numbers of subjects. One study compared adolescents without a psychiatric disorder, but at high risk for MDD by virtue of having an affected parent, with healthy adolescents.[128] The authors reported decreases in FA in number of tracts, including cingulum, corpus callosum, and superior longitudinal fasciculus. Of note, this was a small study, looking at 18 at risk and 13 control subjects, respectively.

GERIATRIC DEPRESSION

Most of the studies conducted in LLD detected the presence of WMHs, and these are discussed in an earlier section of this chapter. Studies analyzing WM microstructure in the elderly population are less numerous. A recent meta-analysis identified 15 studies, of which 11 reported a decrease in FA in at least one region.[129] Frontal lobe, corpus callosum, uncinated fasciculus, and cingulum were reported as the most frequently implicated areas in this analysis. The authors then performed a meta-analysis, focusing on these four regions, and detected a decrease in FA in the

dorsolateral prefrontal cortex and the uncinate fasciculus among patients.

CONCLUSIONS

In summary, the development and recurrence of depressive symptoms have been associated with structural abnormalities in brain regions underlying the regulation of mood and cognitive functions such as the hippocampus, limbic regions, the orbital and medial prefrontal cortex, cingulate cortices, amygdale, striatum, thalamic nuclei, and ventral pallidum. Although structural alterations in the paralimbic circuits have been consistently replicated, other patterns of structural brain alterations have yet to be confirmed. This is due to small sample sizes, the heterogeneous nature of MDD, with subclusters of individuals having different underlying pathophysiology, demographic characteristics, and differences in data acquisition protocols and data analyses. Our review has highlighted the need for longitudinal studies to quantify the role of developmental delays, medication, time to remission, and mood state on the brain structural abnormalities observed in MDD.

Reproducible protocols and appropriately powered statistical methods are critical to inform future scientific investigations, facilitate active transdisciplinary collaborations, and lead to validation of current findings. It is, however, important to consider potential sources of variability across studies such as eligibility criteria, scanners, and acquisition parameters. Along the same line, an increasing number of studies have applied machine learning methods to complex, multidimensional datasets. In the field of psychiatry, current studies are moving toward characterizing a biosignature of mood disorders based on several features such as cortical complexity, curvature, spectral content, and genetic polymorphisms, and inflammatory markers. The findings of these studies are clinically relevant, as they will allow the characterization of subtypes of MDD, with the potential to predict treatment response and identify high-risk individuals.

ABBREVIATIONS

ACC	anterior cingulate cortex
BA	Brodmann area
BD	bipolar disorder
CC	corpus callosum
DTI	diffusion tensor imaging
EOD	early-onset depression
LLD	late-life depression
MDD	major depressive disorder
MRT	magnetic resonance imaging

OFC   orbital frontal cortex
ROI   region of interest
SLF   superior longitudinal fasciculus
SBM   surface-based morphometry
TBSS   tract-based spatial statistics
VBM   voxel-based morphometry
WMHS   white matter hyperintensities
WM   white matter

REFERENCES

1. Kessler RC, et al. Development of lifetime comorbidity in the World Health Organization world mental health surveys. *Arch Gen Psychiatr*. 2011;68(1):90−100.
2. Murray CJ, et al. Disability-adjusted life years (DALYs) for 291 diseases and injuries in 21 regions, 1990−2010: a systematic analysis for the Global Burden of Disease Study 2010. *Lancet*. 2012;380(9859):2197−2223.
3. Cowen PJ. Serotonin and depression: pathophysiological mechanism or marketing myth? *Trends Pharmacol Sci*. 2008;29(9):433−436.
4. Nutt DJ. The role of dopamine and norepinephrine in depression and antidepressant treatment. *J Clin Psychiatry*. 2006;67:3−8.
5. Kim YK, et al. The role of pro-inflammatory cytokines in neuroinflammation, neurogenesis and the neuroendocrine system in major depression. *Prog Neuro Psychopharmacol Biol Psychiatr*. 2016;64:277−284.
6. Bouhuys AL, et al. The association between levels of cortisol secretion and fear perception in patients with remitted depression predicts recurrence. *J Nerv Ment Dis*. 2006;194(7):478−484.
7. Fischer S, Macare C, Cleare AJ. Hypothalamic-pituitary-adrenal (HPA) axis functioning as predictor of antidepressant response—meta-analysis. *Neurosci Biobehav Rev*. 2017;83:200−211.
8. Gerritsen L, et al. HPA axis genes, and their interaction with childhood maltreatment, are related to cortisol levels and stress-related phenotypes. *Neuropsychopharmacology*. 2017;42(12):2446−2455.
9. Phillips ML, et al. Neurobiology of emotion perception II: implications for major psychiatric disorders. *Biol Psychiatry*. 2003;54(5):515−528.
10. Drevets WC, Price JL, Furey ML. Brain structural and functional abnormalities in mood disorders: implications for neurocircuitry models of depression. *Brain Struct Funct*. 2008;213(1−2):93−118.
11. Saleem KS, Kondo H, Price JL. Complementary circuits connecting the orbital and medial prefrontal networks with the temporal, insular, and opercular cortex in the macaque monkey. *J Comp Neurol*. 2008;506(4):659−693.
12. Kondo H, Saleem KS, Price JL. Differential connections of the perirhinal and parahippocampal cortex with the orbital and medial prefrontal networks in macaque monkeys. *J Comp Neurol*. 2005;493(4):479−509.
13. Öngür D, Price J. The organization of networks within the orbital and medial prefrontal cortex of rats, monkeys and humans. *Cerebr Cortex*. 2000;10(3):206−219, 2000.
14. Van Laere K, et al. Metabolic imaging of anterior capsular stimulation in refractory obsessive-compulsive disorder: a key role for the subgenual anterior cingulate and ventral striatum. *J Nucl Med*. 2006;47(5):740−747.
15. Ashburner J, Friston KJ. Why voxel-based morphometry should be used. *Neuroimage*. 2001;14:1238−1243.
16. Uchida RR, et al. Correlation between voxel based morphometry and manual volumetry in magnetic resonance images of the human brain. *Anais da Academia Brasileira de Ciencias*. 2008;80:149−156.
17. Davies RR. Development of an MRI rating scale for multiple brain regions: comparison with volumetrics and with voxel-based morphometry. *NeuroRadiology*. 2009;51:491−503.
18. Yuan Y, et al. Regional gray matter changes are associated with cognitive deficits in remitted geriatric depression: an optimized voxel-based morphometry study. *Biol Psychiatry*. 2008;64(6):541−544, 15.
19. Ribeiz SR, et al. Structural brain changes as biomarkers and outcome predictors in patients with late-life depression: a cross-sectional and prospective study. *PLoS One*. 2013;8(11):e80049, 14.
20. Du MY, et al. Voxelwise meta-analysis of gray matter reduction in major depressive disorder. *Prog Neuro Psychopharmacol Biol Psychiatr*. 2012;36:11−16.
21. Wang W, et al. Conjoint and dissociated structural and functional abnormalities in first-episode drug-naive patients with major depressive disorder: a multimodal meta-analysis. *Nature Sci Rep*. 2017;7(1):10401, 4.
22. Zhao Y, et al. Gray matter abnormalities in non-comorbid medication-naive patients with major depressive disorder or social anxiety disorder. *EBioMedicine*. 2017;21:228−235.
23. Lai CH, Wu YT. Frontal-insula gray matter deficits in first episode medication-naive patients with major depressive disorder. *J Affect Disord*. 2014;160:74−79.
24. Zhao YJ, et al. Brain grey matter abnormalities in medication-free patients with major depressive disorder: a meta-analysis. *Psychol Med*. 2014;44:2927−2937.
25. Peterson BS, et al. Cortical thinning in persons at increased familial risk for major depression. *Proc Natl Acad Sci U S A*. 2009;106:6273−6278.
26. Tu PC, et al. Regional cortical thinning in patients with major depressive disorder: a surface-based morphometry study. *Psychiatr Res Neuroimaging*. 2012;202:206−213.
27. Qiu L, et al. Regional increases of cortical thickness in untreated, first-episode major depressive disorder. *Transl Psychiatry*. 2014;4:e378.
28. Zhang H, et al. Brain gray matter alterations in first episodes of depression: a meta-analysis of whole-brain studies. *Neurosci Biobehav Rev*. 2015;60:43−50, 2016.
29. Niu M, et al. Common and specific abnormalities in cortical thickness in patients with major depressive and bipolar disorders. *EBioMedicine*. 2017;16:162−171.

30. Soriano-Mas C, et al. Cross-sectional and longitudinal assessment of structural brain alterations in melancholic depression. *Biol Psychiatry.* 2011;69:318–325.

31. Chen CH, et al. Brain imaging correlates of depressive symptom severity and predictors of symptom improvement after antidepressant treatment. *Biol Psychiatry.* 2007;62:407–414.

32. Bora E, et al. Gray matter abnormalities in major depressive disorder: a meta-analysis of voxel based morphometry studies. *J Affect Disord.* 2012;138:9–18.

33. Lai CH. Gray matter volume in major depressive disorder: a meta-analysis of voxel-based morphometry studies. *Psychiatr Res.* 2013;211:37–46.

34. Redlich R, et al. Brain morphometric classification approach. *JAMA Psychiatry.* 2014;71:1222–1230.

35. Hajek T, et al. Reduced subgenual cingulate volumes in mood disorders: a meta-analysis. *J Psychiatry Neurosci.* 2008;33:91–99.

36. Koolschijn P, et al. Brain volume abnormalities in major depressive disorder: a meta-analysis of magnetic resonance imaging studies. *Hum Brain Mapp.* 2009;30: 3719–3735.

37. Tang Y, et al. Reduced ventral anterior cingulate and amygdala volumes in medication-naïve females with major depressive disorder: a voxel-based morphometric magnetic resonance imaging study. *Psychiatr Res.* 2007; 156:83–86.

38. Phillips JL, et al. A prospective, longitudinal study of the effect of remission on cortical thickness and hippocampal volume in patients with treatment-resistant depression. *Int J Neuropsychopharmacol.* 2015;18(8), 30.

39. Yang X, et al. Anatomical and functional brain abnormalities in unmedicated major depressive disorder. *Neuropsychiatric Dis Treat.* 2015;11:2415–2423, 18.

40. Stratmann M, et al. Insular and hippocampal gray matter volume reductions in patients with major depressive disorder. *PLoS One.* 2014;9:e102692.

41. Price J, Drevets W. Neurocircuitry of mood disorders. *Neuropsychopharmacology.* 2009;35:192–216.

42. Arnone D, et al. Magnetic resonance imaging studies in unipolar depression: systematic review and metaregression analyses. *Eur Neuropsychopharmacol.* 2012a;22:1–16.

43. Arnone D, et al. State-dependent changes in hippocampal grey matter in depression. *Mol Psychiatr.* 2012b;6: 1265–1272.

44. Steffens DC, et al. Change in hippocampal volume on magnetic resonance imaging and cognitive decline among older depressed and nondepressed subjects in the neurocognitive outcomes of depression in the elderly study. *Am J Geriatr Psychiatry.* 2011;19:4–12.

45. Taylor WD, et al. Hippocampus atrophy and the longitudinal course of late-life depression. *Am J Geriatr Psychiatry.* 2014;22:1504–1512.

46. Egger K, et al. Pattern of brain atrophy in elderly patients with depression revealed by voxel-based morphometry. *Psychiatry Res Neuroimaging.* 2008;164:237–244.

47. MacMaster FP, Kusumakar V. Hippocampal volume in early onset depression. *BMC Med.* 2004;2:2, 29.

48. Hickie I, et al. Reduced hippocampal volumes and memory loss in patients with early- and late-onset depression. *Br J Psychiatry.* 2005;186:197–202.

49. Hou Z, et al. Longitudinal changes in hippocampal volumes and cognition in remitted geriatric depressive disorder. *Behav Brain Res.* 2012;227:30–35.

50. Bell-mcginty S, et al. Brain morphometric abnormalities in geriatric depression: long-term neurobiological effects of illness duration. *Am J Psychiatry.* 2002;159: 1424–1427.

51. Campbell S, et al. Lower hippocampal volume in patients suffering from depression: a meta-analysis. *Am J Psychiatry.* 2004;161:598–607.

52. McKinnon MC, et al. A meta-analysis examining clinical predictors of hippocampal volume in patients with major depressive disorder. *J Psychiatry Neurosci.* 2009; 34:41–54.

53. Videbech P, Ravnkilde B. Hippocampal volume and depression: a meta-analysis of MRI studies. *Am J Psychiatry.* 2004;161:1957–1966.

54. Zou K, et al. Changes of brain morphometry in first-episode, drug-naive, non-late-life adult patients with major depression: an optimized voxel-based morphometry study. *Biol Psychiatry.* 2010;67:186–188.

55. Frodl T, O'Keane V. How does the brain deal with cumulative stress? A review with focus on developmental stress, HPA axis function and hippocampal structure in humans. *Neurobiol Dis.* 2013;52:24–37.

56. Isıklı S, et al. Altered hippocampal formation shape in first-episode depressed patients at 5-year follow-up. *ASJ Psychiatr Res.* 2013;47(1):50–55.

57. Schmaal L, et al. Subcortical brain alterations in major depressive disorder: findings from the ENIGMA Major Depressive Disorder working group. *Mol Psychiatr.* 2016;21(6):806–812.

58. Redlich R, et al. The limbic system in youth depression: brain structural and functional alterations in adolescent in-patients with severe depression. *Neuropsychopharmacology.* 2018;43(3):546–554.

59. Sachs-Ericsson N, et al. A longitudinal study of differences in late and early onset geriatric depression: depressive symptoms and psychosocial, cognitive, and neurological functioning. *Aging Ment Health.* 2013; 17(1):1–11.

60. Frodl T, et al. Reduced hippocampal volume correlates with executive dysfunctioning in major depression. *J Psychiatry Neurosci.* 2006;31:316–323.

61. MacQueen GM, Campbell S, McEwen BS, et al. Course of illness, hippocampal function, and. hippocampal volume in major depression. *Proc Natl Acad Sci U S A.* 2003;3:1387–1392.

62. Shah PJ, et al. Cortical grey matter reductions associated with treatment-resistant chronic unipolar depression. Controlled magnetic resonance imaging study. *Br J Psychiatry.* 1998;172:527–532.

63. van Eijndhoven P, et al. Amygdala volume marks the acute state in the early course of depression. *Biol Psychiatry.* 2009;65:812–818.

64. Hamilton JP, Siemer M, Gotlib IH. Amygdala volume in major depressive disorder:a meta- analysis of magnetic resonance imaging studies. *Mol Psychiatr.* 2008;13: 993−1000.

65. Saleh K, et al. Impact of family history and depression on amygdala volume. *Psychiatr Res.* 2012;203:24−30.

66. Kronenberg G, et al. Reduced amygdala volume in newly admitted psychiatric in-patients with unipolar major depression. *J Psychiatr Res.* 2009;43:1112−1117.

67. Altshuler LL, et al. Amygdala astrocyte reduction in subjects with major depressive disorder but not bipolar disorder. *Bipolar Disord.* 2010;12:541−549.

68. Bowley MP, et al. Low glial numbers in the amygdala in major depressive disorder. *Biol Psychiatry.* 2002;52: 404−412.

69. Lu Y, et al. The volumetric and shape changes of the putamen and thalamus in first episode, untreated major depressive disorder. *Neuroimage Clin.* 2016;11: 658−666, 14.

70. Bielau H, et al. Volume deficits of subcortical nuclei in mood disorders. *Eur Arch Psychiatry Clin Neurosci.* 2005; 255:401−412.

71. Kim M, Hamilton J, Gotlib I. Reduced caudate gray matter volume in women with major depressive disorder. *Psychiatry Res Neuroimaging.* 2008;164:114−122.

72. Peng J, et al. Cerebral and cerebellar gray matter reduction in first-episode patients with major depressive disorder: a voxel-based morphometry study. *Eur J Radiol.* 2011;80(2):395−399.

73. Frodl TS, et al. Depression-related variation in brain morphology over 3 year: effects of stress? *Arch Gen Psychiatr.* 2008;65:1156−1165.

74. Fatemi SH, et al. Glial fibrillary acidic protein is reduced in cerebellum of subjects with major depression, but not schizophrenia. *Schizophr Res.* 2004;69:317−323.

75. Becker G, et al. Reduced echogenicity of brainstem raphe specific to unipolar depression: a transcranial color-coded real-time sonography study. *Biol Psychiatry.* 1995; 38:180−184.

76. Becker G, et al. Echogenicity of the brainstem raphe in patients with major depression. *Psychiatry Res Neuroimaging.* 1994;55:75−84.

77. Steele JD, et al. Possible structural abnormality of the brainstem in unipolar depressive illness: a transcranial ultrasound and diffusion tensor magnetic resonance imaging study. *J Neurol Neurosurg Psychiatry.* 2005;76(11): 1510−1515.

78. Ahdidan J, et al. Longitudinal MR study of brain structure and hippocampus volume in major depressive disorder. *Acta Psychiatr Scand.* 2011;123:211−219.

79. Qi H, et al. Gray matter volume abnormalities in depressive patients with and without anxiety disorders. *Medicine.* 2014;93:e345.

80. Lee HY, et al. Demonstration of decreased gray matter concentration in the midbrain encompassing the dorsal raphe nucleus and the limbic subcortical regions in major depressive disorder: an optimized voxel-based morphometry study. *J Affect Disord.* 2011;133:128−136.

81. Han KM, et al. Alterations in the brainstem volume of patients with major depressive disorder and their relationship with antidepressant treatment. *J Affect Disord.* 2017;208:68−75, 15.

82. Weber K, et al. Personality traits, cognition and volumetric MRI changes in elderly patients with early onset depression: a 2-year follow-up study. *Psychiatr Res.* 2012;198:47−52.

83. Frodl T, et al. Hippocampal and amygdala changes in patients with major depressive disorder and healthy controls during a 1-year follow-up. *J Clin Psychiatry.* 2004; 65(4):492−499.

84. Koch MA, Norris DG, Hund-Georgiadis M. An investigation of functional and anatomical connectivity using magnetic resonance imaging. *Neuroimage.* 2002;16(1): 241−250.

85. Teipel SJ, et al. White matter microstructure underlying default mode network connectivity in the human brain. *Neuroimage.* 2010;49(3):2021−2032.

86. Damoiseaux JS, Greicius MD. Greater than the sum of its parts: a review of studies combining structural connectivity and resting-state functional connectivity. *Brain Struct Funct.* 2009;213(6):525−533.

87. Soares JC, Mann JJ. The anatomy of mood disorders–review of structural neuroimaging studies. *Biol Psychiatry.* 1997;41(1):86−106.

88. Drevets WC. Neuroimaging and neuropathological studies of depression: implications for the cognitive-emotional features of mood disorders. *Curr Opin Neurobiol.* 2001;11(2):240−249.

89. Sexton CE, Mackay CE, Ebmeier KP. A systematic review of diffusion tensor imaging studies in affective disorders. *Biol Psychiatry.* 2009;66(9):814−823.

90. Raz N, et al. Vascular health and longitudinal changes in brain and cognition in middle-aged and older adults. *Neuropsychology.* 2007;21(2):149−157.

91. Herrmann LL, Le Masurier M, Ebmeier KP. White matter hyperintensities in late life depression: a systematic review. *J Neurol Neurosurg Psychiatry.* 2008;79(6): 619−624.

92. Kales HC, Maixner DF, Mellow AM. Cerebrovascular disease and late-life depression. *Am J Geriatr Psychiatry.* 2005;13(2):88−98.

93. Thomas AJ, et al. Pathologies and pathological mechanisms for white matter hyperintensities in depression. *Ann N Y Acad Sci.* 2002;977:333−339.

94. Alexopoulos GS, et al. Frontal white matter microstructure and treatment response of late-life depression: a preliminary study. *Am J Psychiatry.* 2002;159(11):1929−1932.

95. Khalaf A, et al. White matter hyperintensity accumulation during treatment of late-life depression. *Neuropsychopharmacology.* 2015;40(13):3027−3035.

96. Steffens DC, et al. Severity of subcortical gray matter hyperintensity predicts ECT response in geriatric depression. *J ECT.* 2001;17(1):45−49.

97. Lesser IM, et al. Cognition and white matter hyperintensities in older depressed patients. *Am J Psychiatry.* 1996; 153(10):1280−1287.

98. Hybels CF, et al. Late-life depression modifies the association between cerebral white matter hyperintensities and functional decline among older adults. *Am J Geriatr Psychiatry*. 2016;24(1):42−49.

99. Steingard RJ, et al. Smaller frontal lobe white matter volumes in depressed adolescents. *Biol Psychiatry*. 2002; 52(5):413−417.

100. Abe O, et al. voxel-based analyses of gray/white matter volume and diffusion tensor data in major depression. *Psychiatr Res Neuroimaging*. 2010;181(1):64−70.

101. Liao YL, et al. Cortical shape and curvedness analysis of structural deficits in remitting and non-remitting depression. *PLoS One*. 2013a;8:e68625.

102. Liao Y, et al. Is depression a disconnection syndrome? Meta- analysis of diffusion tensor imaging studies in patients with MDD. *J Psychiatry Neurosci*. 2013b;38(1): 49−56.

103. Wise T, et al. Voxel-based meta-analytical evidence of structural disconnectivity in major depression and bipolar disorder. *Biol Psychiatry*. 2016;79(4):293−302.

104. Smith SM, et al. Tract-based spatial statistics: voxelwise analysis of multi-subject diffusion data. *Neuroimage*. 2006;31(4):1487−1505.

105. Bracht T, Linden D, Keedwell P. A review of white matter microstructure alterations of pathways of the reward circuit in depression. *J Affect Disord*. 2015;187(c):45−53.

106. Choi KS, et al. Reconciling variable findings of white matter integrity in major depressive disorder. *Neuropsychopharmacology*. 2014;39(6):1332−1339.

107. Jiang J, et al. Microstructural brain abnormalities in medication-free patients with major depressive disorder: a systematic review and meta-analysis of diffusion tensor imaging. *J Psychiatry Neurosci*. 2017;42(3):150−163.

108. Hofer S, Frahm J. Topography of the human corpus callosum revisited–comprehensive fiber tractography using diffusion tensor magnetic resonance imaging. *Neuroimage*. 2006;32(3):989−994.

109. van Wingen GA, et al. Neural state and trait bases of mood-incongruent memory formation and retrieval in first-episode major depression. *J Psychiatr Res*. 2010; 44(8):527−534.

110. Surguladze S, et al. A differential pattern of neural response toward sad versus happy facial expressions in major depressive disorder. *Biol Psychiatry*. 2005;57(3): 201−209.

111. Vuilleumier P. How brains beware: neural mechanisms of emotional attention. *Trends Cognit Sci*. 2005;9(12): 585−594.

112. Wang X, et al. Subcomponents and connectivity of the superior longitudinal fasciculus in the human brain. *Brain Struct Funct*. 2016;221(4):2075−2092. http://doi.org/10.1007/s00429-015-1028-5.

113. Makris N, et al. Segmentation of subcomponents within the superior longitudinal fascicle in humans: a quantitative, in vivo, DT-MRI study. *Cerebr Cortex*. 2005;15(6): 854−869.

114. Catani M. Occipito-temporal connections in the human brain. *Brain*. 2003;126(9):2093−2107.

115. Fox C, Iaria G, Barton J. Disconnection in prosopagnosia and face processing. *Cortex*. 2008;44(8):996−1009.

116. Ffytche D. The hodology of hallucinations. *Cortex*. 2008; 44(8):1067−1083.

117. Epelbaum S, et al. Pure alexia as a disconnection syndrome: new diffusion imaging evidence for an old concept. *Cortex*. 2008;44(8):962−974.

118. Ross E. Sensory-specific amnesia and hypoemotionality in humans and monkeys: gateway for developing a hodology of memory. *Cortex*. 2008;44(8):1010−1022.

119. Catani M, Mesulam M. The arcuate fasciculus and the disconnection theme in language and aphasia: history and current state. *Cortex*. 2008;44(8):953−961.

120. Catani M. From hodology to function. *Brain*. 2007; 130(3):602−605.

121. Martino J, et al. Anatomic dissection of the inferior fronto-occipital fasciculus revisited in the lights of brain stimulation data. *Cortex*. 2010;46(5):691−699.

122. Almairac F, et al. The left inferior fronto-occipital fasciculus subserves language semantics: a multilevel lesion study. *Brain Struct Funct*. 2015;22(4):1983−1995.

123. Rudrauf D, Mehta S, Grabowski T. Disconnection's renaissance takes shape: formal incorporation in group-level lesion studies. *Cortex*. 2008;44(8):1084−1096.

124. Catani M, de Schotten MT. *Atlas of Human Brain Connections*. Oxford University Press; 2012.

125. Cullen KR, et al. Altered white matter microstructure in adolescents with major depression: a preliminary study. *J Am Acad Child Adolesc Psychiatry*. 2010;49(2):173−183 e1.

126. Henderson SE, et al. A preliminary study of white matter in adolescent depression: relationships with illness severity, anhedonia, and irritability. *Front Psychiatry*. 2013;4:152.

127. LeWinn KZ, et al. White matter correlates of adolescent depression: structural evidence for frontolimbic disconnectivity. *J Am Acad Child Adolesc Psychiatry*. 2014;53(8):899−909, 909.e1−7.

128. Huang H, et al. White matter changes in healthy adolescents at familial risk for unipolar depression: a diffusion tensor imaging study. *Neuropsychopharmacology*. 2011; 36(3):684−691.

129. Wen MC, et al. Diffusion tensor imaging studies in late-life depression: systematic review and meta-analysis. *Int J Geriatr Psychiatry*. 2014;29(12):1173−1184.

130. Shad MU, et al. Gary matter differences between healthy and depressed adolescents: a voxel-based morphometry study. *J Child adolesc Psychopharmacol*. 2012;22(3): 190−197.

131. Sheline YI. 3D MRI studies of neuroanatomic changes in unipolar major depression: the role of stress and medical comorbidity. *Biol Psychiatry*. 2000;48:791−800.

132. Catani M. Occipito-temopral connections in the human brain. *Brain*. 2003;126(9):2093−2017.

CHAPTER 4

Cognitive Deficits in Major Depression: From Mechanisms to Management

ALEXANDRIA S. COLES, BA • YENA LEE, HBSC •
MEHALA SUBRAMANIAPILLAI, MSC • ROGER S. MCINTYRE, MD, FRCP(C)

INTRODUCTION

Major depressive disorder (MDD) is a chronic and pervasive illness characterized by symptoms of persistent low mood, hopelessness, anhedonia, loss of energy, and cognitive dysfunction.[1] According to the World Health Organization (2012), MDD is a leading cause of disability, affecting nearly 350 million individuals worldwide and contributing significantly to the global burden of disease.[2]

Cognitive impairment is a commonly underestimated, albeit core feature of depression. According to the DSM-5, cognitive impairment in depression can be characterized by difficulty in decision making, poor concentration, and psychomotor slowing.[1] Recent research has documented the span of cognitive impairment in MDD across domains of attention, memory, executive functioning, and processing speed, contributing significantly to functional and occupational impairment among individuals with MDD.[3–5] Between 25% and 50% of individuals with MDD demonstrate impairment in one or more domains of cognition at one standard deviation or more below the normative mean.[5] Additional research indicates that neurocognitive deficits are an important determinant of functional recovery in this disorder.[6]

Greater severity of depressive symptoms has been linked to greater cognitive dysfunction.[5] Notably, studies suggest that cognitive deficits in depression persist during periods of euthymia, after recovery from major depressive episodes (MDE) and in subsyndromal manifestations of the disorder, potentially indicating that it represents a trait instead of state in MDD.[5,7] In addition, progression of cognitive deficits in some individuals with depression has been observed.[5] Such residual cognitive impairments represent a significant risk for episode relapse and failure to achieve remission status in this population.[8] Studies examining onset of MDD

have also suggested that cognitive impairments may precede the development of depression in some individuals.[8]

Despite its prevalence, neurobiological mechanisms underlying cognitive deficits in MDD remain relatively unclear. Nevertheless, evidence for neuroanatomical, neurochemical, and functional connectivity abnormalities relating to cognitive dysfunction in MDD has been demonstrated and these abnormalities have been proposed as contributing factors to cognitive dysfunction in depression; hormone imbalances, inflammatory processes, oxidative stress, neurotrophic factors, and metabolism are also hypothesized to play a role.[9–22] It is apparent that multiple integrated and overlapping factors contribute to the presence and persistence of cognitive deficits in individuals with depression.

Importantly, many patients do not experience clinically significant remission from cognitive symptoms with available antidepressant and/or psychosocial treatment, indicating that the critical need for further research in this area is necessary to improve functional outcomes in this illness.[5] Despite this, little research examining potential treatments have been conducted.

The following will evaluate the domains of cognitive dysfunction in depression, the neurobiological evidence underlying its mechanisms, and the currently available data on treatment options for this core deficit of MDD.

COGNITIVE DEFICITS AND RELATED FUNCTIONAL IMPAIRMENT IN DEPRESSION

Types of Cognitive Deficits Observed in Depression

The link between overall cognitive deficits and depression is both robust and consistent. The exact mechanisms underlying these cognitive deficits have been

Major Depressive Disorder. https://doi.org/10.1016/B978-0-323-58131-8.00004-5

thoroughly reviewed elsewhere.[23] Heterogeneity of studied samples (e.g., depressive subtypes and severity, comorbidities, medication use, age, gender, etc.) and types of neuropsychological tests used to evaluate them has led to significant variability among the types of cognitive deficits reported in this population.[5,6] Furthermore, consistent language to describe domains of cognition affected in MDD is lacking. Separate categories of hot and cold cognition are therefore relevant: hot cognition refers to emotionally dependent cognitive processes including negative response bias, rumination, anhedonia, and negative automatic thought processes associated with depression. In contrast, cold cognition refers to processes that are emotionally independent, such as executive function, memory, and attention.[24,25] It is proposed that abnormalities in both hot and cold cognitive domains result in the onset, maintenance, and treatment response of depressive symptoms in individuals with MDD.[24] Cold cognition deficits have been most consistently reported in domains of executive function, attention, memory, and processing speed among depressed individuals.[3-5] Additionally, concentration and general intelligence declines as a result of MDD have also been shown, although they are considered as a result of the previously stated domain-specific deficits.[3] Definitions of cognitive domains affected in depression are presented in Table 4.1.

Measurement of Cognitive Deficits in Depression

Cognitive dysfunction in depression is typically assessed via psychological interview, patient observation, and the administration of a neuropsychological test battery that can be tailored to each situation and individual, as assessed by the researcher or clinician.[3] Subjective cognitive dysfunction does not correlate with objective results.[5] Currently, there is no "gold standard" measure of cognitive dysfunction in MDD that has been accepted by the global psychiatric community, leading to the heterogeneity of tests used in both research and practice. Consistent with this, no measures have been created to specifically assess cognitive deficits in depression. The development of such measures may prove useful in better understanding the presence, impact, and variability of cognitive deficits in depression. A list of commonly used measures to assess cognitive dysfunction in depression is presented in Table 4.1.

Effects of Cognitive Deficits on Depressed Individuals

Subjective complaints of cognitive dysfunction are common in clinical settings.[5] Measures used to assess depressive symptoms in these settings (e.g., Structured Clinical Interview for the DSM-5, Beck Depression Inventory) commonly underestimate the role and impact of such deficits, despite their association with significant functional, psychosocial, and occupational impairments in depressed individuals.[25] However, research examining the mediating effects of cognitive symptoms in MDD on functional disability is currently limited. A cross-sectional study of cognition, mood, and functional outcomes by Baune and Air (2016)[26] indicates that executive functioning was the strongest predictor of function in patients with MDD, a domain with well-established deficits in this population.[26,27] A second study demonstrated that patients with MDD who

TABLE 4.1
Domains of Cognitive Dysfunction in MDD and Commonly Used Measures.

Domains of Cognitive Deficits	Commonly Used Measures
Executive functioning	Wisconsin card sorting task (WCST), trail making test part B (TMT-B), intra/extradimensional shift test (ID/ED), controlled oral word association test (COWAT), Stroop color-word interference test (SCWT), categories test
Attention	Digit symbol substitution test (DSST), continuous performance task (CPT), choice reaction time (CRT), simple reaction time (SRT)
Memory	California verbal learning test (CVLT), Weschler Memory Scale (WMS), Rey auditory verbal learning test (RAVLT), Benton visual retention test (BVRT), Hopkins verbal learning test (HVLT), visual verbal learning test (VVLT)
Processing speed	Digit symbol substitution test (DSST), finger tapping, grooved Pegboard test, Perdue pegs, continuous performance test (CPT), reaction time (RTI from CANTAB), simple reaction time (SRT), choice reaction time (CRT)
General intelligence	Mini mental state exam (MMSE), Weschler test of adult reading (WTAR), Weschler adult intelligence scale revised (WAIS-R), CNS vital signs

presented with both occupational and neurocognitive dysfunction went unchanged or indeed worsened after 1 year of treatment. These deficits were persistent and severe enough to negatively affect daily functioning on a large scale.[28] Cognitive performance may also be a central determinant of an individual's ability to function in the workplace. Employed individuals with MDD are less cognitively impaired compared to their unemployed counterparts.[29] It is estimated that declines in workplace performance due to MDD result in annual costs of approximately 36.6 billion dollars and 27.2 missed workdays per year in the United States alone.[5,30,31] A study of 312 South Korean participants with MDD showed that subjective cognitive dysfunction was associated with lower work-productivity outcomes, as a function of cognitive deficit severity.[32] Cognitive deficits in depression are also significantly associated with decreased quality of life.[30,33] Remission from depressive episodes do not always translate to improvements in cognitive performance: at least 20% of remitted individuals with MDD report outstanding difficulties concentration and decision making.[34] This emphasizes the need for treatments specifically targeting residual cognitive symptoms in MDD to better improve overall functional outcomes and remission rates for all symptoms.

NEUROBIOLOGY OF COGNITIVE DEFICITS IN DEPRESSION

Current models describing the pathophysiology of MDD are well understood and have been described elsewhere[35]; the neurobiological mechanisms underlying cognitive deficits among patients with MDD are less clear. Notwithstanding, several evidence-based hypotheses support the premise of neuroanatomical, neurochemical, functional, and circuitry-related abnormalities in MDD, which may mediate cognitive deficits in this disorder. Each unique category of cognitive dysfunction may have its own separate neurocircuitry and neurobiological mechanisms. It is therefore possible that combinations of these malfunctioning domains will differ between patients, contributing to the heterogeneity of symptoms expressed in depressed individuals.[36]

A combination of neuroanatomical abnormalities based on neuroimaging studies have been well documented in individuals with MDD. Primarily, volumetric decreases in areas of the bilateral hippocampus, amygdala, anterior cingulate cortex (ACC), orbitofrontal cortex, and dorsolateral prefrontal cortex (DLPFC) have been demonstrated in depressed individuals, all of

which play important roles in a variety of cognitive processes.[9-11] Specifically, such areas are implicated as important contributors to processes such as working memory, planning, and executive functioning, and volumetric changes may contribute to deficits in these domains.[10,11] These volumetric and functional changes are said to be dependent on factors of illness severity, duration, and episode frequency, and are thus not present in individuals experiencing their first MDE.[5,9] Additional neuroimaging studies have also reported cortical thinning, decreased dendritic, and neuronal soma size of depressed subjects compared to healthy controls.[9,10,16] Finally, decreased gray matter in the right DLPFC as a function of illness severity is associated with cognitive deficits in executive functioning processes.[37] A hypothesis concerning dysfunctional glutamatergic systems and subsequent altered transmission due to environmental stressors may account for the aforementioned volumetric and structural changes seen in patients with MDD.[38]

Neurochemical abnormalities in individuals with depression have also been well established, particularly within monoamine systems involving neurotransmitters of serotonin, dopamine, and norepinephrine. It is well recognized that monoaminergic neurotransmission wields significant influence on brain circuits concerned with both mood and cognitive performance. As a result, chemical abnormalities within these systems have been implicated as mediators of cognitive dysfunction among depressed individuals.[5,36,39] For instance, Fourrier et al.[20] report dysfunctions in neurotransmission at the synapse and in resulting long-term potentiation in the hippocampus as potentially responsible for the underlying learning and memory deficits in MDD.[20]

Functional connectivity issues between cortical and subcortical structures have also been hypothesized to generate cognitive deficits among depressed individuals within areas of processing speed, memory, attention, and executive functioning. Specifically, alterations in connectivity between networks responsible for aspects of cognition and emotional regulation such as the default mode network and executive control network have been documented in depression and may account for some of the cognitive deficits seen in this disorder.[22,40] Hypoactivity in the prefrontal cortex and increased activation of the ACC have been documented in depressed individuals and have been shown to affect functional and cognitive outcomes within this population.[37,40] Finally, abnormal functional connectivity in the temporal gyrus has been posited to negatively affect working memory in MDD.[40]

Inflammatory processes and immune dysfunction (e.g., elevated cytokine levels and microglial activation) may also play a role in cognitive deficits in MDD via disruption in neurobiological processes.[20] Patients with MDD have been shown to have elevations in inflammatory biomarkers compared to healthy controls.[19] Resulting increases in TNF-α, TNF-R1, and TNF-R2 serum levels seen in MDD have been negatively correlated with cognitive domains of memory, attention, and executive functioning.[20] MDD is also associated with increases in C-reactive protein and IL-6 levels, which are linked to cognitive dysfunction in depressed individuals.[13]

Cognitive dysfunction has also been linked to several other factors observed in MDD. For instance, the association between cognition, depression, and metabolism has been well established and documented.[14] Brain structures that play a key role in both cognition and mood such as the hippocampus and amygdala have an elevated vulnerability to effects of oxidative stress, which may contribute to deficits documented in this area.[15] Finally, hormone imbalances such as insulin resistance and glucocorticoid abnormalities (e.g., Cortisol) and dysregulation of neurotrophins (e.g., Brain-derived neurotrophic factor) have also been associated with impairment of cognition in patients with MDD.[5,12,41]

PHARMACOLOGICAL TREATMENTS FOR COGNITIVE DEFICITS IN DEPRESSION

Currently, very little data exist on the effects of pharmacological interventions on cognitive dysfunction in MDD. Thus far, antidepressants (SSRI's, SNRI's, NRI's), including vortioxetine and duloxetine, have shown the most promising results. A meta-analysis by Rosenblat and colleagues concluded that antidepressant use was significantly associated with improvements in domains of delayed recall and psychomotor processing speed in individuals with MDD.[42] Other pharmacological interventions such as psychostimulants, ketamine, incretins, metabolic regulators (e.g., Liraglutide), and TNF-α antagonists have been investigated for their potential to improve cognitive function among depressed individuals.[14,17,18,43–45] Notably, a paucity of studies has been conducted in this area and evidence to indicate the efficacy of these agents in targeting cognitive symptoms is still uncertain. Further research is necessary to better understand the procognitive potential of these agents in MDD. Refer to Table 4.2 for a breakdown of currently available, randomized controlled trials investigating the effects of pharmacological intervention on cognitive deficits in depression.

Antidepressants

Primarily, antidepressant medications (SSRIs, SNRIs, NRIs) have been most commonly investigated as potential treatments for cognitive dysfunction in MDD. The following are evidence from randomized controlled trials, where cognition was a primary outcome. A comprehensive review of all available studies has been conducted elsewhere.[46]

The antidepressant vortioxetine (Lu AA21004) has been studied for its procognitive effects in patients with MDD and is currently the only FDA-approved agent shown to directly improve cognitive function in this population. This SSRI primarily acts on serotonin receptors, but has been shown to increase dopaminergic, cholinergic, histaminergic, and noradrenergic neurotransmission in brain regions associated with MDD, and demonstrated the ability to exert positive effects on mood symptoms in this disorder.[5] Five studies have investigated the effects of vortioxetine in randomized controlled trials.[47–51] Nirenberg et al. recently compared vortioxetine with placebo in 151 patients with MDD who remained on their previous SSRI treatments. Findings indicate that all treatment groups improved on cognitive measures, but vortioxetine demonstrated trending superiority.[47] Another study by McIntyre compared two doses of vortioxetine (10 vs. 20 mg/day) to placebo with promising results. Both vortioxetine groups performed significantly better than placebo on the DSST and RAVLT (primary outcome measures) in 602 participants with moderate-to-severe depression.[50] Similar results were found in two other studies[49,51] which compared vortioxetine to both duloxetine and placebo groups. In both cases, vortioxetine groups outperformed placebo and duloxetine groups on primary measures of cognition (RAVLT and DSST).[49,51] Finally, a fifth study by Vieta et al. compared vortioxetine to escitalopram in an 8-week study of participants with MDD. Both groups improved significantly on all primary cognitive outcomes, though no statistically significant differences between groups were observed.[48]

Duloxetine, a serotonin norepinephrine reuptake inhibitor (SNRI), has also shown promise. Two studies have investigated the potential of this agent in the treatment of cognitive deficits in depression.[52,53] Raskin et al. compared 60 mg of duloxetine to placebo in an 8-week trial of geriatric participants with MDD. The duloxetine group improved significantly compared to placebo across primary measures of cognitive function.[53] The second study compared duloxetine (60 mg per day) to escitalopram (10 mg per day) in patients with MDD compared to healthy controls, observing increased cognitive functioning in both treatment

TABLE 4.2
Randomized Controlled Trials for Pharmacological Treatments of Cognitive Dysfunction in MDD [a].

Reference	Sample	Study Design	Treatment	Cognitive Measures	Results
ANTIDEPRESSANT TREATMENT STUDIES					
Nirenberg et al., 2019[47]	N = 151 participants with MDD	An 8-week, randomized, placebo-controlled, double-blind study	(1:1:1 randomization) Current SSRI and placebo, current SSRI and vortioxetine (10–20 mg/day) or vortioxetine (10–20 mg/day) and Placebo	DSST, ST, CRT, TMT A and B, SRT, RAVLT	• Patients in all treatment groups improved on cognitive performance measures • Trend toward superiority of vortioxetine, but differences between groups were not statistically significant • All participants improved on subjective measure of cognitive deficits (PDQ)
Vieta et al., 2018[48]	N = 101 participants with MDD	An 8-week, randomized, double-blind, controlled study	(1:1 randomization) Vortioxetine (10–20 mg/day) or Escitalopram (10–20 mg/day)	DSST, UPSA-B, SRT, CRT, RAVLT, TMT A and B, ST	• Significant improvement on all primary outcome cognitive measures were observed across groups, with no significant between group differences
Reddy et al., 2016[56]	N-427 currently employed participants with a primary diagnosis of MDD	A 12-week, randomized, double-blind, placebo-controlled study	(1:1 randomization) Desvenlafaxine (50 mg/day) or placebo	CDR, ST, TMT A and B	• Venlafaxine group improved in domain of working memory significantly, compared to placebo • No between group differences were observed on measures of attention
Gorlyn et al., 2015[57]	N = 64 patients with MDD and current suicidal ideation	An 8-week, randomized, double-blind trial	(1:1 randomization) Paroxetine (25–50 mg/day) or Bupropion XL (150–450 mg/day)	CFQ, CRT, SRT, WAIS-III, TMT A and B, CPT, ST, N-Back, BVRT	• Cognitive function improved across groups, with no significant between group differences noted
Mahableshwarkar et al., 2015[49]	N = 602 participants with MDD and self-reported cognitive deficits	An 8-week, randomized, double-blind, placebo-controlled study	(1:1:1 randomization) Vortioxetine (10–20 mg/day) or Duloxetine (60 mg/day) or Placebo	DSST	• Duloxetine was not significantly different than placebo on DSST • Vortioxetine was statistically superior to both placebo and duloxetine groups on DSST measure

Continued

TABLE 4.2
Randomized Controlled Trials for Pharmacological Treatments of Cognitive Dysfunction in MDD [a].—cont'd

Reference	Sample	Study Design	Treatment	Cognitive Measures	Results
McIntyre et al., 2014[50]	N = 602 participants with moderate to severe MDD	An 8-week, randomized, double-blind, placebo-controlled study	(1:1:1 randomization) Vortioxetine (10 mg/day) or vortioxetine (20 mg/day) or Placebo	DSST, RAVLT, TMT A and B, ST, CRT, SRT	• Both vortioxetine groups performed significantly better than the placebo group on the DSST and RAVLT (primary outcome measures) and most of the secondary outcome measures
Soczynska et al., 2014[54]	N = 38 participants with MDD	An 8-week, randomized, double-blind, flexible dose, controlled study	(1:1 randomization) Bupropion XL (150–300 mg/day) or escitalopram (10–20 mg/day)	CVLT-II, WMS, BVMT-R, SDS, EWPS	• Treatment with either escitalopram or bupropion XL was associated with significant psychosocial and memory improvements, with no differences between groups
Culang-Reinlieb et al., 2012[58]	N = 63 geriatric participants with MDD	A 12-week, randomized, double-blind study	(1:1 randomization) Sertraline (50–150 mg/day) or nortriptyline (1 mg/kg)	MMSE, SRT, CPT, ST, PP, TMT A and B	• Participants in sertraline group improved more than nortriptyline group in verbal learning • No other between group differences were noted
Katona et al., 2012[51]	N = 452 geriatric patients with MDD	An 8-week, randomized, double-blind, placebo-controlled, fixed dose study	(1:1:1 randomization) Vortioxetine (5 mg/day) or duloxetine (60 mg/day) or placebo	RAVLT, DSST	• Vortioxetine and duloxetine groups performed superiorly to placebo groups in measures of processing speed and verbal learning and memory.
Herrera-Guzman et al., 2010[52]	N = 73 participants with MDD and 37 healthy controls	A 24-week, randomized controlled study	(1:1 randomization) Escitalopram (10 mg/day) or duloxetine (60 mg/day)	SOC, ID/ED, ST, MTS, RVIP, SWM, WAIS III (digit span and vocabulary)	• Both duloxetine and escitalopram groups improved significantly on measures of cognition, but not enough to reach level of healthy controls
Culang et al., 2009[59]	N = 174 geriatric participants with MDD	An 8-week, randomized, double-blind, placebo-controlled study	(1:1 randomization) Citalopram (20–40 mg/day) or placebo	MMSE, ST, CRT, WAIS-III, BSRT, JLO	• No significant differences between citalopram and placebo groups on cognitive measures

Study	Sample	Design	Intervention	Measures	Results
Raskin et al., 2007[53]	N = 311 geriatric participants with MDD	An 8-week, randomized, double-blind, placebo-controlled study	(2:1 randomization) Duloxetine (60 mg/day) or placebo	VLRT, LNST, TDCT, SDST	• Duloxetine group significantly improved on cognitive measures compared to placebo group
Trick et al., 2004[61]	N = 43 geriatric participants with MDD	A 26-week, randomized, double-blind, parallel group trial	(1:1 randomization) Venlafaxine (75 mg/day) or dothiepin (75 mg/day)	CFF, CFQ	• Significant improvements on CFF were observed in the venlafaxine group compared to dothiepin
Fergusson et al., 2003[55]	N = 74 participants with MDD	An 8-week, randomized, double-blind, placebo-controlled study	(1:1:1 randomization) Reboxetine (8–10 mg/day), paroxetine (20–40 mg/day) or placebo	SRT, DVT, CRT, NWM	• Reboxetine group showed significant improvements in cognitive functioning, particularly in sustained attention • No differences between paroxetine group and placebo
Nebes et al., 2003[60]	N = 73 geriatric participants with MDD and 21 healthy controls	A 12-week, randomized, controlled study	(1:1 randomization) Paroxetine (dosage NR) or nortriptyline (dosage NR)	DSST, TMT A and B, N-Back	• No significant difference between medication groups
PSYCHOSTIMULANT TREATMENT STUDIES					
Madhoo et al., 2014[62]	N = 143 participants with MDD and executive dysfunction	A 9-week, randomized, double-blind, placebo-controlled study	(1:1 randomization) Lisdexamphetamine (20–70 mg/day) or placebo	BRIEF-A, CNS vital signs	• Treatment difference between baseline and week 9 showed that the Lisdexamphetamine group performed better than the placebo group. Lisdexamphetamine significantly improved executive functioning.
OTHER TREATMENT STUDIES					
Murrough et al., 2014[65]	N = 62 participants with TRD	A randomized, double-blind, controlled trial	(2:1 randomization) Ketamine (0.5 mg/kg) or midazolam (0.045 mg/kg)	HVLT, BVMT, TMT A, WMS	• Neurocognitive performance improved in both treatment groups with no between group differences

BSRT, Buschke selective reminding test; *BVMT*, brief visual memory test; *BVMT-R*, brief visuospatial memory test revised; *CDR*, computerized cognitive battery; *CFF*, critical flicker fusion test; *CFQ*, cognitive failure questionnaire; *CPFQ*, cognitive and physical functioning test; *CRT*, choice reaction time task; *CVLT-II*, California verbal learning test (II); *DSST*, digit symbol substitution test; *DVT*, digit vigilance task; *EWPS*, Endicott Work Productivity Scale; *ID/ED*, intra/extradimensional set shift; *IU*, international units; *JLO*, judgment of line orientation test; *LNST*, letter number sequencing test; *MDD*, major depressive disorder; *MDE*, major depressive episode; *MMSE*, mini mental status exam; *MTS*, match to sample visual search; *NMW*, numeric working memory; *NR*, not reported; *PDQ*, perceived deficits questionnaire; *PP*, Perdue pegboard task; *RAVLT*, Rey verbal learning test; *RVIP*, rapid visual information processing; *SDS*, Sheehan Disability Scale; *SDST*, symbol digit substitution test; *SOC*, Stockings of Cambridge; *SRT*, simple reaction time task; *ST*, Stroop test; *SWM*, spatial working memory; *TDCT*, two digit cancellation test; *TMT A and B*, trail making test A and B; *TRD*, treatment-resistant depression; *UPSA-B*, performance-based skills assessment; *VLRT*, verbal learning and recall test; *WAIS-III*, Wechsler Adult Intelligence Scale; *WMS*, Wechsler Memory Scale; *XL*, extended release
[a] Only studies with cognitive measures listed as primary outcomes have been included in this table.

groups. Despite this, patient performance levels did not improve enough to reach those of healthy control subjects.[52]

Several other studies have investigated the use of antidepressant agents as potential treatments for cognitive dysfunction. Soczynska et al. studied the effects of escitalopram (an SSRI) compared to bupropion extended release (a dopamine modulator) in a small sample of patients with MDD. Both treatment groups saw clinically significant improvements in psychosocial and memory domains, though no significant between group differences were observed.[54] A different study compared the agent reboxetine (a norepinephrine inhibitor) to paroxetine (an SSRI) and placebo with positive results. The reboxetine group showed clinically significant improvements across domains of cognition, particularly in measures of sustained attention.[55]

Several other preliminary studies have investigated the use of antidepressants such as venlafaxine, paroxetine, citalopram, nortriptyline, and dothiepin in the treatment of cognitive deficits in MDD populations with less favorable results.[56–61] Refer to Table 4.2 for a detailed description of each randomized controlled trial.

Psychostimulants

Historically, psychostimulants as adjunct treatments to antidepressants or antipsychotic medication have proven modestly useful in the treatment of unipolar and bipolar depression.[43] Their psychodynamic profile also indicates that this class of medication may be a promising treatment avenue for cognitive dysfunction.[5] In this regard, studies examining their potential efficacy are warranted. Despite this fact, there is a prominent lack of trials investigating this category of medications. Madhoo and colleagues have conducted the only randomized placebo-controlled study examining the effects of lisdexamfetamine on cognition in depressed individuals, with encouraging results. Individuals in the lisdexamfetamine group performed better compared to placebo, particularly on measures of executive functioning.[62]

Other Pharmacological Agents

Ketamine, a dissociative anesthetic and NMDA receptor agonist, has the ability to exert rapid antidepressant effects in patients with MDD, mitigating depressive symptoms even among those with treatment-resistant depression who have failed to respond to traditional pharmacological interventions.[45,63,64] In contrast, its reported effects on cognition have been mixed: although chronic use of ketamine at high doses is associated with significant impairment across cognitive domains, low dose ketamine does not demonstrate the same negative effects. Moreover, it has been posited that the antidepressant effects of ketamine may be partially due to the targeting of neural circuits that are relevant to various cognitive processes, including executive functioning.[63] A study by Murrough et al. investigated the use of ketamine compared to midazolam in participants with treatment-resistant depression. Results revealed improvements across neurocognitive domains in both groups.[65] Notably, these may be because of depressive symptom alleviation, and further studies to investigate its potential precognitive effects are needed.

Other pharmacological agents such as incretins, metabolic regulators (e.g., Liraglutide), and TNF-α antagonists also have the potential to improve cognitive function among individuals with MDD, as they may address underlying pathophysiology of cognitive deficits in this disorder. Studies investigating these agents are warranted.[18,21,25,44]

NONPHARMACOLOGICAL TREATMENTS FOR COGNITIVE DEFICITS IN DEPRESSION

Several nonpharmacological treatment options for cognitive dysfunction in MDD have been proposed, including cognitive remediation therapy (CRT), brain stimulation, and aerobic exercise. Cognitive remediation therapy involves the use of behavioral strategies to improve a span of cognitive processes and overcome-related cognitively challenging tasks.[25,66] The positive effects of CRT have been shown in other disorders such as schizophrenia and bipolar disorder.[66,67] A study by Bowie and colleagues (2013) examines the effects of a 10-week CRT protocol in treatment-resistant individuals with MDD. Improvements were observed in domains of attention, processing speed, and verbal memory, consistent with previous studies.[66,67] As such, CRT may be useful with adjunct pharmacological agents in the treatment of cognitive dysfunction in MDD.

Different brain stimulation modalities have also indicated procognitive effects in patients with MDD. Studies on the cognitive enhancing potential of noninvasive repetitive transcranial magnetic stimulation (rTMS) have demonstrated modest improvements in areas of language, visuospatial function, episodic memory, psychomotor speed, attention, and task switching.[68,69] Deep brain stimulation (DBS), a surgically invasive treatment modality, has also shown promise. In a meta-analysis by Bergfeld et al. patients with MDD who underwent DBS treatment improved in cognitive domains of verbal memory, working memory, sustained attention, motor speed, and cognitive flexibility.[70] Thus, brain stimulation modalities of rTMS and DBS may prove beneficial for cognitive deficits in MDD, and continued research into their potential to mitigate these deficits is justified.

Finally, several studies have demonstrated incontrovertible evidence for the positive effects of aerobic exercise in patients with MDD.[71,72] In contrast, no studies to our knowledge have been conducted on the effects of exercise on cognition. Research in this area is also warranted.

DISCUSSION

Cognitive deficits and overall dysfunction represent a core trait of MDD that commonly remains unimpacted by traditional pharmacological and psychosocial treatment interventions. Moreover, the presence of these cognitive impairments, during periods of remission from depressive episodes and at times before the development of MDD, suggests that they may represent an endophenotype of the disorder, rather than a mood-state-related issue.[5,7] As previously discussed, cognitive deficits in MDD are highly associated with impairments in functional and occupational disability, workplace productivity, and quality-of-life reductions, as well as increased risk of depressive episode relapse.[4,5,8] Consequently, treatments to improve cognitive deficits among individuals with depression are essential to improve overall remission rates and functional outcomes in this population. Greater emphasis on the role and impact of cognition and related disability must also permeate clinical practice, as their role in recovery is commonly underestimated.

Several hypotheses for the underlying pathophysiology of cognitive deficits in depression stipulate the existence of abnormalities in neuroanatomical, neurochemical, functional, and circuitry-related domains. Volumetric reductions in brain regions of the bilateral hippocampus and amygdala, as well as monoamine neurotransmission abnormalities were most commonly reported.[9,11,19] Similarly, several hypotheses also posit the dysfunction of metabolic, inflammatory, and oxidative stress mechanisms as contributing factors.[13–15] A clearer understanding of underlying mechanisms and related factors involved in the presentation of cognitive deficits in depression are critical to formulate more specialized and potentially successful treatment targets. In this regard, there is also an unmet requirement for standardized language and specific measures that can properly identify cognitive deficits in the MDD population. Standardization will allow for increased homogeneity and generalizability in research in addition to routine identification of cognitive dysfunction.

Efficacious, safe, and tolerable treatments (both pharmacological and other) that specifically address the range of cognitive deficits prevalent in depression are currently lacking. This is primarily due to the lack empirically derived evidence from randomized controlled trials evaluating the potential effects of various interventions on this subject. Nevertheless, the existing data points to antidepressant treatments, which act on monoamine systems in the brain (e.g., vortioxetine and duloxetine), as showing the most promise. Additionally, the mitigation of external factors that may contribute to the extent of cognitive dysfunction in depression such as psychiatric and medical comorbidities, substance use, and environmental stressors should be emphasized and made priority in clinical practice.

Future research should focus on the conduction of randomized controlled trials to investigate both pharmacological and nonpharmacological treatment options. Furthermore, combinations of treatment options, for instance, vortioxetine and cognitive remediation therapy together, are worth investigating as successful treatment of cognitive dysfunction may involve addressing multiple contributing factors simultaneously. Investigators should also aim for more uniform and discrete samples of MDD participants when conducting research. Stratifying participant groups based on MDD subtype, current treatments, illness duration, severity, and any present psychiatric comorbidities will provide a platform for better understanding of cognitive deficits in depression.

REFERENCES

1. Association AP. *Diagnostic and Statistical Manual of Mental Disorders: DSM-5*. 5th ed. Arlington, VA: American Psychiatric Publishing; 2013.
2. Organization WH. *Depression: A Global Public Health Concern*. 2012.
3. Marazziti D, Consoli G, Picchetti M, Carlini M, Faravelli L. Cognitive impairment in major depression. *Eur J Pharmacol*. 2010;626(1):83–86.
4. MacQueen GM, Memedovich KA. Cognitive dysfunction in major depression and bipolar disorder: Assessment and treatment options. *Psychiatr Clin Neurosci*. 2017; 71(1):18–27.
5. McIntyre RS, Cha DS, Soczynska JK, et al. Cognitive deficits and functional outcomes in major depressive disorder: determinants, substrates, and treatment interventions. *Depress Anxiety*. 2013;30(6):515–527.

6. Jaeger J, Berns S, Uzelac S, Davis-Conway S. Neurocognitive deficits and disability in major depressive disorder. *Psychiatr Res*. 2006;145(1):39–48.

7. Conradi HJ, Ormel J, de Jonge P. Presence of individual (residual) symptoms during depressive episodes and periods of remission: a 3-year prospective study. *Psychol Med*. 2011;41(6):1165–1174.

8. Lee RS, Hermens DF, Porter MA, Redoblado-Hodge MA. A meta-analysis of cognitive deficits in first-episode Major Depressive Disorder. *J Affect Disord*. 2012;140(2):113–124.

9. MacQueen GM, Campbell S, McEwen BS, et al. Course of illness, hippocampal function, and hippocampal volume in major depression. *Proc Natl Acad Sci USA*. 2003;100(3):1387–1392.

10. Malykhin NV, Carter R, Seres P, Coupland NJ. Structural changes in the hippocampus in major depressive disorder: contributions of disease and treatment. *J Psychiatry Neurosci*. 2010;35(5):337–343.

11. Kheirbek MA, Hen R. Dorsal vs ventral hippocampal neurogenesis: implications for cognition and mood. *Neuropsychopharmacology*. 2011;36(1):373–374.

12. Keller J, Gomez R, Williams G, et al. HPA axis in major depression: cortisol, clinical symptomatology and genetic variation predict cognition. *Mol Psychiatr*. 2017;22(4):527–536.

13. Li M, Soczynska JK, Kennedy SH. Inflammatory biomarkers in depression: an opportunity for novel therapeutic interventions. *Curr Psychiatr Rep*. 2011;13(5):316–320.

14. McIntyre RS, Rasgon NL, Kemp DE, et al. Metabolic syndrome and major depressive disorder: co-occurrence and pathophysiologic overlap. *Curr Diabetes Rep*. 2009;9(1):51–59.

15. van Velzen LS, Wijdeveld M, Black CN, et al. Oxidative stress and brain morphology in individuals with depression, anxiety and healthy controls. *Prog Neuropsychopharmacol Biol Psychiatry*. 2017;76:140–144.

16. Schmaal L, Hibar DP, Samann PG, et al. Cortical abnormalities in adults and adolescents with major depression based on brain scans from 20 cohorts worldwide in the ENIGMA Major Depressive Disorder Working Group. *Mol Psychiatr*. 2017;22(6):900–909.

17. Raison CL, Rutherford RE, Woolwine BJ, et al. A randomized controlled trial of the tumor necrosis factor antagonist infliximab for treatment-resistant depression: the role of baseline inflammatory biomarkers. *JAMA psychiatry*. 2013;70(1):31–41.

18. McIntyre RS, Vagic D, Swartz SA, et al. Insulin, insulin-like growth factors and incretins: neural homeostatic regulators and treatment opportunities. *CNS Drugs*. 2008;22(6):443–453.

19. Haase J, Brown E. Integrating the monoamine, neurotrophin and cytokine hypotheses of depression–a central role for the serotonin transporter? *Pharmacol Ther*. 2015;147:1–11.

20. Fourrier C, Singhal G, Baune BT. Neuroinflammation and cognition across psychiatric conditions. *CNS Spectrums*. 2019:1–12.

21. Bortolato B, Carvalho AF, Soczynska JK, Perini GI, McIntyre RS. The involvement of TNF-alpha in cognitive dysfunction associated with major depressive disorder: an opportunity for domain specific treatments. *Curr Neuropharmacol*. 2015;13(5):558–576.

22. Albert KM, Potter GG, Boyd BD, Kang H, Taylor WD. Brain network functional connectivity and cognitive performance in major depressive disorder. *J Psychiatr Res*. 2019;110:51–56.

23. Galecki P, Talarowska M, Anderson G, Berk M, Maes M. Mechanisms underlying neurocognitive dysfunctions in recurrent major depression. *Med Sci Mon Int Med J Exp Clin Res*. 2015;21:1535–1547.

24. Roiser JP, Sahakian BJ. Hot and cold cognition in depression. *CNS Spectrums*. 2013;18(3):139–149.

25. Pan Z, Park C, Brietzke E, et al. Cognitive impairment in major depressive disorder. *CNS Spectrums*. 2018:1–8.

26. Baune BT, Air T. Clinical, functional, and biological correlates of cognitive dimensions in major depressive disorder - rationale, design, and characteristics of the cognitive function and mood study (CoFaM-Study). *Front Psychiatry*. 2016;7:150.

27. Knight MJ, Air T, Baune BT. The role of cognitive impairment in psychosocial functioning in remitted depression. *J Affect Disord*. 2018;235:129–134.

28. Godard J, Baruch P, Grondin S, Lafleur MF. Psychosocial and neurocognitive functioning in unipolar and bipolar depression: a 12-month prospective study. *Psychiatr Res*. 2012;196(1):145–153.

29. McIntyre RS, Xiao HX, Syeda K, et al. The prevalence, measurement, and treatment of the cognitive dimension/domain in major depressive disorder. *CNS Drugs*. 2015;29(7):577–589.

30. Woo YS, Rosenblat JD, Kakar R, Bahk WM, McIntyre RS. Cognitive deficits as a mediator of poor occupational function in remitted major depressive disorder patients. *Clinical Psychopharmacol Neurosci*. 2016;14(1):1–16.

31. Kessler RC, Akiskal HS, Ames M, et al. Prevalence and effects of mood disorders on work performance in a nationally representative sample of U.S. workers. *Am J Psychiatry*. 2006;163(9):1561–1568.

32. Kim JM, Chalem Y, di Nicola S, Hong JP, Won SH, Milea D. A cross-sectional study of functional disabilities and perceived cognitive dysfunction in patients with major depressive disorder in South Korea: the PERFORM-K study. *Psychiatr Res*. 2016;239:353–361.

33. McCall WV, Dunn AG. Cognitive deficits are associated with functional impairment in severely depressed patients. *Psychiatr Res*. 2003;121(2):179–184.

34. Trivedi MH, Greer TL. Cognitive dysfunction in unipolar depression: implications for treatment. *J Affect Disord*. 2014;152–154:19–27.

35. Krishnan V, Nestler EJ. Linking molecules to mood: new insight into the biology of depression. *Am J Psychiatry.* 2010;167(11):1305–1320.

36. Stahl SM, Zhang L, Damatarca C, Grady M. Brain circuits determine destiny in depression: a novel approach to the psychopharmacology of wakefulness, fatigue, and executive dysfunction in major depressive disorder. *J Clin Psychiatry.* 2003;64(suppl 14):6–17.

37. Pizzagalli DA. Frontocingulate dysfunction in depression: toward biomarkers of treatment response. *Neuropsychopharmacology.* 2011;36(1):183–206.

38. Sanacora G, Treccani G, Popoli M. Towards a glutamate hypothesis of depression: an emerging frontier of neuropsychopharmacology for mood disorders. *Neuropharmacology.* 2012;62(1):63–77.

39. Hamon M, Blier P. Monoamine neurocircuitry in depression and strategies for new treatments. *Prog Neuropsychopharmacol Biol Psychiatry.* 2013;45:54–63.

40. Zeng LL, Shen H, Liu L, et al. Identifying major depression using whole-brain functional connectivity: a multivariate pattern analysis. *Brain.* 2012;135(Pt 5):1498–1507.

41. Hamer JA, Testani D, Mansur RB, Lee Y, Subramaniapillai M, McIntyre RS. Brain insulin resistance: a treatment target for cognitive impairment and anhedonia in depression. *Exp Neurol.* 2019;315:1–8.

42. Rosenblat JD, Kakar R, McIntyre RS. The cognitive effects of antidepressants in major depressive disorder: a systematic review and meta-analysis of randomized clinical trials. *Int J Neuropsychopharmacol.* 2015;19(2).

43. McIntyre RS, Lee Y, Zhou AJ, et al. The efficacy of psychostimulants in major depressive episodes: a systematic review and meta-analysis. *J Clin Psychopharmacol.* 2017; 37(4):412–418.

44. Mansur RB, Ahmed J, Cha DS, et al. Liraglutide promotes improvements in objective measures of cognitive dysfunction in individuals with mood disorders: a pilot, open-label study. *J Affect Disord.* 2017;207:114–120.

45. Vidal S, Gex-Fabry M, Bancila V, et al. Efficacy and safety of a rapid intravenous injection of ketamine 0.5 mg/kg in treatment-resistant major depression: an open 4-week longitudinal study. *J Clin Psychopharmacol.* 2018;38(6): 590–597.

46. Salagre E, Sole B, Tomioka Y, et al. Treatment of neurocognitive symptoms in unipolar depression: a systematic review and future perspectives. *J Affect Disord.* 2017;221: 205–221.

47. Nirenberg AA, Loft H, Olsen CK. Treatment effects on residual cognitive symptoms among partially or fully remitted patients with major depressive disorder: a randomized, double-blinded, exploratory study with vortioxetine. *J Affect Disord.* 2019;250:35–42.

48. Vieta E, Sluth LB, Olsen CK. The effects of vortioxetine on cognitive dysfunction in patients with inadequate response to current antidepressants in major depressive disorder: a short-term, randomized, double-blind, exploratory study versus escitalopram. *J Affect Disord.* 2018;227: 803–809.

49. Mahableshwarkar AR, Zajecka J, Jacobson W, Chen Y, Keefe RS. A randomized, placebo-controlled, active-reference, double-blind, flexible-dose study of the efficacy of vortioxetine on cognitive function in major depressive disorder. *Neuropsychopharmacology.* 2016; 41(12):2961.

50. McIntyre RS, Lophaven S, Olsen CK. A randomized, double-blind, placebo-controlled study of vortioxetine on cognitive function in depressed adults. *Int J Neuropsychopharmacol.* 2014;17(10):1557–1567.

51. Katona C, Hansen T, Olsen CK. A randomized, double-blind, placebo-controlled, duloxetine-referenced, fixed-dose study comparing the efficacy and safety of Lu AA21004 in elderly patients with major depressive disorder. *Int Clin Psychopharmacol.* 2012;27(4):215–223.

52. Herrera-Guzman I, Herrera-Abarca JE, Gudayol-Ferre E, et al. Effects of selective serotonin reuptake and dual serotonergic-noradrenergic reuptake treatments on attention and executive functions in patients with major depressive disorder. *Psychiatr Res.* 2010;177(3):323–329.

53. Raskin J, Wiltse CG, Siegal A, et al. Efficacy of duloxetine on cognition, depression, and pain in elderly patients with major depressive disorder: an 8-week, double-blind, placebo-controlled trial. *Am J Psychiatry.* 2007;164(6): 900–909.

54. Soczynska JK, Ravindran LN, Styra R, et al. The effect of bupropion XL and escitalopram on memory and functional outcomes in adults with major depressive disorder: results from a randomized controlled trial. *Psychiatr Res.* 2014;220(1–2):245–250.

55. Ferguson JM, Wesnes KA, Schwartz GE. Reboxetine versus paroxetine versus placebo: effects on cognitive functioning in depressed patients. *Int Clin Psychopharmacol.* 2003; 18(1):9–14.

56. Reddy S, Fayyad R, Edgar CJ, Guico-Pabia CJ, Wesnes K. The effect of desvenlafaxine on cognitive functioning in employed outpatients with major depressive disorder: a substudy of a randomized, double-blind, placebo-controlled trial. *J Psychopharmacol.* 2016;30(6):559–567.

57. Gorlyn M, Keilp J, Burke A, Oquendo M, Mann JJ, Grunebaum M. Treatment-related improvement in neuropsychological functioning in suicidal depressed patients: paroxetine vs. bupropion. *Psychiatr Res.* 2015;225(3): 407–412.

58. Culang-Reinlieb ME, Sneed JR, Keilp JG, Roose SP. Change in cognitive functioning in depressed older adults following treatment with sertraline or nortriptyline. *Int J Geriatr Psychiatry.* 2012;27(8):777–784.

59. Culang ME, Sneed JR, Keilp JG, et al. Change in cognitive functioning following acute antidepressant treatment in late-life depression. *Am J Geriatr Psychiatry.* 2009;17(10): 881–888.

60. Nebes RD, Pollock BG, Houck PR, et al. Persistence of cognitive impairment in geriatric patients following antidepressant treatment: a randomized, double-blind clinical trial with nortriptyline and paroxetine. *J Psychiatr Res.* 2003;37(2):99–108.

61. Trick L, Stanley N, Rigney U, Hindmarch I. A double-blind, randomized, 26-week study comparing the cognitive and psychomotor effects and efficacy of 75 mg (37.5 mg b.i.d.) venlafaxine and 75 mg (25 mg mane, 50 mg nocte) dothiepin in elderly patients with moderate major depression being treated in general practice. *J Psychopharmacol.* 2004;18(2):205–214.

62. Madhoo M, Keefe RS, Roth RM, et al. Lisdexamfetamine dimesylate augmentation in adults with persistent executive dysfunction after partial or full remission of major depressive disorder. *Neuropsychopharmacology.* 2014;39(6):1388–1398.

63. Lee Y, Syeda K, Maruschak NA, et al. A new perspective on the anti-suicide effects with ketamine treatment: a procognitive effect. *J Clin Psychopharmacol.* 2016;36(1):50–56.

64. Caddy C, Amit BH, McCloud TL, et al. Ketamine and other glutamate receptor modulators for depression in adults. *Cochrane Database Syst Rev.* 2015;(9):Cd011612.

65. Murrough JW, Burdick KE, Levitch CF, et al. Neurocognitive effects of ketamine and association with antidepressant response in individuals with treatment-resistant depression: a randomized controlled trial. *Neuropsychopharmacology.* 2015;40(5):1084–1090.

66. Bowie CR, Gupta M, Holshausen K, Jokic R, Best M, Milev R. Cognitive remediation for treatment-resistant depression: effects on cognition and functioning and the role of online homework. *J Nerv Ment Dis.* 2013;201(8):680–685.

67. Naismith SL, Redoblado-Hodge MA, Lewis SJ, Scott EM, Hickie IB. Cognitive training in affective disorders improves memory: a preliminary study using the NEAR approach. *J Affect Disord.* 2010;121(3):258–262.

68. Martin DM, McClintock SM, Forster JJ, Lo TY, Loo CK. Cognitive enhancing effects of rTMS administered to the prefrontal cortex in patients with depression: a systematic review and meta-analysis of individual task effects. *Depress Anxiety.* 2017;34(11):1029–1039.

69. Nadeau SE, Bowers D, Jones TL, Wu SS, Triggs WJ, Heilman KM. Cognitive effects of treatment of depression with repetitive transcranial magnetic stimulation. *Cogn Behav Neurol.* 2014;27(2):77–87.

70. Bergfeld IO, Mantione M, Hoogendoorn ML, Denys D. Cognitive functioning in psychiatric disorders following deep brain stimulation. *Brain Stimul.* 2013;6(4):532–537.

71. Kvam S, Kleppe CL, Nordhus IH, Hovland A. Exercise as a treatment for depression: a meta-analysis. *J Affect Disord.* 2016;202:67–86.

72. Mammen G, Faulkner G. Physical activity and the prevention of depression: a systematic review of prospective studies. *Am J Prev Med.* 2013;45(5):649–657.

CHAPTER 5

Neuroendocrine Alterations in Major Depressive Disorder

FARIYA ALI, BS, MD • CHARLES B. NEMEROFF, MD, PHD

INTRODUCTION

A considerable body of research suggests dysfunction of neuroendocrine systems in major depression, particularly those modulating the stress response. Much of this research was driven by the neuroendocrine window hypothesis that suggested that central nervous system (CNS) alterations in depression were reflected in alterations in neuroendocrine activity as originally assessed by measurement of pituitary and peripheral end organ hormones in the general circulation. In this chapter, we review the major findings of hypothalamic–pituitary–adrenal (HPA), hypothalamic–pituitary–thyroid (HPT), and hypothalamic–pituitary–gonadal axes activity and the role they play in the development, manifestation, and maintenance of major depression.

OVERVIEW OF NORMAL HPA AXIS PHYSIOLOGY

The primary regulator of the mammalian stress response is the HPA axis.

Environmental stress has been shown to increase susceptibility for the development of depression and triggers activation of the HPA axis. Corticotropin-releasing factor (CRF) (or corticotropin-releasing hormone (CRH)) is the major physiological regulator of HPA axis activity and thereby the preeminent mediator of the mammalian stress response. CRF is synthesized in the parvocellular neurons of the paraventricular nucleus (PVN) of the hypothalamus that project mainly to the median eminence, from where CRF is secreted into the hypothalamic-hypophyseal portal system.[1] This portal system connects the hypothalamus to the anterior pituitary where CRF acts upon CRF 1 receptors to stimulate the anterior pituitary corticotropes to produce and release adrenocorticotrophic hormone (ACTH), thereby controlling HPA axis activity.[2] ACTH secreted from the anterior pituitary is released

into the systemic circulation and in turn acts on the adrenal cortex to stimulate the production and release of glucocorticoids, mainly cortisol. Cortisol is the key systemic mediator of the stress response and activates glucocorticoid receptors (GR) and mineralocorticoid receptors, mobilizing energy stores in response to a threat[3] thereby initiating the intracellular response to stress. Additionally, cortisol in turn regulates the release of CRF and ACTH via negative feedback on the hypothalamus and pituitary, respectively. Not only does CRF locally regulate noradrenergic and adrenergic tone through its regulation of adrenal steroid and catecholamine synthesis and release,[4] but through their projections to the locus coeruleus, CRF regulates the central noradrenergic and sympathetic response to stress.[5]

HPA AXIS PATHOPHYSIOLOGY IN DEPRESSION

As previously stated, it is well known that stressful life events can trigger episodes of psychiatric illness,[6] particularly mood disorders. However, different individuals may exhibit varying degrees of resilience when exposed to similar stressful events and thereby vary in the degree to which they are vulnerable to developing psychiatric illness in response to those stressors. Some individuals may be more resilient and thereby able to maintain homeostatic mechanisms in response to prolonged stress. However, a constitutional predisposition may render others very vulnerable to developing a stress-induced illness. This predisposition to illness or diathesis is the basis of the diathesis-stress hypothesis of depression.[7,8]

Over 5 decades ago, depressed patients were found to exhibit hyperactivity of the HPA axis, arguably one of the most reproducible findings in biological psychiatry. This was demonstrated by findings of higher circulating levels of ACTH and cortisol[9–11] and its

Major Depressive Disorder. https://doi.org/10.1016/B978-0-323-58131-8.00005-7

metabolites in the plasma of depressed patients as well as increases in urinary-free 24-hour cortisol concentrations.[12] Additionally, patients with Cushing's disease or Cushing's syndrome with chronically elevated levels of ACTH and/or cortisol often experience significant comorbid anxiety and depression.[13] This taken together with more sensitive HPA axis function tests showing hyperactivity in depressed patients and increased production and secretion of cortisol in healthy people exposed to stress led to the modern diathesis-stress hypothesis of depression.[10]

Several endocrine challenge tests have been used to assess HPA axis function including the dexamethasone suppression test (DST). The DST was originally developed to aid in the diagnostic assessment of Cushing's syndrome. Dexamethasone, a synthetic analogue of cortisol but several folds more potent, acts via negative feedback at the level of the anterior pituitary corticotropes to suppress ACTH secretion and consequently decrease the synthesis and release of cortisol. In the standardized DST, a small dose (1 mg) of dexamethasone is administered orally at 11 p.m., and plasma cortisol levels are obtained at 23 time points the following day. In healthy individuals, dexamethasone suppresses HPA axis activity as illustrated by lower levels of serum cortisol, so-called dexamethasone suppression. In contrast, in many depressed patients, dexamethasone failed to suppress cortisol release, termed dexamethasone nonsuppression (NS), suggesting that either the HPA axis is hyperactive and/or the negative feedback mechanisms are disrupted in these patients.[10,14,15] DST-NS status was more commonly found in more severe forms of depression including psychotic depression and mixed bipolar states and also predicted a more severe course of illness.[16,17] A meta-analysis assessing the use of the DST as a predictor of outcomes in depression found that although baseline DST status did not predict response to treatment, posttreatment DST-NS is a significant risk factor for relapse and poorer outcomes.[18–20] A subsequent meta-analysis confirmed the association of hypercortisolemia and psychotic depression using the DST.[21] Early suggestions for the use of DST as a screening tool for depression[22,23] were criticized due to its lack of specificity.[24,25] Likely of greater consequence, however, was the DST findings that revealed the robust correlation between HPA axis hyperactivity and clinical severity of depression.[26–28] Thus, it has served as an impetus for numerous subsequent studies to further focus on the pathophysiology of depression as it relates to the HPA axis.

THE CRF NEUROPEPTIDE SYSTEM

The discovery of CRF as a 41 amino-acid containing peptide in 1981,[29,30] paved the way for numerous clinical and laboratory studies that demonstrated the pivotal role that CRF and three related neuropeptides, Urocortins (Ucn), played in mediating the behavioral, cognitive, autonomic, neuroendocrine, and immunologic responses to stress through their actions on two major CRF receptor subtypes.[31–33] CRF-expressing cells are widely distributed throughout both the CNS (higher levels in the PVN of the hypothalamus, locus coeruleus (LC), amygdala, bed nucleus of stria terminalis (BNST), hippocampus, neocortex, and spinal cord) and periphery (skin, lung, testes, ovaries, blood vessels, and placenta).[2,34] Ucn1, Ucn2, and Ucn3 are the three CRF-related neuropeptides, and CRF1R and CRF2R are the major CRF receptor subtypes.

Ucn1 is found in the centrally projecting Edinger-Westphal nucleus, not to be confused with the preganglionic Edinger-Westphal nucleus (a cholinergic parasympathetic nucleus known for its oculomotor function).[35,36] Ucn2 (stresscopin-related peptide) is expressed in the hypothalamus (PVN, supraoptic nucleus, arcuate nucleus), brainstem, and spinal cord and has overlapping expression with CRF2R.[37,38] Ucn3 (stresscopin) is expressed primarily in the hypothalamus, medial nucleus of amygdala, and brainstem areas including lateral septum (LS) and BNST.[39,40]

Both CRF1R and CRF2R are found in the CNS, but have varying substrate affinities and tissue distribution. Centrally, CRF1 receptor distribution is more pervasive and is found throughout the neocortical, limbic, and brainstem regions of the CNS[41]; peripherally, it is limited to skin, ovaries, testes, and adrenal gland. CRF2 receptors are limited to discrete brain regions including the dorsal raphe nucleus, periaqueductal gray, and LS,[42] but are widely expressed in peripheral tissues (heart, GI, lungs, muscle, and blood vessels). Although the role of CRF2 receptors in the stress response is less clear than that of CRF1 receptors, it typically acts to counteract stress responses initiated by CRF1 stimulation.[33,43] This contrast in the roles of the two receptor subtypes is reflected in their differential localization. Both comprise 7-transmembrane G-protein coupled receptors and share nearly 70% homology in their amino acid sequences. CRF has a 10-fold higher affinity for CRF1R than CRF2R.[44] Both CRF and Ucn1 bind with high affinity to CRF1R and all three urocortins bind with a high affinity to the CRF2R.[32]

The biological activity of all four peptides is regulated by a nonreceptor CRF-binding protein (CRF-BP), a soluble circulating glycoprotein, which upon binding to the neuropeptides reduces their bioavailability and prevents their binding to CRF receptors. In the CNS, CRF-BP is present in all CRF pathways and pituitary and its expression is partially colocalized with CRF and CRF receptors in the CNS.[45]

CRF HYPOTHESIS OF DEPRESSION

As outlined earlier, because CRF is the major regulator of the HPA axis and the mammalian response to environmental stress, it has been hypothesized to play an important role in the pathogenesis of mood and anxiety disorders.[46] The CRF stimulation test is another endocrine challenge test in which synthetic CRF is administered intravenously to stimulate HPA activity and is now recognized to be a very sensitive test of the HPA axis. Synthetic human or ovine CRF is administered intravenously and ACTH and cortisol concentrations are measured at 30 minute intervals over a 2–3 hour period.[47] In healthy controls, CRF infusion results in increased secretion of ACTH and cortisol, whereas in depressed patients a blunted ACTH response but normal cortisol levels is observed.[48–50] In line with these findings, a blunted ACTH response to CRF is seen in DST-NS depressed patients but not in those with normal DST suppression.[51] This blunted ACTH response to CRF challenge seen in depressed patients may be explained by a downregulation of CRF1 receptors in the anterior pituitary, presumably secondary to chronic CRF hypersecretion and/or chronic hypercortisolemia.[52]

A growing body of evidence suggests that CRF hypersecretion is likely the cause of HPA axis hyperactivity in depressed patients.[53,54] CRH hypersecretion in depression is likely to be state dependent, that is, a disease phase-specific phenomenon, rather than a more enduring or trait dependent phenomenon.[55] This state-dependent hypothesis of HPA axis disruption is supported by normalization of HPA axis disruption including elevated CSF CRF concentrations,[56] plasma cortisol concentrations,[12] DST-NS,[28] blunted ACTH response to CRH stimulation test,[57] and adrenal hypertrophy[58] following resolution of depressive symptoms. In addition, the association of elevated levels of CSF CRF and earlier relapse of depression following symptomatic improvement[59] may serve as a biomarker for depressive vulnerability.

CRF-containing circuits in extrahypothalamic brain regions have projections to limbic areas including the amygdala and LC. Many clinical and preclinical studies have demonstrated how the extrahypothalamic CRF containing neuronal circuits play a key role in modulating autonomic, immune, and behavioral response to stress.[60] Intracerebral administration of CRF into specific extrahypothalamic brain regions of laboratory animals produces behavioral effects homologous to those seen in major depression in humans, including reduced slow wave sleep, decreased appetite, and diminished sexual drive.[61,62] Postmortem studies revealed increased hypothalamic CRF concentrations[63–65] and increased number of CRF expressing neurons in the hypothalamus[66] of depressed patients. Increased CRF secretion should plausibly result in a reduced density of CRF receptor binding sites via downregulation. Postmortem studies of depressed patients who completed suicide showed increased PVN and LC CRF mRNA expression,[65,67] downregulation of cortical CRF1R (but not CRF2R),[68] increased CRF concentration, and reduced expression of CRF1R in the frontal cortex[69] when compared to controls. Successful treatment with either ECT[56] or antidepressants[70,71] lowers CSF CRF concentrations. In addition, persistent elevations in CSF CRF levels in a euthymic state were found to increase patients' risk of an earlier relapse of their depression.[59] These findings are all indicative of over activity of the CRF/CRF1R system in both hypothalamic and extrahypothalamic brain areas in depression. CRF1R seems to play an important role in the behavioral response to stress, while CRF2R exerts a modulating effect on the CRF1R.

Cortisol exerts differential effects on CRF gene expression in the hypothalamus and in extrahypothalamic brain areas thought to be involved in depression. It is hypothesized that the finding of elevated CRF in LC of depressed patients may originate from the central nucleus of the amygdala (CeA), via the amygdalar/LC pathway. Increased levels of glucocorticoids have been shown to decrease CRF mRNA expression in the hypothalamic PVN via hippocampal inhibition,[72] and contrastingly increase CRF mRNA expression in the CeA.[53] The increased expression of CRF in the CeA might be responsible for the increases in emotionality and anxiety that is often associated with major depression.[73]

The dexamethasone-CRF test, a combination of the DST and CRF stimulation test devised by Holsboer and colleagues, was found to be a highly sensitive diagnostic measure for depression.[74] In this test, patients are pretreated with 1.5 mg of oral dexamethasone at 11 p.m. and given a 100 µg CRF infusion at 3 p.m. the following day. Depressed patients with HPA axis dysfunction exhibit increased (as opposed to blunted) secretion of ACTH and cortisol relative to controls. Furthermore, asymptomatic nondepressed first-degree relatives of depressed patients at high familial risk for affective disorders show disturbed HPA axis activity as assessed by this test[75] that are maintained over time.[76] These findings together support the possibility of a genetically transmissible defect in HPA axis dysregulation that may render individuals more vulnerable to development of depression. The dex-CRF stimulation test may be a potential biomarker to predict antidepressant response, as suggested by the finding that patients with symptomatic improvement of depression without a simultaneous normalization of the dex-CRF response were more likely to relapse.[77] Depressed patients who showed an improvement in the dex-CRF response after 2 weeks of hospitalization were found to have better outcomes with remission 3 weeks later.[15] Additionally, the magnitude of decrease in cortisol as measured by the dex-CRF test from pretreatment baseline to 5 weeks posttreatment with citalopram was found to correlate with the degree of symptom improvement in a 16-week study.[78] In another study, abnormal dex-CRF responses before discharge, despite symptomatic improvement, was associated with a 4–6-fold increase in the likelihood of relapsing; and therefore may be able to predict the relapse and recurrence of depression.[79]

EARLY-LIFE STRESS AND DEPRESSION: HPA AXIS INVOLVEMENT

Childhood trauma is a significant risk factor for developing depression and other psychotic disorders later in adulthood. A CDC study involving 8667 HMO members found a strong dose-response relationship between the number of adverse childhood experiences (ACEs) and adult mental health scores[80] and also between the number of ACEs and the presence of a depressive episode in the past year, suicide attempts or lifetime chronic depression.[81] A seminal study conducted with a cohort of 1900 women from four internal medicine practices found childhood, but not adulthood, sexual, or physical abuse to be associated with increased depression and/or anxiety.[82]

Several studies of early-life stress (ELS) in animals (rodent and nonhuman primates) and humans have shown that such exposure leads to persistent increases in HPA axis activity and extrahypothalamic CRF neuronal activity [80]. ELS that can include any number of adverse experiences including early physical or sexual abuse, neglect, early parental loss, or permanent separation is associated with sensitization of the central CRF-containing stress response systems, thereby persistently enhancing the HPA regulated neuroendocrine, autonomic, behavioral, and immune responsiveness to stress. Bonnet macaques reared under stressful conditions exhibited higher CSF CRF concentrations than those reared in nonstressful conditions.[83] In rodents, ELS results in increased CRF concentrations, increased CRF mRNA expression, and altered CRF receptor expression and binding.[84,85] These preclinical findings are consistent with those in humans that show early-life trauma to be a strong predictor of higher CSF CRF concentrations in adulthood.[86] This chronic upregulation of the stress response increases the risk of developing mood-related disorders later in life.[87,88]

HPA AXIS AND RESPONSE TO PSYCHOLOGICAL STRESS

In our 2008 study of a possible link between childhood abuse, disruptions in the HPA axis, and depression, we used a standardized psychosocial stress protocol, the Trier Social Stress Test, which included public speaking and performing a mental arithmetic task before an audience. ACTH and cortisol levels along with heart rate were measured before, during and after induction of the stress. Four groups of women were studied that included those with (1) no history of ELS and no psychiatric disorder, (2) a history of ELS without current depression, (3) a history of ELS and current depression, and (4) no history of ELS but current major depression. We found that when compared to controls, abused women with depression exhibited increases in both ACTH (6-fold) and cortisol in response to the stress. Abused women not currently depressed exhibited an elevated ACTH but a normal cortisol response, which may be an indicator of their resilience to depression in spite of ELS. Depressed women who did not have a history of ELS exhibited a normal neuroendocrine response. Together these findings suggest that CRF driven hyperactivity of the HPA axis after ELS may persist into adulthood and thereby serve as a diathesis for the development of depression.[89]

A multiple regression analysis that examined the effect of ACEs on central CRF sensitization, found childhood abuse to be the strongest predictor of ACTH responsiveness, followed by the number of abusive events, number of adulthood trauma and then depression.[90] This finding suggests that ACTH and thus HPA axis stress reactivity is strongly correlated with childhood and adulthood traumas, and the authors hypothesized that childhood trauma sensitizes the HPA stress response to subsequent stress later in life as evidenced by significantly higher ACTH levels in women with childhood and adulthood trauma. Additionally, when comparing the subgroups, the authors found that ACTH responses in women with a history of childhood trauma but no depression and those with ELS and depression to be similar. This is significant as it suggests that a history of ELS confers a discernible biological risk factor for development of depression in adulthood, even in the absence of lifetime psychopathology.

CHILDHOOD TRAUMA AND HPA AXIS CHALLENGE TESTS

The CRF stimulation test and ACTH 1–24 stimulation tests were performed to further assess HPA axis disruption in these patients. They used high doses of ACTH1-24 to evaluate for the maximal responsiveness of the adrenal cortex. The authors hypothesized that if women with ELS showed a difference in the CRF stimulation test this would be indicative of changes in the anterior pituitary corticotrophs likely secondary to changes in the "PVN-median eminence-CRF circuit." As previously mentioned, a blunted ACTH response is a consistent finding in depressed patients.[91] The study showed high levels of ACTH responsiveness in women who had ELS without depression, which was similar to their response in the psychological stressor protocol. Depressed women with and without ELS both showed a blunted response to CRF simulation. Women with ELS with and without depression had the lowest levels of cortisol in response to the ACTH1-24 stimulation test. These findings suggest that ELS may decrease cortisol availability, thereby disrupting the central stress response. Upon subsequent exposure to stress in adulthood these women likely hypersecrete CRF contributing to the depressive symptoms linked to excess CRF activity in extrahypothalamic brain circuits.

GLUCOCORTICOID INVOLVEMENT

The pathological enhancement of the stress response subsequent to ELS may be further exacerbated by changes in GR-mediated feedback of the HPA axis. As previously noted, the dex-CRF stimulation test is the most sensitive measure of HPA axis activity. Pathological elevations in ACTH and cortisol levels in depressed patients due to CRF-induced escape from suppression reflects impaired glucocorticoid-mediated feedback control of the HPA axis under conditions of increased hypothalamic drive. The dex-CRF stimulation test was used to examine HPA axis activity in abused and nonabused men with and without concurrent depression. Men with a history of ELS showed a marked increase in ACTH response regardless of current depression. Only those men with ELS and concurrent depression exhibited increased cortisol responses. These findings suggest that childhood trauma is associated with impaired glucocorticoid-mediated feedback control of the HPA axis. Impaired glucocorticoid effects may contribute to enhanced reactivity to acute stress in adulthood and subsequently promote symptoms of depression.[89]

CSF CRF IN CHILDHOOD TRAUMA AND DEPRESSION

The earlier findings of enhanced stress responsiveness, blunted ACTH response to CRF stimulation, and impaired glucocorticoid-mediated feedback in individuals with ELS are all consistent with central CRF hypersecretion. CRF1R antagonists and CRF1R knockout mice both showed an attenuated response to stress.[53] As cited previously, postmortem studies of depressed patients revealed increased CRF concentrations and increased CRF mRNA expression in the hypothalamic PVN, LC, and frontal cortex. In line with these findings is the higher CSF CRF concentrations in women with a history of childhood abuse compared to controls. Additionally, women who had experienced sexual and physical abuse in childhood had significantly higher CSF CRF concentrations than those with no history of abuse or sexual abuse alone. The CRF concentrations correlated with the severity and duration of physical and sexual abuse. Women who had experienced physical or sexual abuse at an older age (>6 years old) had higher CSF CRF concentrations when compared with those who experienced abuse at an earlier age.[89]

THYROTROPIN-RELEASING HORMONE, THE HYPOTHALAMIC–PITUITARY–THYROID AXIS, AND DEPRESSION

Dysfunction of the HPT axis is known to be associated with a wide array of mood alterations ranging from mild depression or anxiety to overt psychosis. Similar to the HPA axis, the HPT axis is organized hierarchically. Thyrotropin-releasing hormone (TRH), a tripeptide synthesized by hypothalamic PVN neurons, is stored in median eminence nerve terminals and subsequently released into the hypothalamic-hypophyseal portal system. TRH binds to and stimulates TRH receptors on thyrotropes in the anterior pituitary to release thyroid-stimulating hormone (TSH) into the systemic circulation. TSH, a large peptide hormone, in turn binds to receptors on the thyroid gland to induce iodine uptake and increased synthesis and release of the thyroid hormones, tri-iodothyronine (T_3) and thyroxine (T_4). Once in the general circulation, T_3 and T_4 are found largely bound to plasma proteins including thyroid binding globulin and transthyretin. Free T_3 and T_4 are major regulators of cellular metabolism. Circulating T3 and T4 exert negative feedback at the level of the hypothalamus and adenohypophysis, decreasing HPT activity. Thyroid hormones are extraordinarily important for neurodevelopment, as highlighted by the devastating effects of hypothyroidism on the developing CNS.

In the CNS, thyroid hormones act on thyroid hormone receptors, which are part of a large superfamily of nuclear hormone receptors. Both T_3 and T_4 are transported across the blood-brain barrier, but the brain only contains T_3 receptors. T_4 in the brain must therefore be converted to T_3 by a deiodinase enzyme. Like steroid hormones, thyroid hormones diffuse across the cell membrane and enter the nucleus where they bind to the thyroid hormone receptor. Once bound to its receptor, the thyroid hormone/receptor complex mediates gene transcription by binding to thyroid hormone response elements in the promoter. Animal studies have shown a relatively high density of thyroid hormone receptors in the cortex, hippocampus, hypothalamus, and olfactory bulbs.

PSYCHIATRIC MANIFESTATIONS OF THYROID DYSFUNCTION

Thyroid hormone abnormalities are associated with many psychiatric disturbances, ranging from mild depression to mania and psychosis. Irrespective of etiology, hypothyroidism can lead to several clinical manifestations many of which overlap with symptoms of depression including depressed mood, slowed mentation, fatigue, cognitive disturbance, forgetfulness, and constipation. Patients suffering from hypothyroidism usually have high rates of comorbid depression and cognitive disturbances. This along with the presence of several overlapping symptoms makes it imperative to always rule out thyroid hormone abnormalities when evaluating patients suffering from depression. Although depression is strongly associated with hypothyroidism, it is also the most commonly seen psychiatric symptom in hyperthyroidism. Hypothyroidism is the leading medical cause of depression and remarkably remains undetected in many patients.

TRH stimulation test abnormalities have been repeatedly observed in major depression. Studies in the 1970s showed that approximately 25% of euthyroid patients with major depression had a blunted TSH response in the TRH stimulation test,[92] in which a fixed dose of TRH (200–500 µg) is administered intravenously, usually in the morning, and TSH levels are obtained every 30 minutes for 2–3 hours. The blunted response is thought to be a result of TRH hypersecretion from the median eminence, leading to downregulation of TRH receptors in the pituitary. This is supported by findings of elevated CSF TRH concentrations in depressed patients.[93] Conversely, 15% of depressed patients exhibited an exaggerated TSH response to TRH stimulation. Interestingly, depressed patients have also been found to have an abnormally high rate of antithyroglobulin and/or antimicrosomal thyroid antibodies manifested as symptomless autoimmune thyroiditis.

Augmentation with T_3 has been shown to be effective in improving and accelerating antidepressant treatment response in depression. A meta-analysis on combination of TCAs and thyroid hormone supported their efficacy in refractory depression.[94] However, TCAs have largely been replaced by SSRIs as first-line treatment of depression. A placebo-controlled RCT assessing at the ability of T_3 to augment or enhance response to SSRI did not find any clinical benefit.[95] The STAR*D trial, a large placebo-controlled multicenter study compared lithium and T_3 augmentation in 142 patients who failed to respond to two sequential trials with antidepressants. During the 14-week follow-up, 24.7% of patients receiving T_3 attained clinical remission compared with only 15.9% in the lithium augmentation group.[96] Although T_3 augmentation has a lower side effect burden and ease of use as compared to lithium, the remission rate of 24.7% was not significantly better than other options and prolonged use of adjunctive T_3 use is not free of safety concerns including osteopenia.[97] Finally, augmentation with both T_3 and T_4 has also been studied and the combination improved results on both neuropsychological and mood scales in patients with hypothyroidism.[98] However, subsequent placebo-controlled studies did not show clinically significant improvement of T_3 augmentation in patients treated with T_4.[99,100]

GROWTH HORMONE, SOMATOSTATIN, AND DEPRESSION

Growth hormone (GH) is synthesized and secreted by anterior pituitary somatotrophs. Its release is regulated by two hypothalamic peptide hormones; growth hormone-releasing factor (GHRF) and somatostatin, which are in turn regulated by secondary neurotransmitters including dopamine (DA), norepinephrine (NE), and 5-hydroxytryptamine (5-HT). Somatostatin or growth hormone-release inhibiting hormone is a tetradecapeptide synthesized in periventricular and paraventricular neurons of hypothalamus, is released into the median eminence and inhibits GH release. It is widely distributed in various extrahypothalamic sites including the limbic system, cortex, and hippocampus. GHRF containing neurons are limited to the infundibular and arcuate nuclei of the hypothalamus and stimulate the synthesis and release of GH. Neurons containing DA, NE, and 5HT innervate the GHRF neurons and thereby modulate GH release. GH in turn exerts negative feedback by stimulating the release of somatostatin.

GH dysregulation in depression has been demonstrated as evidenced by a blunted nocturnal GH surge and daytime hypersecretion of GH in both unipolar and bipolar depression.[101] Some studies have reported a blunted GH response to dopamine agonists (apomorphine) and drugs that increase noradrenergic activity (clonidine, desipramine). A GHRF stimulation test similar to the CRF and TRH stimulation tests has been developed. Although some studies showed a blunted GH response to the GHRF stimulation test, these results have not been reliably replicated. Large variations owing to patient age and body weight may have contributed to these discrepant findings. Additional studies to standardize the GHRF stimulation test for assessment of the GH response in depression are needed.

HYPOTHALAMIC–PROLACTIN AXIS AND DEPRESSION

In contrast to other hormones of the anterior pituitary, prolactin (PRL) release is regulated via constitutive inhibition by a prolactin-inhibitory factor that has been identified as the neurotransmitter DA. DA is released from hypothalamic periventricular and arcuate neurons and secreted from nerve terminals of the median eminence. It directly inhibits PRL release from anterior pituitary lactotrophs. Additionally, PRL regulates its own release via a short negative feedback loop back to the hypothalamus. PRL stimulates breast growth and lactation and is thought to play a role in certain of the behavioral aspects of infant care and reproduction.

Hyperprolactinemia leads to reduced testosterone secretion in men, and gynecomastia, lactation and reduced libido in both men and women. It can also cause amenorrhea in women. Patients can experience psychiatric symptoms including depression, anxiety, stress intolerance, and increased irritability that often resolve with treatment with a DA agonist and resulting reduction in PRL serum levels.

Drugs that increase serotonergic neurotransmission and thereby PRL secretion have been used in endocrine challenge tests in depressed patients. The PRL response to agents such as L-tryptophan, 5-HTP and fenfluramine that increase serotonergic activity was found to be blunted in depression. However, another study showed an exaggerated PRL response to L-tryptophan. It is possible that concurrent use of antidepressants or persistent hypercortisolemia contributes to hyperprolactinemia and may have confounded the data from earlier studies.[102]

CONCLUSIONS

It is clear from the literature reviewed in this chapter that many patients with depression exhibit clear and reproducible alterations in neuroendocrine systems that is likely due to the pathophysiological involvement in CNS circuits that regulate pituitary and endocrine target organ activity. The most prominent findings involve the HPA and HPT axes. What is unclear is how these alterations in individual patients modify the disease course and most importantly treatment response. Adequately powered studies that would scrutinize such alterations, coupled with genetic variations in the components of these axes and how these interact with environmental factors such as early-life adversity are urgently needed.

FINANCIAL DISCLOSURES

Research/Grants: National Institutes of Health (NIH), Stanley Medical Research Institute. *Consulting (last 3 years):* Xhale, Takeda, Taisho Pharmaceutical Inc., Bracket (Clintara), Sunovion Pharmaceuticals Inc., Janssen Research & Development LLC, Magstim, Inc., Navitor Pharmaceuticals, Inc., TC MSO, Inc., Intra-Cellular Therapies, Inc. *Stockholder:* Xhale, Celgene, Seattle Genetics, Abbvie, OPKO Health, Inc., Antares, BI Gen Holdings, Inc., Corcept Therapeutics Pharmaceuticals Company. *Scientific Advisory Boards:* American Foundation for Suicide Prevention (AFSP), Brain and Behavior Research Foundation (BBRF), Xhale, Anxiety and Depression Association of America (ADAA), Skyland Trail, Bracket (Clintara), Laureate Institute for Brain Research (LIBR), Inc. *Board of Directors:* AFSP, Gratitude America, ADAA. *Income sources or equity of $10,000 or more:*

American Psychiatric Publishing, Xhale, Bracket (Clintara), CME Outfitters, Intra-Cellular Therapies, Inc., EMA Wellness, Magstim. *Patents:* Method and devices for transdermal delivery of lithium (US 6,375,990B1). Method of assessing antidepressant drug therapy via transport inhibition of monoamine neurotransmitters by ex vivo assay (US 7,148,027B2). *Speakers Bureau:* None.

REFERENCES

1. Owens MJ, Nemeroff CB. Physiology and pharmacology of corticotropin-releasing factor. *Pharmacol Rev.* 1991; 43(4):425−473. http://www.ncbi.nlm.nih.gov/pubmed/1775506.
2. Swanson LW, Sawchenko PE, Rivier J, Vale WW. Organization of ovine corticotropin-releasing factor immunoreactive cells and fibers in the rat brain: an immunohistochemical study. *Neuroendocrinology.* 1983;36(3):165−186. http://www.ncbi.nlm.nih.gov/pubmed/6601247.
3. Martin EI, Nemeroff CB. The role of corticotropin-releasing factor in the pathophysiology of depression: implications for antidepressant mechanisms of action. *Psychiatr Ann.* 2008;38(4):260−266. https://doi.org/10.3928/00485713-20080401-02.
4. Heim C, Bradley B, Mletzko TC, et al. Effect of childhood trauma on adult depression and neuroendocrine function: sex-specific moderation by CRH receptor 1 gene. *Front Behav Neurosci.* 2009;3:41. https://doi.org/10.3389/neuro.08.041.2009.
5. Valentino RJ, Foote SL, Aston-Jones G. Corticotropin-releasing factor activates noradrenergic neurons of the locus coeruleus. *Brain Res.* 1983;270(2):363−367. http://www.ncbi.nlm.nih.gov/pubmed/6603889.
6. Kendler KS, Karkowski LM, Prescott CA. Causal relationship between stressful life events and the onset of major depression. *Am J Psychiatry.* 1999;156(6):837−841. https://doi.org/10.1176/ajp.156.6.837.
7. Robins CJ, Block P. Cognitive theories of depression viewed from a diathesis-stress perspective: evaluations of the models of Beck and of Abramson, Seligman, and Teasdale. *Cogn Ther Res.* 1989;13(4):297−313. https://doi.org/10.1007/BF01173475.
8. Nemeroff CB. The neurobiology of depression. *Sci Am.* 1998;278(6):42−49. http://www.ncbi.nlm.nih.gov/pubmed/9608732.
9. Gibbons jl, Mchugh PR. Plasma cortisol in depressive illness. *J Psychiatr Res.* 1962;1:162−171. http://www.ncbi.nlm.nih.gov/pubmed/13947658.
10. Gillespie CF, Nemeroff CB. Hypercortisolemia and depression. *Psychosom Med.* 2005;67:S26−S28. https://doi.org/10.1097/01.psy.0000163456.22154.d2.
11. Carpenter WT, Bunney WE. Adrenal cortical activity in depressive illness. *Am J Psychiatry.* 1971;128(1):31−40. https://doi.org/10.1176/ajp.128.1.31.
12. Sachar EJ, Hellman L, Fukushima DK, Gallagher TF. Cortisol production in depressive illness. A clinical and biochemical clarification. *Arch Gen Psychiatr.* 1970; 23(4):289−298. http://www.ncbi.nlm.nih.gov/pubmed/4918519.
13. Gutman DA, Nemeroff CB. Corticotropin-releasing factor circuitry in the brain − relevance for affective disorders and anxiety. In: *Encyclopedia of Stress.* Elsevier; 2007: 630−634. https://doi.org/10.1016/B978-012373947-6.00454-2.
14. Newport DJ, Nemeroff CB. Axis: normal physiology and disturbances in depression. 1-22.
15. Ising M, Künzel HE, Binder EB, Nickel T, Modell S, Holsboer F. The combined dexamethasone/CRH test as a potential surrogate marker in depression. *Prog Neuro-Psychopharmacol Biol Psychiatry.* 2005;29(6): 1085−1093. https://doi.org/10.1016/j.pnpbp.2005.03.014.
16. Schatzberg AF, Rothschild AJ, Bond TC, Cole JO. The DST in psychotic depression: diagnostic and pathophysiologic implications. *Psychopharmacol Bull.* 1984;20(3): 362−364. http://www.ncbi.nlm.nih.gov/pubmed/6473631.
17. Evans DL, Nemeroff CB. The dexamethasone suppression test in mixed bipolar disorder. *Am J Psychiatry.* 1983; 140(5):615−617. https://doi.org/10.1176/ajp.140.5.615.
18. Ribeiro SC, Tandon R, Grunhaus L, Greden JF. The DST as a predictor of outcome in depression: a meta-analysis. *Am J Psychiatry.* 1993;150(11):1618−1629. https://doi.org/10.1176/ajp.150.11.1618.
19. Greden JF, Albala AA, Haskett RF, et al. Normalization of dexamethasone suppression test: a laboratory index of recovery from endogenous depression. *Biol Psychiatry.* 1980;15(3):449−458. http://www.ncbi.nlm.nih.gov/pubmed/7378518.
20. Nemeroff CB, Evans DL. Correlation between the dexamethasone suppression test in depressed patients and clinical response. *Am J Psychiatry.* 1984;141(2): 247−249. https://doi.org/10.1176/ajp.141.2.247.
21. Nelson JC, Davis JM. DST studies in psychotic depression: a meta-analysis. *Am J Psychiatry.* 1997;154(11): 1497−1503. https://doi.org/10.1176/ajp.154.11.1497.
22. Carroll BJ, Martin FI, Davies B. Pituitary-adrenal function in depression. *Lancet.* 1968;1(7556):1373−1374. http://www.ncbi.nlm.nih.gov/pubmed/4172674.
23. Carroll BJ. Use of the dexamethasone suppression test in depression. *J Clin Psychiatry.* 1982;43(11 Pt 2):44−50. http://www.ncbi.nlm.nih.gov/pubmed/7174632.
24. Krishnan KRR, Davidson JRT, Rayasam K, Tanas KS, Shope FS, Pelton S. Diagnostic utility of the dexamethasone suppression test. *Biol Psychiatry.* 1987;22(5):618−628. https://doi.org/10.1016/0006-3223(87)90189-2.
25. Arana GW, Mossman D. The dexamethasone suppression test and depression. Approaches to the use of a laboratory test in psychiatry. *Neurol Clin.* 1988;6(1):21−39. http://www.ncbi.nlm.nih.gov/pubmed/2837633.

26. Evans DL, Nemeroff CB, Haggerty JJ, Pedersen CA. Use of the dexamethasone suppression test with DSM-III criteria in psychiatrically hospitalized adolescents. *Psychoneuroendocrinology*. 1987;12(3):203−209. http://www.ncbi.nlm.nih.gov/pubmed/3615749.

27. Krishnan KR, France RD, Pelton S, McCann UD, Manepalli AN, Davidson JR. What does the dexamethasone suppression test identify? *Biol Psychiatry*. 1985; 20(9):957−964. http://www.ncbi.nlm.nih.gov/pubmed/4027315.

28. Arana GW, Baldessarini RJ, Ornsteen M. The dexamethasone suppression test for diagnosis and prognosis in psychiatry. Commentary and review. *Arch Gen Psychiatr*. 1985;42(12):1193−1204. http://www.ncbi.nlm.nih.gov/pubmed/3000317.

29. Spiess J, Rivier J, Rivier C, Vale W. Primary structure of corticotropin-releasing factor from ovine hypothalamus. *Proc Natl Acad Sci U S A*. 1981;78(10):6517−6521. http://www.ncbi.nlm.nih.gov/pubmed/6273874.

30. Vale W, Spiess J, Rivier C, Rivier J. Characterization of a 41-residue ovine hypothalamic peptide that stimulates secretion of corticotropin and beta-endorphin. *Science*. 1981;213(4514):1394−1397. http://www.ncbi.nlm.nih.gov/pubmed/6267699.

31. Hauger RL, Grigoriadis DE, Dallman MF, Plotsky PM, Vale WW, Dautzenberg FM. International Union of Pharmacology. XXXVI. Current status of the nomenclature for receptors for corticotropin-releasing factor and their ligands. *Pharmacol Rev*. 2003;55(1):21−26. https://doi.org/10.1124/pr.55.1.3.

32. Hauger RL, Risbrough V, Brauns O, Dautzenberg FM. Corticotropin releasing factor (CRF) receptor signaling in the central nervous system: new molecular targets. *CNS Neurol Disord - Drug Targets*. 2006;5(4):453−479. http://www.ncbi.nlm.nih.gov/pubmed/16918397.

33. Bale TL, Vale WW. CRF and CRF receptors: role in stress responsivity and other behaviors. *Annu Rev Pharmacol Toxicol*. 2004;44(1):525−557. https://doi.org/10.1146/annurev.pharmtox.44.101802.121410.

34. Boorse GC, Denver RJ. Widespread tissue distribution and diverse functions of corticotropin-releasing factor and related peptides. *Gen Comp Endocrinol*. 2006;146(1): 9−18. https://doi.org/10.1016/j.ygcen.2005.11.014.

35. Ryabinin AE, Tsivkovskaia NO, Ryabinin SA. Urocortin 1-containing neurons in the human Edinger-Westphal nucleus. *Neuroscience*. 2005;134(4):1317−1323. https://doi.org/10.1016/j.neuroscience.2005.05.042.

36. Kozicz T, Bittencourt JC, May PJ, et al. The Edinger-Westphal nucleus: a historical, structural, and functional perspective on a dichotomous terminology. *J Comp Neurol*. 2011;519(8):1413−1434. https://doi.org/10.1002/cne.22580.

37. Reyes TM, Lewis K, Perrin MH, et al. Urocortin II: a member of the corticotropin-releasing factor (CRF) neuropeptide family that is selectively bound by type 2 CRF receptors. *Proc Natl Acad Sci Unit States Am*. 2001;98(5): 2843−2848. https://doi.org/10.1073/pnas.051626398.

38. Vaughan J, Donaldson C, Bittencourt J, et al. Urocortin, a mammalian neuropeptide related to fish urotensin I and to corticotropin-releasing factor. *Nature*. 1995; 378(6554):287−292. https://doi.org/10.1038/378287a0.

39. Li C, Vaughan J, Sawchenko PE, Vale WW. Urocortin III-immunoreactive projections in rat brain: partial overlap with sites of type 2 corticotrophin-releasing factor receptor expression. *J Neurosci*. 2002;22(3): 991−1001. http://www.ncbi.nlm.nih.gov/pubmed/11826127.

40. Lewis K, Li C, Perrin MH, et al. Identification of urocortin III, an additional member of the corticotropin-releasing factor (CRF) family with high affinity for the CRF2 receptor. *Proc Natl Acad Sci U S A*. 2001; 98(13):7570−7575. https://doi.org/10.1073/pnas.121165198.

41. Potter E, Sutton S, Donaldson C, et al. Distribution of corticotropin-releasing factor receptor mRNA expression in the rat brain and pituitary. *Proc Natl Acad Sci U S A*. 1994;91(19):8777−8781. http://www.ncbi.nlm.nih.gov/pubmed/8090722.

42. Van Pett K, Viau V, Bittencourt JC, et al. Distribution of mRNAs encoding CRF receptors in brain and pituitary of rat and mouse. *J Comp Neurol*. 2000;428(2):191−212. https://doi.org/10.1002/1096-9861(20001211)428:2<191::AID-CNE1>3.0.CO;2-U.

43. Lee K-F, Bale TL, Contarino A, et al. Mice deficient for corticotropin-releasing hormone receptor-2 display anxiety-like behaviour and are hypersensitive to stress. *Nat Genet*. 2000;24(4):410−414. https://doi.org/10.1038/74263.

44. Perrin M, Donaldson C, Chen R, et al. Identification of a second corticotropin-releasing factor receptor gene and characterization of a cDNA expressed in heart. *Proc Natl Acad Sci U S A*. 1995;92(7):2969−2973. http://www.ncbi.nlm.nih.gov/pubmed/7708757.

45. Potter E, Behan DP, Linton EA, Lowry PJ, Sawchenko PE, Vale WW. The central distribution of a corticotropin-releasing factor (CRF)-binding protein predicts multiple sites and modes of interaction with CRF. *Proc Natl Acad Sci U S A*. 1992;89(9):4192−4196. http://www.ncbi.nlm.nih.gov/pubmed/1315056.

46. Binder EB, Nemeroff CB. The CRF system, stress, depression and anxiety-insights from human genetic studies. *Mol Psychiatr*. 2010;15(6):574−588. https://doi.org/10.1038/mp.2009.141.

47. Hermus AR, Pieters GF, Smals AG, Benraad TJ, Kloppenborg PW. Plasma adrenocorticotropin, cortisol, and aldosterone responses to corticotropin-releasing factor: modulatory effect of basal cortisol levels. *J Clin Endocrinol Metab*. 1984;58(1):187−191. https://doi.org/10.1210/jcem-58-1-187.

48. Gold PW, Loriaux DL, Roy A, et al. Responses to corticotropin-releasing hormone in the hypercortisolism of depression and Cushing's disease. *N Engl J Med*. 1986; 314(21):1329−1335. https://doi.org/10.1056/NEJM198605223142101.

49. Kathol RG, Jaeckle RS, Lopez JF, Meller WH. Consistent reduction of ACTH responses to stimulation with CRH, vasopressin and hypoglycaemia in patients with major depression. *Br J Psychiatry.* 1989;155:468–478. http://www.ncbi.nlm.nih.gov/pubmed/2558771.

50. Heim C, Newport DJ, Bonsall R, Miller AH, Nemeroff CB. Altered pituitary-adrenal axis responses to provocative challenge tests in adult survivors of childhood abuse. *Am J Psychiatry.* 2001;158(4):575–581. https://doi.org/10.1176/appi.ajp.158.4.575.

51. Krishnan KRR, Rayasam K, Reed D, et al. The corticotropin releasing factor stimulation test in patients with major depression: relationship to dexamethasone suppression test results. *Depression.* 1993;1(3):133–136. https://doi.org/10.1002/depr.3050010303.

52. Gold PW, Chrousos G, Kellner C, et al. Psychiatric implications of basic and clinical studies with corticotropin-releasing factor. *Am J Psychiatry.* 1984;141(5):619–627. https://doi.org/10.1176/ajp.141.5.619.

53. Arborelius L, Owens MJ, Plotsky PM, Nemeroff CB. The role of corticotropin-releasing factor in depression and anxiety disorders. *J Endocrinol.* 1999;160(1):1–12. http://www.ncbi.nlm.nih.gov/pubmed/9854171.

54. Plotsky PM, Owens MJ, Nemeroff CB. Psychoneuroendocrinology of depression. Hypothalamic-pituitary-adrenal axis. *Psychiatr Clin.* 1998;21(2):293–307. http://www.ncbi.nlm.nih.gov/pubmed/9670227.

55. Lloyd RB, Nemeroff CB. The role of corticotropin-releasing hormone in the pathophysiology of depression: therapeutic implications. *Curr Top Med Chem.* 2011;11(6):609–617. http://www.ncbi.nlm.nih.gov/pubmed/21261589.

56. Nemeroff CB, Bissette G, Akil H, Fink M. Neuropeptide concentrations in the cerebrospinal fluid of depressed patients treated with electroconvulsive therapy. Corticotrophin-releasing factor, beta-endorphin and somatostatin. *Br J Psychiatry.* 1991;158:59–63. http://www.ncbi.nlm.nih.gov/pubmed/1673078.

57. Amsterdam JD, Maislin G, Winokur A, Berwish N, Kling M, Gold P. The oCRH stimulation test before and after clinical recovery from depression. *J Affect Disord.* 14(3):213-222. http://www.ncbi.nlm.nih.gov/pubmed/2838538. Accessed December 30, 2017.

58. Rubin RT, Phillips JJ, Sadow TF, McCracken JT. Adrenal gland volume in major depression. Increase during the depressive episode and decrease with successful treatment. *Arch Gen Psychiatr.* 1995;52(3):213–218. http://www.ncbi.nlm.nih.gov/pubmed/7872849.

59. Banki CM, Karmacsi L, Bissette G, Nemeroff CB. CSF corticotropin-releasing hormone and somatostatin in major depression: response to antidepressant treatment and relapse. *Eur Neuropsychopharmacol.* 1992;2(2):107–113. http://www.ncbi.nlm.nih.gov/pubmed/1352999.

60. Heim C, Newport DJ, Heit S, et al. Pituitary-adrenal and autonomic responses to stress in women after sexual and physical abuse in childhood. *J Am Med Assoc.* 2000; 284(5):592–597. http://www.ncbi.nlm.nih.gov/pubmed/10918705.

61. Dunn AJ, Berridge CW. Physiological and behavioral responses to corticotropin-releasing factor administration: is CRF a mediator of anxiety or stress responses? *Brain Res Brain Res Rev.* 15(2):71-100. http://www.ncbi.nlm.nih.gov/pubmed/1980834. Accessed December 15, 2017.

62. Kormos V, Gaszner B. Role of neuropeptides in anxiety, stress, and depression: from animals to humans. *Neuropeptides.* 2013;47(6):401–419. https://doi.org/10.1016/j.npep.2013.10.014.

63. Nemeroff CB, Widerlöv E, Bissette G, et al. Elevated concentrations of CSF corticotropin-releasing factor-like immunoreactivity in depressed patients. *Science.* 1984; 226(4680):1342–1344. http://www.ncbi.nlm.nih.gov/pubmed/6334362.

64. Banki CM, Bissette G, Arato M, O'Connor L, Nemeroff CB. CSF corticotropin-releasing factor-like immunoreactivity in depression and schizophrenia. *Am J Psychiatry.* 1987;144(7):873–877. https://doi.org/10.1176/ajp.144.7.873.

65. Hartline KM, Owens MJ, Nemeroff CB. Postmortem and cerebrospinal fluid studies of corticotropin-releasing factor in humans. *Ann N Y Acad Sci.* 1996;780: 96–105. http://www.ncbi.nlm.nih.gov/pubmed/8602742.

66. Raadsheer FC, Hoogendijk WJ, Stam FC, Tilders FJ, Swaab DF. Increased numbers of corticotropin-releasing hormone expressing neurons in the hypothalamic paraventricular nucleus of depressed patients. *Neuroendocrinology.* 1994;60(4):436–444. http://www.ncbi.nlm.nih.gov/pubmed/7824085.

67. Arató M, Bánki CM, Bissette G, Nemeroff CB. Elevated CSF CRF in suicide victims. *Biol Psychiatry.* 1989;25(3):355–359. http://www.ncbi.nlm.nih.gov/pubmed/2536563.

68. Nemeroff CB, Owens MJ, Bissette G, Andorn AC, Stanley M. Reduced corticotropin releasing factor binding sites in the frontal cortex of suicide victims. *Arch Gen Psychiatr.* 1988;45(6):577–579. http://www.ncbi.nlm.nih.gov/pubmed/2837159.

69. Merali Z, Du L, Hrdina P, et al. Dysregulation in the suicide brain: mRNA expression of corticotropin-releasing hormone receptors and GABAA receptor subunits in frontal cortical brain region. *J Neurosci.* 2004;24(6): 1478–1485. https://doi.org/10.1523/JNEUROSCI.4734-03.2004.

70. De Bellis MD, Gold PW, Geracioti TD, Listwak SJ, Kling MA. Association of fluoxetine treatment with reductions in CSF concentrations of corticotropin-releasing hormone and arginine vasopressin in patients with major depression. *Am J Psychiatry.* 1993;150(4):656–657. https://doi.org/10.1176/ajp.150.4.656.

71. Heuser I, Bissette G, Dettling M, et al. Cerebrospinal fluid concentrations of corticotropin-releasing hormone, vasopressin, and somatostatin in depressed patients and healthy controls: response to amitriptyline treatment. *Depress Anxiety.* 1998;8(2):71–79. http://www.ncbi.nlm.nih.gov/pubmed/9784981.

72. Kageyama K, Suda T. Regulatory mechanisms underlying corticotropin-releasing factor gene expression in the hypothalamus. *Endocr J.* 2009;56(3):335−344. http://www.ncbi.nlm.nih.gov/pubmed/19352056.

73. Reul JMHM, Holsboer F. Corticotropin-releasing factor receptors 1 and 2 in anxiety and depression. *Curr Opin Pharmacol.* 2002;2(1):23−33. http://www.ncbi.nlm.nih.gov/pubmed/11786305.

74. Holsboer F, von Bardeleben U, Wiedemann K, Müller OA, Stalla GK. Serial assessment of corticotropin-releasing hormone response after dexamethasone in depression. Implications for pathophysiology of DST nonsuppression. *Biol Psychiatry.* 1987; 22(2):228−234. http://www.ncbi.nlm.nih.gov/pubmed/3028512.

75. Holsboer F, Lauer CJ, Schreiber W, Krieg JC. Altered hypothalamic-pituitary-adrenocortical regulation in healthy subjects at high familial risk for affective disorders. *Neuroendocrinology.* 1995;62(4):340−347. http://www.ncbi.nlm.nih.gov/pubmed/8544947.

76. Modell S, Lauer CJ, Schreiber W, Huber J, Krieg JC, Holsboer F. Hormonal response pattern in the combined DEX-CRH test is stable over time in subjects at high familial risk for affective disorders. *Neuropsychopharmacology.* 1998;18(4):253−262. https://doi.org/10.1016/S0893-133X(97)00144-9.

77. Schüle C, Baghai TC, Eser D, et al. Time course of hypothalamic-pituitary-adrenocortical axis activity during treatment with reboxetine and mirtazapine in depressed patients. *Psychopharmacology.* 2006;186(4): 601−611. https://doi.org/10.1007/s00213-006-0382-7.

78. Nikisch G, Mathé AA, Czernik A, et al. Long-term citalopram administration reduces responsiveness of HPA axis in patients with major depression: relationship with S-citalopram concentrations in plasma and cerebrospinal fluid (CSF) and clinical response. *Psychopharmacology.* 2005;181(4):751−760. https://doi.org/10.1007/s00213-005-0034-3.

79. Zobel AW, Nickel T, Sonntag A, Uhr M, Holsboer F, Ising M. Cortisol response in the combined dexamethasone/CRH test as predictor of relapse in patients with remitted depression. a prospective study. J Psychiatr Res. 35(2):83-94. http://www.ncbi.nlm.nih.gov/pubmed/11377437. Accessed December 30, 2017.

80. Edwards VJ, Holden GW, Felitti VJ, Anda RF. Relationship between multiple forms of childhood maltreatment and adult mental health in community respondents: results from the adverse childhood experiences study. *Am J Psychiatry.* 2003;160(8):1453−1460. https://doi.org/10.1176/appi.ajp.160.8.1453.

81. Chapman DP, Whitfield CL, Felitti VJ, Dube SR, Edwards VJ, Anda RF. Adverse childhood experiences and the risk of depressive disorders in adulthood. *J Affect Disord.* 2004;82(2):217−225. https://doi.org/10.1016/j.jad.2003.12.013.

82. McCauley J, Kern DE, Kolodner K, et al. Clinical characteristics of women with a history of childhood abuse: unhealed wounds. *J Am Med Assoc.* 1997;277(17): 1362−1368. http://www.ncbi.nlm.nih.gov/pubmed/9134941.

83. Coplan JD, Andrews MW, Rosenblum LA, et al. Persistent elevations of cerebrospinal fluid concentrations of corticotropin-releasing factor in adult nonhuman primates exposed to early-life stressors: implications for the pathophysiology of mood and anxiety disorders. *Proc Natl Acad Sci U S A.* 1996;93(4):1619−1623. http://www.ncbi.nlm.nih.gov/pubmed/8643680.

84. Plotsky PM, Thrivikraman KV, Nemeroff CB, Caldji C, Sharma S, Meaney MJ. Long-Term consequences of neonatal rearing on central corticotropin-releasing factor systems in adult male rat offspring. *Neuropsychopharmacology.* 2005;30(12):2192−2204. https://doi.org/10.1038/sj.npp.1300769.

85. Ladd CO, Huot RL, Thrivikraman KV, Nemeroff CB, Meaney MJ, Plotsky PM. Long-term behavioral and neuroendocrine adaptations to adverse early experience. *Prog Brain Res.* 2000;122:81−103. http://www.ncbi.nlm.nih.gov/pubmed/10737052.

86. Carpenter LL, Tyrka AR, McDougle CJ, et al. Cerebrospinal fluid corticotropin-releasing factor and perceived early-life stress in depressed patients and healthy control subjects. *Neuropsychopharmacology.* 2004;29(4):777−784. https://doi.org/10.1038/sj.npp.1300375.

87. Nemeroff CB, Binder E. The preeminent role of childhood abuse and neglect in vulnerability to major psychiatric disorders: toward elucidating the underlying neurobiological mechanisms. *J Am Acad Child Adolesc Psychiatry.* 2014;53(4):395−397. https://doi.org/10.1016/j.jaac.2014.02.004.

88. Heim C, Nemeroff CB. The role of childhood trauma in the neurobiology of mood and anxiety disorders: preclinical and clinical studies. *Biol Psychiatry.* 2001;49(12): 1023−1039. http://www.ncbi.nlm.nih.gov/pubmed/11430844.

89. Heim C, Newport DJ, Mletzko T, Miller AH, Nemeroff CB. The link between childhood trauma and depression: insights from HPA axis studies in humans. *Psychoneuroendocrinology.* 2008;33(6):693−710. https://doi.org/10.1016/j.psyneuen.2008.03.008.

90. Heim C, Newport DJ, Wagner D, Wilcox MM, Miller AH, Nemeroff CB. The role of early adverse experience and adulthood stress in the prediction of neuroendocrine stress reactivity in women: a multiple regression analysis. *Depress Anxiety.* 2002;15(3):117−125. https://doi.org/10.1002/da.10015.

91. Holsboer F, Von Bardeleben U, Gerken A, Stalla GK, Müller OA. Blunted corticotropin and normal cortisol response to human corticotropin-releasing factor in depression. *N Engl J Med.* 1984;311(17):1127. https://doi.org/10.1056/NEJM198410253111718, 1127.

92. Prange AJ, Lara PP, Wilson IC, Alltop LB, Breese GR. Effects of thyrotropin-releasing hormone in depression. *Lancet.* 1972;2(7785):999−1002. http://www.ncbi.nlm.nih.gov/pubmed/4116985.

93. Fraser SA, Kroenke K, Callahan CM, Hui SL, Williams JW, Unützer J. Low yield of thyroid-stimulating hormone testing in elderly patients with depression. *Gen Hosp Psychiatry.* 2004;26(4):302—309. https://doi.org/10.1016/j.genhosppsych.2004.03.007.

94. Aronson R, Offman HJ, Joffe RT, Naylor CD. Triiodothyronine augmentation in the treatment of refractory depression. A meta-analysis. *Arch Gen Psychiatr.* 1996; 53(9):842—848. http://www.ncbi.nlm.nih.gov/pubmed/8792761.

95. Joffe RT, Sokolov ST, Levitt AJ. Lithium and triiodothyronine augmentation of antidepressants. *Can J Psychiatr.* 2006;51(12):791—793. https://doi.org/10.1177/070674370605101209.

96. Nierenberg AA, Fava M, Trivedi MH, et al. A comparison of lithium and T$_3$ augmentation following two failed medication treatments for depression: a STAR*D report. *Am J Psychiatry.* 2006;163(9):1519—1530. https://doi.org/10.1176/ajp.2006.163.9.1519.

97. Connolly KR, Thase ME. If at first you Don't succeed. *Drugs.* 2011;71(1):43—64. https://doi.org/10.2165/11587620-000000000-00000.

98. Bunevičius R, Kažanavičius G, Žalinkevičius R, Prange AJ. Effects of thyroxine as compared with thyroxine plus triiodothyronine in patients with hypothyroidism. *N Engl J Med.* 1999;340(6):424—429. https://doi.org/10.1056/NEJM199902113400603.

99. Musselman DL, Nemeroff CB. Depression and endocrine disorders: focus on the thyroid and adrenal system. *Br J Psychiatr Suppl.* 1996;(30):123—128. http://www.ncbi.nlm.nih.gov/pubmed/8864158.

100. Gutman DA, Nemeroff CB. Neuroendocrinology of affective disorders. In: *Encyclopedia of Neuroscience.* Elsevier; 2009:355—366. https://doi.org/10.1016/B978-008045046-9.01185-2.

101. Mendlewicz J, Linkowski P, Kerkhofs M, et al. Diurnal hypersecretion of growth hormone in depression*. *J Clin Endocrinol Metab.* 1985;60(3):505—512. https://doi.org/10.1210/jcem-60-3-505.

102. Faron-Górecka A, Kuśmider M, Solich J, et al. Involvement of prolactin and somatostatin in depression and the mechanism of action of antidepressant drugs. *Pharmacol Rep.* 2013;65(6):1640—1646. http://www.ncbi.nlm.nih.gov/pubmed/24553012.

CHAPTER 6

Inflammatory Abnormalities in Major Depressive Disorder

GAURAV SINGHAL, M.TROP.V.SC., B.V.SC. & A.H. •
BERNHARD T. BAUNE, PHD, MD, MPH, FRANZCP

INTRODUCTION

Mental disorders are affecting a large population around the globe. Depression is foremost among them, affecting more than 300 million people worldwide.[1] State of low mood, sense of lost-self, sadness, irritability, loss of interest in all activities, and psychophysiological changes are common symptoms associated with depression.[2] Depression has been shown to decrease lifespan and impairs quality of life.[3,4] In addition, it poses a heavy burden on the public health sector with reported estimated economic burden more than 83 billion dollars in the United States alone in 2000.[5]

The external factors, such as substance abuse, lack of peer support, marital problems, low socioeconomic status, and stressful life events have been shown to result in neurobiological such as chronic neuroinflammation, neurodegeneration, loss of neuroplasticity, neuroprotection, and cellular resilience,[6–11] as well as molecular, such as noradrenergic and serotonergic neurotransmission deficiencies,[12,13] immunological insult,[14–16] altered levels of growth factors,[17–20] and impaired hypothalamic–pituitary–adrenal (HPA) axis metabolism[21,22] changes in the brain that play a significant role in the onset of depression. Evidently, functional causes of depression go hand in hand with anatomic alterations at the cellular level.[23]

The wide array of causative factors associated with depression, therefore, pose difficulties in treating patients with major depressive disorder (MDD). Nonetheless, depression is associated with inflammatory abnormalities, either central nervous system (CNS) or systemic, or both. This inflammatory basis provides opportunities to treat depression among the subset of patients with inflammation. Hence, neurobiological changes during depression, such as neuroinflammation with resultant neurodegeneration, and loss of

neuroplasticity and neuroprotection, have been under extensive investigation lately.[6,8,9] In this chapter, we aim to provide an insight into the common inflammatory pathophysiology of depression and various metabolic disorders, as well as the current pharmacological and nonpharmacological treatment strategies that alter inflammatory pathways both in the CNS and the periphery, associated with depression.

INFLAMMATION AND DEPRESSION: CAUSE AND EFFECT RELATIONSHIP, AND THE ROLE OF CYTOKINES

Accumulating evidence suggests a role of neuroinflammation in the pathophysiology of several psychiatric disorders. Important immune mediators that mediate mental illness include proinflammatory and antiinflammatory cytokines, chemokines, T and B lymphocytes, the complement system, natural killer (NK) cells, prostaglandins, and acute phase reactive proteins, such as C-reactive protein (CRP). Glial cells, microglia, and astrocytes become dysfunctional and lose neuroprotective properties releasing excess proinflammatory cytokines in the aging brain.[24–26] Proinflammatory cytokines are involved in a variety of immune reactions associated with the initiation, regulation, and maintenance of inflammation.[27,28] Neuroinflammation when chronic has been shown to result in neurodegeneration, in turn causing long-term neuropsychiatric disorders, including depression and dementia.[29]

Furthermore, the cumulative meta-analysis to assess observational evidence on systemic inflammation in individuals with major depressive disorder has shown that the higher mean levels of IL-6 and CRP in the serum of patients is related to major depression compared to nondepressed controls.[30] Another meta-analysis has confirmed that the magnitude and

Major Depressive Disorder. https://doi.org/10.1016/B978-0-323-58131-8.00006-9

direction of depression, and CRP, IL-1, and IL-6 are positively associated in the community and clinical samples.[31] Similarly, the overexpression of TNF-α could result in hippocampal degeneration and microglial apoptosis, both being important contributing mechanisms of depression.[32,33] Kronfol and Remick who reviewed the literature on the biology of cytokines during CNS disorders concluded that specific cytokines play a role in signaling the brain to produce neurochemical, neuroendocrine, neuroimmune, and behavioral changes, and that cytokines play a role in the pathophysiology of major depression.[34]

Interestingly, age may significantly affect the level of proinflammatory cytokines in the brain. As such, peripheral infections during old age could, therefore, be an important etiology for the onset of major depression. For example, a study on aged BALB/c mice has shown that exposure to peripheral infections enhanced age-associated reactivity of the brain cytokine. The authors suggested that this could be the pathophysiology for the increased prevalence of depression observed in the elderly.[35]

Mechanism of cytokine action: Proinflammatory cytokines, such as TNF-α and IL-1β attract leukocytes and enhance their proliferation, stimulate cytotoxicity and release of proteolytic enzymes, increase synthesis of prostaglandins, and initiate synthesis and secretion of secondary cytokines, in turn promoting inflammation and raising the thermoregulatory set point.[36] In addition, TNF-α and IL-1β enhance secretion of adhesion molecules that attach to the endothelium of blood vessels in the brain facilitating migration of leukocytes from blood to the brain tissues.[37] Another proinflammatory cytokine, interferon (IFN)-α, promotes expression of proinflammatory surface markers class II major histocompatibility complex (MHC) antigens, CD86, and CD54 (M1 polarization), causing neuroinflammation, subsequently depression.[4] Conversely, antiinflammatory cytokines regulate inflammatory response by suppressing genes that induce production of proinflammatory cytokines. For example, transgenic mice knocked out for genes transcribing antiinflammatory cytokines, such as IL-1ra, IL-10, and transforming growth factor (TGF)-β1 showed enhanced inflammatory reactions.[27]

Activated T cells can cross blood-brain barrier and are present at all times in the brain along with macrophages/monocytes for immune surveillance.[38,39] During immune insult, the CD4+ T helper (Th)1 cells secrete proinflammatory cytokines such as IL-2, TNF-α, and IFN-γ in the brain, in turn activating macrophages and microglia-driven cell-mediated immune response resulting in inflammatory condition.[27,40] Subsequently, CD4+ Th2 cells secrete antiinflammatory cytokines, including IL-4, IL-5, IL-6, IL-10, and IL-13, which activate the humoral immune system and suppress production of proinflammatory cytokines TNF-α and IL-1β from Th1 cells, as well as chemokines such as IL-8 and vascular adhesion molecules, thereby reducing inflammation.[27,40]

MACROPHAGE THEORY OF DEPRESSION

In mammals, macrophages are cells of myeloid cell lineage and derived from the yolk sac, fetal liver, and bone marrow.[41] During fetal life, myeloid progenitors from the yolk sac migrate to all tissues and develop into resident tissue macrophages, for example, Langerhans cells in the skin, Kupffer cells in liver, and microglia in the CNS. After birth, myeloid cells derived from the bone marrow become the main source of circulating monocytes, dendritic cells, and macrophages.[42] Together, macrophages and macrophage-derived cells play a role in development, tissue repair, immunity, as well as maintenance of homeostasis in organ systems. However, in the presence of a chronic immune insult, macrophages have been shown to be associated with inflammatory diseased states.[41] They trigger specific immune responses and function to clear pathogens and damaged cells, eventually allowing tissue remodeling and repair.[43]

The population of brain macrophages includes microglia, perivascular cells, meningeal and choroid plexus macrophages, and pericytes.[44] Under basal conditions, brain macrophages help to maintain homeostasis by supporting the functioning of neural cells and preserving the neuronal network.[42] However, brain macrophages also play a key role in the pathophysiology of MDD. Pathogen and stress-associated proteins, both in the CNS and in the periphery, attract macrophages and macrophage-derived cells, creating sustained inflammatory states that also alter the neurotransmitter systems in the brain.[45] In the presence of a sustained external or internal pathogenic stimulus, neuroinflammation may turn chronic that could result in the degeneration of brain regions, thereby leading to symptoms, such as the cognitive and behavioral deficit, dementia, and depression.[46] Overexpression of brain and systemic macrophages and excessive secretion of macrophage monokines, for example, cytokines and interleukins, have been shown to be the cause of depression and associated coronary heart disease, atherosclerosis, rheumatoid arthritis, stroke, Crohn's disease, obesity, and other systemic illnesses.[47−49]

Upon stimulation, macrophages release proinflammatory mediators in the CNS, thereby mediating a wide range of neurobiological processes leading to sickness- and depressive-like behavior. These processes include disturbances in the synthesis and metabolism of neurotransmitters, and alterations in neurogenesis, neural plasticity, and neurotoxicity.[42] For example, proinflammatory cytokines and prostaglandins induce microglia to produce an enzyme called indoleamine 2, 3-dioxygenase (IDO), which is essential for the conversion of tryptophan to kynurenine. The overexpressed IDO causes serotonin depletion, subsequently amplifying glutamatergic neurotransmission, increasing oxidative stress, and inducing inflammation-associated depression.[50,51] The additional metabolites of this kynurenine pathway, 3-hydroxykynurenine, and quinolinic acid are a strong agonist of the glutamatergic N-methyl-D-aspartate receptor, hence potentially neurotoxic and, thereby also contributing to depression.[42]

ROLE OF MICROGLIA IN DEPRESSION

Microglia, the primary innate immune effector cells of the brain, recognize and react to extrinsic and intrinsic pathologies by creating a sustained inflammatory state that in turn helps to eliminate the causative factor.[52] Microglia phagocytose dead cells and pathogens and expresses various immune proteins and cell adhesion molecules required for the initiation of the innate immune response.[53–55] They are phenotypically similar to blood monocytes and tissue macrophages[15,56] and are important for the rescue of the CNS from pathologies such as infectious diseases, trauma, ischemia, brain tumors, neuroinflammation, and neurodegeneration.[57] In addition, microglia along with cytotoxic T cells enhance neurogenesis, adult brain plasticity, and spatial memory.[58] Conversely, overexpression of microglia may result in enhanced production of proinflammatory cytokines (e.g., TNF-α and IL-1β)[59,60] and increased expression of class I and II MHC antigens[61] in the brain, which in turn, may result in neuroinflammation, neurodegeneration, and subsequent cognitive dysfunction and depression.

Microglia are categorized phenotypically into M1 and M2 types based on their activation state.[62] The M1 phenotype of microglia release proinflammatory cytokines and attract chemokines and circulating immune cells that induce neuroinflammation. Once the pathology is eliminated, the M2 phenotype of microglia release antiinflammatory factors that help to alleviate neuroinflammation and initiate tissue reconstruction. However, sustained stimulation of M1 phenotype and diminished activity of M2 phenotype of microglia may result in chronic neuroinflammation, in turn resulting in neurodegenerative changes. During aging, microglia become progressively dysfunctional, lose neuroprotective properties, and release excessive quantities of proinflammatory cytokines. This, in association with genetic factors and acquired environmental risks, increases the chances of developing psychiatric disorders, including depression.[24,26,63,64]

Microglia become deramified, get primed with class II MHC antigens, and overexpress proinflammatory cytokines after traumatic brain injury, as reported in BALB/c mice eliciting depressive-like behavior.[65] Similarly, in humans, high concentrations of the proinflammatory cytokines TNF-α, IL-1β, and IL-6 have been reported in depressed subjects than controlled subjects,[66] which may be associated with the hyperactivity of microglia in the brain.[60,67,68] Moreover, TNF-α, a product of microglial hyperactivity has been shown to cause hippocampal degeneration and microglial apoptosis,[32] the findings characteristic of unipolar depression.[33]

ROLE OF INFLAMMASOMES IN DEPRESSION

Neuroinflammation often results in dementia, cognitive impairment, and decline in spatial memory function that are associated with MDD. The cytosolic protein complexes known as inflammasomes that activate the proinflammatory caspase-1, in turn leading to the activation of proinflammatory cytokines IL-1β, IL-18, and IL-33,[69,70] have been shown to play an instrumental role in the pathophysiology of neuroinflammation (see Fig. 6.1) and associated neurodegenerative diseases, cognitive impairment, depression, and dementia.[69,71–73]

An attack by pathogens and rise in stress-associated proteins after trauma and with aging activates the NOD-like receptor family, pyrin domain containing 3 (NLRP3) inflammasomes that in turn induces the secretion of activated IL-1 family cytokines from the glial cells and neurons, leading to neuroinflammation and aging-associated depression.[35,74–76] Many studies have reported chronic mild stress as a possible etiology of depression through the NLRP3 inflammasomes pathway.[77–80] Mice injected with lipopolysaccharide (LPS) showed activation of NLRP3 inflammasomes with resulting neuroinflammation and subsequent depression-like behavior.[77,81] The finding of the caspase-1 knocked out mice being resistant to LPS-induced depression-like behavior[82] further added supports to an inflammasomes pathway of

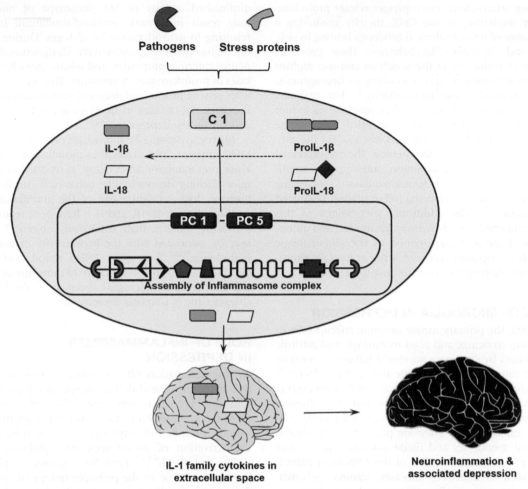

FIG. 6.1 Activation of NLRP3 inflammasomes in the brain: Pathogens and stress-associated proteins are recognized by intracellular pathogen recognition receptors and Toll-like receptors. This triggers assembly of NLRP3 inflammasome complex within the cytoplasm of glial cells, subsequently activating caspase 1 (C1) enzyme. The latter cleaves inactive proforms of proinflammatory IL1 cytokines IL-1β and IL-18 into their active forms. These IL1 cytokines in addition to TNF-α initiate an inflammatory reaction in the extracellular space resulting in neuroinflammation and associated depression: PC1 and PC5, Procaspases 1 and 5.

neuroinflammation and subsequent development of depression-like behavior. These preclinical studies have established a cause–effect relationship between NLRP3 inflammasomes, neuroinflammation, and subsequent development of depressive-like behavior.

Comparable results were found in human studies that reported a significant increase in the levels of caspase-1 and NLRP3 proteins, as well as NLRP3 mRNA expression in the peripheral blood mononuclear cells of depressive patients compared to nondepressed subjects.[83] Moreover, IL-1β and IL-18 were also elevated in the serum of patients with MDD and positively

correlated with the patients' Beck Depression Inventory scores.[83] Similarly, a study reported higher expression levels of NLRP3 and ASC in the mitochondrial fractions derived from the frontal cortex of patients with bipolar disorder,[84] therefore strengthening the idea that NLRP3 inflammasomes have a role to play in mood disorders. The increase in the levels of IL-1 cytokines and neuroinflammation in the brain of depressed patients could, therefore, be regarded as indicators of an enhanced inflammasomes activity playing a role in the pathophysiology of MDD.[85] More research with larger sample sizes and longitudinal designs is required to establish the causative association between NLRP3 inflammasomes, neuroinflammation, and depression in humans.

INFLAMMATORY SYSTEMIC DISEASES AND DEPRESSION

Considerable evidence supports an association between depression and metabolic disorders, such as Type II diabetes and cardiovascular disease (CVD),[86,87] central obesity,[88,89] Crohn's disease,[90] rheumatoid arthritis,[91] osteoarthritis,[92] and cancer,[93] with the prevalence of depression higher by 50% in individuals with the metabolic syndrome.[87] Moreover, significant and independent associations have been shown between large waist circumference and low HDL cholesterol with depression,[87] the defined quantitative criteria's for the diagnosis of metabolic disorders.[94,95]

A significant association between depression and metabolic disorders, therefore, suggests shared mechanisms of pathogenesis. Indeed, the pathophysiology of inflammation is common to both, which affects not just the neurobiological systems, but also disrupts neuroregulatory systems (e.g., serotonergic and dopaminergic) and dysregulates HPA axis.[88] Serotonin[96] and dopamine[97] are established regulators of mood and behavior. Similarly, the HPA axis controls mood is also well known.[98] A common feature of various chronic systemic inflammatory diseases such as osteoarthritis,[99] cancer,[100] diabetes,[101] central obesity,[102] and CVD,[103] as well as aging-associated depression[35] is an increase in the level of proinflammatory cytokines such as IL-1β, TNF-α, and IL-6, and acute phase proteins (e.g., CRP) in the peripheral blood and the brain. There is also evidence to suggest that proinflammatory cytokines TNF-α, IL-1β, IL-6, and IFN-γ can cross the BBB into the systemic circulation and hence play a vital role in the bidirectional relationship between depression and Type II diabetes.[104] Similarly, the three-way association between proinflammatory cytokines, depression, and metabolic syndromes CVD,[105,106] Crohn's disease,[107] rheumatoid arthritis,[108,109] and cancer[110,111] has also been reported.

Central obesity acts as a predisposing factor in the development of metabolic disorders and their comorbidity with depression. High-fat diet consumption with resultant obesity has been reported to elicit an inflammatory response, which in turn was found to be associated with the onset of depression.[102] This is because adipose tissue secretes proinflammatory cytokines including TNF-α, IL-1β, IL-6 IL-8, and monocyte chemoattractant protein-1, resulting in the onset of inflammatory states. Proinflammatory cytokines also recruit various immune cells, including macrophages and T cells, in turn, further promoting inflammation of the adipose tissues.[112] Moreover, IFN-γ which is predominantly expressed on T cells stimulates the expression of chemokines and proinflammatory cytokines in adipocytes as well as cause M1 polarization of macrophages.[112] Taken together, this suggests that obesity may initiate a never-ending and self-propagating cycle of both systemic and CNS inflammatory states.

Both the periphery and the CNS communicate with each other (see Fig. 6.2) in a bidirectional manner: a review has reported that three pathways are relevant for the migration of proinflammatory cytokines from the systemic circulation into the brain and vice versa, namely cellular, humoral, and neural pathways,[76] this supports the inflammation hypothesis for the clinically often found comorbidity between depression and chronic systemic illnesses. A recent review proposed an inflammasome hypothesis, which states that the inflammasome is a central mediator by which psychological and physical stressors contribute to the development of depression and its comorbidity with systemic illnesses.[113] As metabolic disorders such as the development of Type II diabetes,[114,115] central obesity,[116] CVD,[117−119] or cancer[120,121] are known to predispose to the development of psychiatric disorders, alongside depression, microglia-associated cytosolic inflammasome-driven inflammatory pathways may have a role to play in this metabolic-psychiatric comorbidity. The activation of inflammasomes in microglia, particularly NLRP3, therefore could be indirectly related to the pathophysiology of depression and its comorbidity with other systemic diseases through an inflammatory response in the brain. Hence, awareness of depressive symptoms as part of metabolic syndrome and vice versa could be useful in the clinical management of both MDD and metabolic diseases.

INFLAMMATION GENES AND DEPRESSION

As previously reported, proinflammatory cytokines at constitutive levels are relevant for various molecular and cellular neuroimmune mechanisms, such as monoamine metabolism, neuronal genesis and survival, and HPA axis sensitivity to cortisol, all of which are important contributors to the molecular processes of learning and memory.[29,122] On the contrary, antiinflammatory cytokines suppress the gene expression of proinflammatory cytokines production and thereby diminish the proinflammatory response. A study has shown enhanced inflammatory reactions in gene knockout mice of various antiinflammatory cytokines (IL-1ra,

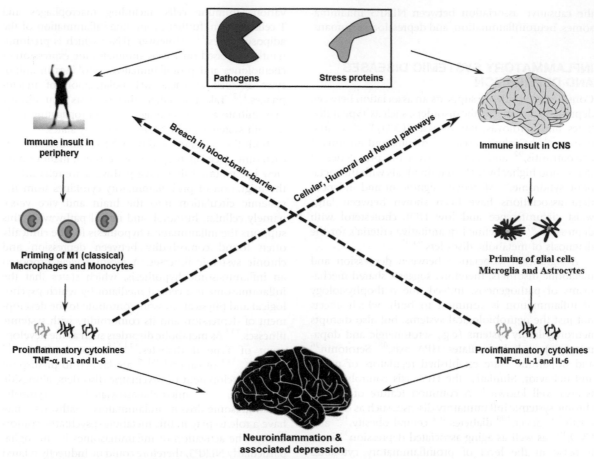

FIG. 6.2 Role of proinflammatory cytokines in neuroinflammation, associated depression and its comorbidity with metabolic illnesses: Pathogens and stress-associated proteins prime M1 macrophages and monocytes in the periphery, and glial cells (microglia and astrocytes) in the CNS. These primed cells then secrete proinflammatory cytokines TNF-α, IL-1β, and IL-6 that can travel between the periphery and CNS in both directions. Three pathways have been proposed for the migration of proinflammatory cytokines from the systemic circulation to the brain: cellular, humoral, and neural. Similarly, proinflammatory cytokines in the CNS finds a way to periphery through breaching blood-brain barrier. These cytokines when constantly overexpressed contribute to the pathophysiology of neuroinflammation. Chronic neuroinflammation could result in neurodegeneration and associated depression.

IL-10, and TGF-1β).[27] Similarly, it has been reported that several genes, for example, thioredoxin-interacting protein, *P2X7* and pannexins, as well as those that signal activation of toll-like receptors (TLRs) and inflammasomes, such as *CD14, TLR2, TLR4, TLR7, TOLLIP, and MYD88*, are upregulated in different regions of the brain such as the hippocampus, postcentral gyrus, and superior frontal gyrus during aging.[123] There was also an increase in the monocytes

gene expression profiles of MDD patients with experiences of childhood maltreatment.[124] A recent review has summarized the functional allelic variants of immune-related genes as well as genetic variations affecting T-cell function, which may have a role in increasing the risk for depression and reduced responsiveness to antidepressant therapy.[125] Taken together, the evidence is suggestive of the importance of genes associated with inflammation in MDD.

MECHANISTIC INSIGHTS INTO NEUROINFLAMMATION AND RELATED PATHWAYS DURING DEPRESSION

Various neuroimmune processes, both humoral and cellular, mediate neuroplastic processes during depression. Pro and antiinflammatory cytokines, monocyte-derived macrophages, in particular, microglia and T reg cells are vital to physiological processes of neuroplasticity such as long-term potentiation, neural stem cells survival, neurocircuitry, synaptic branching, neurotrophin regulation, and neurogenesis.[126] The same factors have also been shown to be responsible for neurodegenerative changes and reduced neuroplasticity during pathophysiological processes, such as psychological stress, some of which are have been shown to reverse with antidepressant treatments, physical exercise, and omega-3 polyunsaturated fatty acids ($\Omega3$ PUFA).[126] Nevertheless, several other factors such as monoamine dysfunction[127] and the HPA axis dysregulation[128] may also contribute to neurodegenerative changes and therefore play a role in the pathophysiology of depression.

Monoamine dysregulation has been a known etiology for the development of depression. The expression levels and functioning of aminergic pathway enzymes and transporter proteins in the extracellular spaces are altered during depression. For example, significantly lower plasma glycine values with a higher serine/glycine ratio, decreased plasma concentration of the excitatory amino acids glutamate, and increased plasma concentration of the inhibitory amino acids taurine have been reported from the depressed group in a clinical trial.[129] Similarly, significantly elevated levels of the enzyme monoamine oxidase A, a biological catalyst that metabolizes monoamines, that is, serotonin, norepinephrine, and dopamine in the brain, were observed in depressed individuals.[127] The functioning of the dopamine transporter and serotonin transporter proteins that primarily regulate the extracellular concentrations of dopamine and serotonin respectively is also affected during depression. For example, a study has shown that the serotonin transporter gene (5-HTT) polymorphism is involved in the pathophysiology of depression and anxiety disorders.[130] Similarly, the development of depressive-like behavior has been reported in the 5-HTT KO mice.[131] Dysregulation in monoamine pathway may, therefore, result in oxidative and nitrosative stress leading to neurodegeneration and subsequently depression.

Psychological stress is a known etiology of depression.[132] HPA axis mediates the cellular mechanisms in response to stress, which includes neural inputs from catecholaminergic, serotonergic and cholinergic brain nuclei.[133] In response to a stress stimulus, the cells in the paraventricular nucleus secrete corticotropin-releasing hormone (CRH). CRH, in turn, acts on the anterior pituitary stimulating the proopiomelanocortin-producing cells to release adrenocorticotrophin, which then migrates through the systemic circulation to the adrenal cortical receptors where it promotes the secretion of catecholamines and glucocorticoids. The sustained overexpression of these end products in plasma is characteristic of the stress response.[133] Although glucocorticoids are considered to be antiinflammatory and immunosuppressive, there is evidence to indicate that they can also show proinflammatory effects in the CNS.[134] Indeed, the chronic release of glucocorticoids could result in the atrophy of certain brain areas[135] and damage to the hippocampus.[136] Moreover, excess glucocorticoids may also inhibit glucose transport in neurons and glia, as well as induce oxidative and nitrosative damage in the brain through interfering with glutamate reuptake and increasing calcium mobilization inside the cells,[133,137] eventually causing neurodegenerative changes and subsequent depression.

ANTIINFLAMMATORY PROPERTIES OF VARIOUS INTERVENTIONS IN THE TREATMENT OF DEPRESSION

The etiology for depression is multifactorial and heterogeneous. This makes it difficult to understand the key mechanisms that are translatable into treatment approaches. However, the role of inflammation and immune activation in depression pathophysiology received far more attention than other likely etiologies, and potential treatment approaches are being formulated to modulate immune function and alleviating inflammation. As mentioned previously, the enhanced expression of proinflammatory cytokines TNF-α, IL-1β, IL-6, and IFN-γ, both in the periphery and CNS play a major role in the pathophysiology of depression. Besides affecting the neurobiological system, proinflammatory cytokines also affect nonimmune pathways, for example, monoamine metabolism and HPA axis functions, adding to the etiologies of depression. As such, regulating chronic overexpression of proinflammatory cytokines received widespread attention of researchers worldwide and hence has been explored largely during the last decade. To achieve the desired results, both selective cyclooxygenase

(COX)-2 and nonselective COX inhibitor nonsteroidal antiinflammatory drugs (NSAIDs) have been investigated as possible adjuncts in the treatment of depression with antidepressants.[138–151] Their antiinflammatory properties are primarily due to inhibition of prostaglandin synthesis. NSAIDs are indeed widely used to control inflammation and are increasingly discussed for their clinical relevance in the treatment of depression.[152,153]

The results, however, varied from study to study. Although some studies reported positive effects of NSAIDs as antidepressants,[138,142,144,145] some reported no effects,[139,140,146] and others reported that NSAIDs reduce the antidepressant effect of selective serotonin reuptake inhibitors (SSRIs).[141,147] This variance in results could be explained through nonmatching factors among the studies, for example, the composition of NSAIDs (selective COX-2 and/or nonselective COX inhibitor), study design, and study population differences (age, varying degrees of depressive symptomatology and presence of comorbid medical conditions). Moreover, the functions and efficacy of selective COX-2 versus nonselective COX inhibitor differ, for example, while COX-1 mediate proinflammatory microglial activation[154] and hence could be averse to the brain functions,[155] COX-2 can exert both beneficial and detrimental effects on the brain.[156] In addition, a study reported a reduction in the recruitment of leukocytes into the inflamed CNS when COX-1 activity was inhibited, and vice versa when COX-2 activity was inhibited.[157] This suggests differential chemotactic effects of these enzymes on the brain. The evidence mentioned here, therefore, may explain the reason for the inconsistent effects of NSAIDs in the clinical treatment of depression, and hence emphasize on the necessity of considering different pharmacological properties of NSAIDs while formulating the design of clinical trials. Moreover, there is evidence that suggests a phase-specific profile of immune-mediated dysfunction,[158] hence the phase of depression during which NSAIDs are administered needs to be carefully considered. Indeed, antiinflammatory treatments used outside the acute clinical phase have been shown to cause more harm.[158]

Aspirin, the most commonly used NSAID, is an irreversible inhibitor of both COX-1 and COX-2, making it a potent antidepressant. In addition, it is a proven anticoagulant, reducing the occurrence of ischemic strokes and other vascular events. Although the use of aspirin in depression is still hypothetical, there is clinical evidence suggesting that aspirin could be beneficial in the treatment of mood disorders through a shortened onset of action of antidepressants.[159] NSAIDs, such as Indomethacin and Ibuprofen, and fusion proteins produced from recombinant DNA, such as Etanercept,[160] when used to block the inflammatory response, considerably improved neurogenesis[161] and reduced depressive-like behavior.[152] Similarly, antidepressant, such as imipramine and minocycline, has been shown to reduce IFN-γ levels by inhibiting microglial proliferation and activation, and subsequently attenuate depressive-like symptoms.[162–164]

The benefits of NSAIDs as antidepressants, however, are not without any side effects. Gastric ulceration and damage to kidneys have been reported after long-term use of NSAIDs.[165,166] Similarly, there are case reports of neurological symptoms including ataxia, vertigo, dizziness, recurrent falls, nystagmus, headache, encephalopathy, seizures, aseptic meningitis, and disorientation after an overdose of NSAIDs. Rofecoxib (Vioxx) and Valdecoxib (Bextra) that are selective COX-2 inhibitors cause specific inhibition of synthesis of prostaglandins participating in inflammation and can increase the risk of stroke.[167]

Further research is required to address this important gap in clinical research in depression-associated inflammation. A transgenic proinflammatory cytokines receptor antagonist, such as IL-1 receptor antagonist, has been reported to reduce microglial apoptosis, subsequently neuroinflammation and depressive-like behavior in rodents.[168–170] This approach could potentially be translated into clinical trials as alternatives to NSAIDs. In addition to antidepressants, interventions such as physical exercise and use of Ω-3 PUFA are increasingly used in the treatment of depression, either as standalone therapies or in combination with antidepressants. Physical exercise elicits immunomodulatory and antiinflammatory effects. It has been shown to cause a decrease in the levels of TNF-α both in serum and CSF,[171,172] induce neurogenesis[173] and an increase in the leukocyte blood levels.[174,175] An increase in the concentration of neutrophilic granulocytes, lymphocytes, monocytes, the blood mononuclear cell subsets (CD3$^+$, CD4$^+$, CD8$^+$, CD16$^+$, CD19$^+$, and CD14$^+$), the NK cell activity, and plasma IL-6 has been reported in the peripheral blood after physical exercise during clinical trials.[176,177] Similarly, Ω3 PUFA has been reported to elicit antiinflammatory effects and shows improvement in patients with depression.[178] Together, it suggests that antiinflammatory therapies in various combinations could be used to modify low-grade inflammation in the treatment of depression.

DISCUSSION

Neuroinflammation has an important role to play in the pathophysiology of depression. When chronic, it results in degeneration of several brain areas, especially the hippocampal regions, predisposing to and potentially causing mood disorders.[29] Several immune factors, for example, proinflammatory and antiinflammatory cytokines, chemokines, T and B cells, the complement system, NK cells, prostaglandins and acute phase reactive proteins (e.g., CRP) participate in inducing and sustaining neuroinflammation in response to external nonfavorable stimuli, such as pathogens and stress proteins.[27,28] Glial cells may lose neuroprotective properties and release excess proinflammatory cytokines under stressful conditions and during aging.[24–26] Moreover, cytosolic inflammasomes in the brain activate the proinflammatory caspase-1, releasing proinflammatory cytokines interleukin IL-1β, IL-18, and IL-33,[69,70] resulting in neuroinflammation and associated neurodegenerative changes, cognitive impairment, depression, and dementia.[69,71–73]

Although macrophages and macrophage-derived cells, especially microglia, in the CNS are important for tissue repair, immunity, and maintenance of homeostasis in the basal state, they may be triggered by pathogens to elicit an innate immune response and produce proinflammatory cytokines.[41] Hence, overexpression of brain and systemic macrophages and excessive secretion of macrophage monokines, for example, cytokines and interleukins, may result in sustained neuroinflammation with resultant depression and could be the reason for comorbidity of depression with systemic inflammatory diseases, such as coronary heart disease, atherosclerosis, rheumatoid arthritis, stroke, Crohn's disease, and obesity.[47–49] However, macrophage activation in the CNS alone may not be sufficient to induce neuroinflammation. Indeed, proinflammatory cytokines produced by macrophages have also been shown to migrate from the peripheral blood into the brain and vice versa, through three pathways namely cellular, humoral, and neural pathways.[76] This suggests that systemic inflammatory illnesses associated with aging may also result in the onset of depression in the absence of pathogenic stimuli in the brain.

Macrophages mediate inflammatory diseases affecting the outcome, alleviate sickness behavior, and improve cognitive function. Antidepressants transform peripheral and brain macrophages to the antiinflammatory M2 phenotype. This evidence suggests that the effects of antidepressive treatments may be, at least in part, mediated by changes in macrophage activity.[28]

Conversely, infection, tissue injury, respiratory allergies, and antigens found in food have been shown to enhance the activity of proinflammatory M1 phenotype macrophage triggering depression.[42]

The efficacy of antidepressants (e.g., SSRI, SNRI, TCAs) is proven, but not all patients benefit from such a pharmacological intervention. Given the contribution of inflammation to depression, various antiinflammatory drug interventions such as NSAIDs have been trialed, some with promising results. Nonpharmacological approaches such as physical exercise that has shown to induce neurogenesis and enhance immune functions in the brain have shown to exert antidepressant properties[173] and are increasingly discussed as adjuvant interventions in combination with antidepressants for treating depression or as standalone prevention interventions. Similarly, fish oil has been proposed as a prophylactic intervention against depression.[179]

In conclusion, chronic inflammation in depressive patients may be an effect of persistent psychosocial stressor or early-life stressful events.[180] Both peripheral macrophages and microglia play important roles in the inflammatory signaling pathways associated with depression. In CNS, psychological stress can prime microglia for subsequent exposure to a similar stressor, which may remain in the quiescent state for a long time but respond excessively to even the slightest of repeating stress stimuli.[181] However, it is important to note that neuroinflammation alone may not be the sole cause for neurodegenerative changes and several other factors, such as monoamine dysfunction[127] and HPA axis dysregulation,[128] which can result in the presence of chronic inflammatory state[88] may also contribute to neurodegeneration and hence to the pathophysiology of depression.

CONFLICT OF INTEREST STATEMENT

The presented work is supported by the National Health and Medical Research Council Australia (APP 1043771 to BTB). The funders had no role in study design, data collection and analysis, decision to publish, or preparation of the manuscript.

REFERENCES

1. WHO. *WHO | Depression*; 2017. http://www.who.int/mediacentre/factsheets/fs369/en/.
2. Belmaker R, Agam G. Major depressive disorder. *N Engl J Med.* 2008;358(1):55–68.
3. Bosnyák E, Kamson DO, Behen ME, Barger GR, Mittal S, Juhász C. Imaging cerebral tryptophan metabolism in

brain tumor-associated depression. *EJNMMI Res.* 2015; 5(1):1.

4. Wachholz S, Eßlinger M, Plümper J, Manitz M-P, Juckel G, Friebe A. Microglia activation is associated with IFN-α induced depressive-like behavior. *Brain Behav Immun.* 2016;55:105−113.

5. Donohue JM, Pincus HA. Reducing the societal burden of depression. *Pharmacoeconomics.* 2007;25(1):7−24.

6. Pittenger C, Duman RS. Stress, depression, and neuroplasticity: a convergence of mechanisms. *Neuropsychopharmacology.* 2008;33(1):88−109.

7. Fuchs E, Czéh B, Kole MH, Michaelis T, Lucassen PJ. Alterations of neuroplasticity in depression: the hippocampus and beyond. *Eur Neuropsychopharmacol.* 2004;14: S481−S490.

8. Player MJ, Taylor JL, Weickert CS, et al. Neuroplasticity in depressed individuals compared with healthy controls. *Neuropsychopharmacology.* 2013;38(11):2101−2108.

9. Malykhin N, Coupland N. Hippocampal neuroplasticity in major depressive disorder. *Neuroscience.* 2015;309: 200−213.

10. Haarman BCB, Riemersma-Van der Lek RF, de Groot JC, et al. Neuroinflammation in bipolar disorder—A [11 C]-(R)-PK11195 positron emission tomography study. *Brain Behav Immun.* 2014;40:219−225.

11. Manji HK, Moore GJ, Rajkowska G, Chen G. Neuroplasticity and cellular resilience in mood disorders. *Mol Psychiatr.* 2000;5(6):578.

12. López-Figueroa AL, Norton CS, López-Figueroa MO, et al. Serotonin 5-HT 1A, 5-HT 1B, and 5-HT 2A receptor mRNA expression in subjects with major depression, bipolar disorder, and schizophrenia. *Biol Psychiatry.* 2004; 55(3):225−233.

13. Tsai S-J, Hong C-J, Hsu C-C, et al. Serotonin-2A receptor polymorphism (102T/C) in mood disorders. *Psychiatr Res.* 1999;87(2):233−237.

14. Schipper HM. Astrocytes, brain aging, and neurodegeneration. *Neurobiol Aging.* 1996;17(3): 467−480.

15. Conde JR, Streit WJ. Microglia in the aging brain. *J Neuropathol Exp Neurol.* 2006;65(3):199−203.

16. Ortiz-Domínguez A, Hernández ME, Berlanga C, et al. Immune variations in bipolar disorder: phasic differences. *Bipolar Disorders.* 2007;9(6):596−602.

17. Svenningsson P, Chergui K, Rachleff I, et al. Alterations in 5-HT1B receptor function by p11 in depression-like states. *Science.* 2006;311(5757):77−80.

18. Duman RS, Heninger GR, Nestler EJ. A molecular and cellular theory of depression. *Arch Gen Psychiatr.* 1997; 54(7):597−606.

19. Thase ME. Molecules that mediate mood. *N Engl J Med.* 2007;357(23):2400.

20. Hill MN, Gorzalka BB. Impairments in endocannabinoid signaling and depressive illness. *JAMA.* 2009;301(11): 1165−1166.

21. Vreeburg SA, Hoogendijk WJ, van Pelt J, et al. Major depressive disorder and hypothalamic-pituitary-adrenal axis activity: results from a large cohort study. *Arch Gen Psychiatr.* 2009;66(6):617−626.

22. Gillespie CF, Nemeroff CB. Hypercortisolemia and depression. *Psychosom Med.* 2005;67:S26−S28.

23. Rajkowska G, Miguel-Hidalgo J. Gliogenesis and glial pathology in depression. *CNS Neurol Disord Drug Targets.* 2007;6(3):219−233.

24. Dilger RN, Johnson RW. Aging, microglial cell priming, and the discordant central inflammatory response to signals from the peripheral immune system. *J Leukoc Biol.* 2008;84(4):932−939.

25. Rozovsky I, Finch C, Morgan T. Age-related activation of microglia and astrocytes: in vitro studies show persistent phenotypes of aging, increased proliferation, and resistance to down-regulation. *Neurobiol Aging.* 1998;19(1): 97−103.

26. Mrak RE, Griffin WST. Glia and their cytokines in progression of neurodegeneration. *Neurobiol Aging.* 2005;26(3): 349−354.

27. Dinarello CA. Proinflammatory cytokines. *CHEST Journal.* 2000;118(2):503−508.

28. Dantzer R, O'Connor JC, Freund GG, Johnson RW, Kelley KW. From inflammation to sickness and depression: when the immune system subjugates the brain. *Nat Rev Neurosci.* 2008;9(1):46−56.

29. McAfoose J, Baune B. Evidence for a cytokine model of cognitive function. *Neurosci Biobehav Rev.* 2009;33(3): 355−366.

30. Haapakoski R, Mathieu J, Ebmeier KP, Alenius H, Kivimäki M. Cumulative meta-analysis of interleukins 6 and 1β, tumour necrosis factor α and C-reactive protein in patients with major depressive disorder. *Brain Behav Immun.* 2015;49:206−215.

31. Howren MB, Lamkin DM, Suls J. Associations of depression with C-reactive protein, IL-1, and IL-6: a meta-analysis. *Psychosom Med.* 2009;71(2):171−186.

32. Cacci E, Claasen JH, Kokaia Z. Microglia-derived tumor necrosis factor-α exaggerates death of newborn hippocampal progenitor cells in vitro. *J Neurosci Res.* 2005; 80(6):789−797.

33. Videbech P, Ravnkilde B. Hippocampal volume and depression: a meta-analysis of MRI studies. *American Journal of Psychiatry.* 2004;161(11):1957−1966.

34. Kronfol Z, Remick DG. Cytokines and the brain: implications for clinical psychiatry. *Am J Psychiatry.* 2014;157(5): 683−694.

35. Godbout JP, Moreau M, Lestage J, et al. Aging exacerbates depressive-like behavior in mice in response to activation of the peripheral innate immune system. *Neuropsychopharmacology.* 2008;33(10):2341−2351.

36. Cannon JG. Inflammatory cytokines in nonpathological states. *Physiology.* 2000;15(6):298−303.

37. Kim JS. Cytokines and adhesion molecules in stroke and related diseases. *J Neurol Sci.* 1996;137(2):69−78.

38. Hickey W, Hsu B, Kimura H. T-lymphocyte entry into the central nervous system. *J Neurosci Res.* 1991;28(2): 254−260.

39. Engelhardt B. Molecular mechanisms involved in T cell migration across the blood–brain barrier. *J Neural Transm.* 2006;113(4):477–485.

40. Fiorentino DF, Bond MW, Mosmann T. Two types of mouse T helper cell. IV. Th2 clones secrete a factor that inhibits cytokine production by Th1 clones. *J Exp Med.* 1989;170(6):2081–2095.

41. Wynn TA, Chawla A, Pollard JW. Macrophage biology in development, homeostasis and disease. *Nature.* 2013; 496(7446):445.

42. Roman A, Kreiner G, Nalepa I. Macrophages and depression–a misalliance or well-arranged marriage? *Pharmacol Rep.* 2013;65(6):1663–1672.

43. Geissmann F, Manz MG, Jung S, Sieweke MH, Merad M, Ley K. Development of monocytes, macrophages, and dendritic cells. *Science.* 2010;327(5966):656–661.

44. Prinz M, Priller J, Sisodia SS, Ransohoff RM. Heterogeneity of CNS myeloid cells and their roles in neurodegeneration. *Nat Neurosci.* 2011;14(10):1227.

45. Leonard BE. Impact of inflammation on neurotransmitter changes in major depression: an insight into the action of antidepressants. *Prog Neuro Psychopharmacol Biol Psychiatr.* 2014;48:261–267.

46. Singhal G, Jaehne EJ, Corrigan F, Toben C, Baune BT. Inflammasomes in neuroinflammation and changes in brain function: a focused review. *Front Neurosci.* 2014;8:315.

47. Smith RS. The macrophage theory of depression. *Med Hypotheses.* 1991;35(4):298–306.

48. Soczynska JK, Kennedy SH, Woldeyohannes HO, et al. Mood disorders and obesity: understanding inflammation as a pathophysiological nexus. *NeuroMolecular Med.* 2011;13(2):93–116.

49. Uzun S, Kozumplik O, Topić R, Jakovljević M. Depressive disorders and comorbidity: somatic illness vs. side effect. *Psychiatr Danub.* 2009;21(3):391–398.

50. Dantzer R. Role of the Kynurenine metabolism pathway in inflammation-induced depression: preclinical approaches. In: *Inflammation-Associated Depression: Evidence, Mechanisms and Implications.* Springer; 2016:117–138.

51. Sanacora G, Treccani G, Popoli M. Towards a glutamate hypothesis of depression: an emerging frontier of neuropsychopharmacology for mood disorders. *Neuropharmacology.* 2012;62(1):63–77. Psychother Psychosom. 2014;83:70-88.

52. Tremblay M-È, Stevens B, Sierra A, Wake H, Bessis A, Nimmerjahn A. The role of microglia in the healthy brain. *J Neurosci.* 2011;31(45):16064–16069.

53. Kitamura Y, Nomura Y. Stress proteins and glial functions: possible therapeutic targets for neurodegenerative disorders. *Pharmacol Ther.* 2003;97(1):35–53.

54. Bunge RP. The role of the Schwann cell in trophic support and regeneration. *J Neurol.* 1994;242(1):S19–S21.

55. Zhang S-C. Defining glial cells during CNS development. *Nat Rev Neurosci.* 2001;2(11):840–843.

56. McGeer PL, Kawamata T, Walker DG, Akiyama H, Tooyama I, McGeer EG. Microglia in degenerative neurological disease. *Glia.* 1993;7(1):84–92.

57. Kreutzberg GW. Microglia: a sensor for pathological events in the CNS. *Trends Neurosci.* 1996;19(8):312–318.

58. Ziv Y, Ron N, Butovsky O, et al. Immune cells contribute to the maintenance of neurogenesis and spatial learning abilities in adulthood. *Nat Neurosci.* 2006;9(2):268–275.

59. Sawada M, Kondo N, Suzumura A, Marunouchi T. Production of tumor necrosis factor-alpha by microglia and astrocytes in culture. *Brain Research.* 1989;491(2): 394–397.

60. Hanisch UK. Microglia as a source and target of cytokines. *Glia.* 2002;40(2):140–155.

61. Tooyama I, Kimura H, Akiyama H, McGeer P. Reactive microglia express class I and class II major histocompatibility complex antigens in Alzheimer's disease. *Brain Research.* 1990;523(2):273–280.

62. Tang Y, Le W. Differential roles of M1 and M2 microglia in neurodegenerative diseases. *Mol Neurobiol.* 2016; 53(2):1181–1194.

63. Streit WJ. Microglia and neuroprotection: implications for Alzheimer's disease. *Brain Research Reviews.* 2005; 48(2):234–239.

64. Norden DM, Godbout JP. Review: microglia of the aged brain: primed to be activated and resistant to regulation. *Neuropathol Appl Neurobiol.* 2013;39(1): 19–34.

65. Fenn AM, Gensel JC, Huang Y, Popovich PG, Lifshitz J, Godbout JP. Immune activation promotes depression 1 month after diffuse brain injury: a role for primed microglia. *Biol Psychiatry.* 2014;76(7):575–584.

66. Dowlati Y, Herrmann N, Swardfager W, et al. A meta-analysis of cytokines in major depression. *Biol Psychiatry.* 2010;67(5):446–457.

67. Smith JA, Das A, Ray SK, Banik NL. Role of pro-inflammatory cytokines released from microglia in neurodegenerative diseases. *Brain Research Bulletin.* 2012;87(1):10–20.

68. Schroeter ML, Abdul-Khaliq H, Krebs M, Diefenbacher A, Blasig IE. Serum markers support disease-specific glial pathology in major depression. *J Affect Disord.* 2008;111(2): 271–280.

69. Chakraborty S, Kaushik DK, Gupta M, Basu A. Inflammasome signaling at the heart of central nervous system pathology. *J Neurosci Res.* 2010;88(8):1615–1631.

70. Arend WP, Palmer G, Gabay C. IL-1, IL-18, and IL-33 families of cytokines. *Immunol Rev.* 2008;223(1): 20–38.

71. Liu L, Chan C. The role of inflammasome in Alzheimer's disease. *Ageing Res Rev.* 2014;15:6–15.

72. Simi A, Lerouet D, Pinteaux E, Brough D. Mechanisms of regulation for interleukin-1β in neurodegenerative disease. *Neuropharmacology.* 2007;52(8):1563–1569.

73. Mawhinney LJ, de Rivero Vaccari JP, Dale GA, Keane RW, Bramlett HM. Heightened inflammasome activation is linked to age-related cognitive impairment in Fischer 344 rats. *BMC Neuroscience.* 2011;12(1):123.

74. Sparkman NL, Johnson RW. Neuroinflammation associated with aging sensitizes the brain to the effects of

infection or stress. *Neuroimmunomodulation.* 2008; 15(4–6):323–330.

75. Wager-Smith K, Markou A. Depression: a repair response to stress-induced neuronal microdamage that can grade into a chronic neuroinflammatory condition? *Neurosci Biobehav Rev.* 2011;35(3):742–764.

76. Capuron L, Miller AH. Immune system to brain signaling: neuropsychopharmacological implications. *Pharmacol Ther.* 2011;130(2):226–238.

77. Zhang Y, Liu L, Peng YL, et al. Involvement of inflamma-some activation in lipopolysaccharide-induced mice depressive-like behaviors. *CNS Neurosci Ther.* 2014; 20(2):119–124.

78. Farooq RK, Isingrini E, Tanti A, et al. Is unpredictable chronic mild stress (UCMS) a reliable model to study depression-induced neuroinflammation? *Behav Brain Res.* 2012;231(1):130–137.

79. Alcocer-Gómez E, Ulecia-Morón C, Marín-Aguilar F, et al. Stress-induced depressive behaviors require a functional NLRP3 inflammasome. *Mol Neurobiol.* 2016;53(7): 4874–4882.

80. Velasquez S, Rappaport J. Inflammasome activation in major depressive disorder: a pivotal linkage between psychological stress, purinergic signaling, and the kynurenine pathway. *Biol Psychiatry.* 2016;80(1):4–5.

81. Zhu W, Cao F-S, Feng J, et al. NLRP3 inflammasome activation contributes to long-term behavioral alterations in mice injected with lipopolysaccharide. *Neuroscience.* 2017;343:77–84.

82. Moon M, McCusker R, Lawson M, Dantzer R, Kelley K. Mice lacking the inflammasome component caspase-1 are resistant to central lipopolysaccharide-induced depressive-like behavior. *Brain Behav Immun.* 2009;23: S50.

83. Alcocer-Gómez E, de Miguel M, Casas-Barquero N, et al. NLRP3 inflammasome is activated in mononuclear blood cells from patients with major depressive disorder. *Brain Behav Immun.* 2014;36:111–117.

84. Kim HK, Andreazza AC, Elmi N, Chen W, Young LT. Nod-like receptor pyrin containing 3 (NLRP3) in the post-mortem frontal cortex from patients with bipolar disorder: a potential mediator between mitochondria and immune-activation. *J Psychiatr Res.* 2016;72:43–50.

85. Schwarz MJ, Chiang S, Müller N, Ackenheil M. T-helper-1 and T-helper-2 responses in psychiatric disorders. *Brain Behav Immun.* 2001;15(4):340–370.

86. Halaris A. Comorbidity between depression and cardio-vascular disease. *Int Angiol.* 2009;28(2):92–99.

87. Dunbar JA, Reddy P, Davis-Lameloise N, et al. Depression: an important comorbidity with metabolic syndrome in a general population. *Diabetes Care.* 2008; 31(12):2368–2373.

88. Nousen EK, Franco JG, Sullivan EL. Unraveling the mechanisms responsible for the comorbidity between metabolic syndrome and mental health disorders. *Neuroendocrinology.* 2013;98(4):254–266.

89. Beydoun MA, Beydoun H, Wang Y. Obesity and central obesity as risk factors for incident dementia and its

subtypes: a systematic review and meta-analysis. *Obes Rev.* 2008;9(3):204–218.

90. Loftus Jr EV, Guérin A, Andrew PY, et al. Increased risks of developing anxiety and depression in young patients with Crohn's disease. *Am J Gastroenterol.* 2011;106(9): 1670.

91. Mella LFB, Bértolo MB, Dalgalarrondo P. Depressive symptoms in rheumatoid arthritis. *Rev Bras Psiquiatr.* 2010;32(3):257–263.

92. Axford J, Butt A, Heron C, et al. Prevalence of anxiety and depression in osteoarthritis: use of the Hospital Anxiety and Depression Scale as a screening tool. *Clin Rheumatol.* 2010;29(11):1277–1283.

93. Krebber A, Buffart L, Kleijn G, et al. Prevalence of depression in cancer patients: a meta-analysis of diagnostic interviews and self-report instruments. *Psycho Oncol.* 2014;23(2):121–130.

94. Alberti KG, Zimmet P, Shaw J. Metabolic syndrome–a new world-wide definition. A consensus statement from the international diabetes federation. *Diabet Med.* 2006; 23(5):469–480.

95. Third report of the national cholesterol education program (NCEP) expert panel on detection, evaluation, and treatment of high blood cholesterol in adults (adult treatment panel III) final report. *Circulation.* 2002; 106(25):3143–3421.

96. Golden RN, Gilmore JH. Serotonin and mood disorders. *Psychiatr Ann.* 1990;20(10):580–586.

97. Diehl DJ, Gershon S. The role of dopamine in mood disorders. *Compr Psychiatr.* 1992;33(2):115–120.

98. Watson S, Mackin P. HPA axis function in mood disorders. *Psychiatry.* 2006;5(5):166–170.

99. Stannus OP, Jones G, Blizzard L, Cicuttini FM, Ding C. Associations between serum levels of inflammatory markers and change in knee pain over 5 years in older adults: a prospective cohort study. *Ann Rheum Dis.* 2013;72(4):535–540.

100. Il'yasova D, Colbert LH, Harris TB, et al. Circulating levels of inflammatory markers and cancer risk in the health aging and body composition cohort. *Cancer Epidemiol Biomark Prev.* 2005;14(10):2413–2418.

101. De Rekeneire N, Peila R, Ding J, et al. Diabetes, hyperglycemia, and inflammation in older individuals the health, aging and body composition study. *Diabetes Care.* 2006; 29(8):1902–1908.

102. Kiecolt-Glaser JK, Derry HM, Fagundes CP. Inflammation: depression fans the flames and feasts on the heat. *Am J Psychiatry.* 2015;172(11):1075–1091.

103. Volpato S, Guralnik JM, Ferrucci L, et al. Cardiovascular disease, interleukin-6, and risk of mortality in older women the women's health and aging study. *Circulation.* 2001;103(7):947–953.

104. Stuart MJ, Baune BT. Depression and type 2 diabetes: inflammatory mechanisms of a psychoneuroendocrine co-morbidity. *Neurosci Biobehav Rev.* 2012;36(1): 658–676.

105. Torre-Amione G, Kapadia S, Benedict C, Oral H, Young JB, Mann DL. Proinflammatory cytokine levels

in patients with depressed left ventricular ejection fraction: a report from the Studies of Left Ventricular Dysfunction (SOLVD). *J Am Coll Cardiol.* 1996;27(5): 1201–1206.

106. Miller GE, Stetler CA, Carney RM, Freedland KE, Banks WA. Clinical depression and inflammatory risk markers for coronary heart disease. *Am J Cardiol.* 2002; 90(12):1279–1283.

107. Guloksuz S, Wichers M, Kenis G, et al. Depressive symptoms in Crohn's disease: relationship with immune activation and tryptophan availability. *PLoS One.* 2013;8(3): e60435.

108. Bruce TO. Comorbid depression in rheumatoid arthritis: pathophysiology and clinical implications. *Curr Psychiatr Rep.* 2008;10(3):258–264.

109. Malemud CJ, Miller AH. Pro-inflammatory cytokine-induced SAPK/MAPK and JAK/STAT in rheumatoid arthritis and the new anti-depression drugs. *Expert Opinion on Therapeutic Targets.* 2008;12(2):171–183.

110. Illman J, Corringham R, Robinson D, et al. Are inflammatory cytokines the common link between cancer-associated cachexia and depression? *J Support Oncol.* 2005;3(1):37–50.

111. Myers JS. Proinflammatory cytokines and sickness behavior: implications for depression and cancer-related symptoms. In: *Paper Presented at: Oncology Nursing Forum.* 2008.

112. Choe SS, Huh JY, Hwang IJ, Kim JI, Kim JB. Adipose tissue remodeling: its role in energy metabolism and metabolic disorders. *Front Endocrinol.* 2016;7:30.

113. Iwata M, Ota KT, Duman RS. The inflammasome: pathways linking psychological stress, depression, and systemic illnesses. *Brain Behav Immun.* 2013;31:105–114.

114. Grant RW, Dixit VD. Mechanisms of disease: inflammasome activation and the development of type 2 diabetes. *Front Immunol.* 2013;4:50.

115. Lee HM, Kim JJ, Kim HJ, Shong M, Ku BJ, Jo EK. Upregulated NLRP3 inflammasome activation in patients with type 2 diabetes. *Diabetes.* 2013;62(1):194–204.

116. Stienstra R, van Diepen JA, Tack CJ, et al. Inflammasome is a central player in the induction of obesity and insulin resistance. *Proc Natl Acad Sci U S A.* 2011;108(37): 15324–15329.

117. Connat JL. Inflammasome and cardiovascular diseases. *Ann Cardiol Angeiol.* 2011;60(1):48–54.

118. Carney RM, Freedland KE. NLRP3 inflammasome as a mechanism linking depression and cardiovascular diseases. *Nat Rev Cardiol.* 2017;14(2).

119. Garg NJ. Inflammasomes in cardiovascular diseases. *Am J Cardiovas Dis.* 2011;1(3):244.

120. Fallowfield L, Ratcliffe D, Jenkins V, Saul J. Psychiatric morbidity and its recognition by doctors in patients with cancer. *Br J Canc.* 2001;84(8):1011.

121. Zitvogel L, Kepp O, Galluzzi L, Kroemer G. Inflammasomes in carcinogenesis and anticancer immune responses. *Nat Immunol.* 2012;13(4):343–351.

122. Eyre H, Baune BT. Neuroimmunological effects of physical exercise in depression. *Brain Behav Immun.* 2012; 26(2):251–266.

123. Cribbs DH, Berchtold NC, Perreau V, et al. Extensive innate immune gene activation accompanies brain aging, increasing vulnerability to cognitive decline and neurodegeneration: a microarray study. *J Neuroinflammation.* 2012;9:179.

124. Grosse L, Ambrée O, Jörgens S, et al. Cytokine levels in major depression are related to childhood trauma but not to recent stressors. *Psychoneuroendocrinology.* 2016;73:24–31.

125. Bufalino C, Hepgul N, Aguglia E, Pariante CM. The role of immune genes in the association between depression and inflammation: a review of recent clinical studies. *Brain Behav Immun.* 2013;31:31–47.

126. Eyre H, Baune BT. Neuroplastic changes in depression: a role for the immune system. *Psychoneuroendocrinology.* 2012;37(9):1397–1416.

127. Meyer JH, Ginovart N, Boovariwala A, et al. Elevated monoamine oxidase a levels in the brain: an explanation for the monoamine imbalance of major depression. *Arch Gen Psychiatr.* 2006;63(11):1209–1216.

128. Gotlib IH, Joormann J, Minor KL, Hallmayer J. HPA axis reactivity: a mechanism underlying the associations among 5-HTTLPR, stress, and depression. *Biol Psychiatry.* 2008;63(9):847–851.

129. Altamura C, Maes M, Dai J, Meltzer H. Plasma concentrations of excitatory amino acids, serine, glycine, taurine and histidine in major depression. *Eur Neuropsychopharmacol.* 1995;5:71–75.

130. Caspi A, Hariri AR, Holmes A, Uher R, Moffitt TE. Genetic sensitivity to the environment: the case of the serotonin transporter gene and its implications for studying complex diseases and traits. *Focus.* 2010;8(3):398–416.

131. Kalueff A, Olivier J, Nonkes L, Homberg J. Conserved role for the serotonin transporter gene in rat and mouse neurobehavioral endophenotypes. *Neurosci Biobehav Rev.* 2010;34(3):373–386.

132. Monroe SM, Slavich GM, Georgiades K. *The Social Environment and Depression: The Roles of Life Stress.* 2014.

133. Munhoz C, Garcia-Bueno B, Madrigal J, Lepsch L, Scavone C, Leza J. Stress-induced neuroinflammation: mechanisms and new pharmacological targets. *Braz J Med Biol Res.* 2008;41(12):1037–1046.

134. Sorrells SF, Sapolsky RM. An inflammatory review of glucocorticoid actions in the CNS. *Brain Behav Immun.* 2007;21(3):259–272.

135. Sapolsky RM. Why stress is bad for your brain. *Science.* 1996;273(5276):749–750.

136. Bremner JD, Vythilingam M, Vermetten E, et al. Reduced volume of orbitofrontal cortex in major depression. *Biol Psychiatry.* 2002;51(4):273–279.

137. McEwen BS, Sapolsky RM. Stress and cognitive function. *Curr Opin Neurobiol.* 1995;5(2):205–216.

138. Akhondzadeh S, Jafari S, Raisi F, et al. Clinical trial of adjunctive celecoxib treatment in patients with major

depression: a double blind and placebo controlled trial. *Depress Anxiety*. 2009;26(7):607–611.

139. Almeida OP, Alfonso H, Jamrozik K, Hankey GJ, Flicker L. Aspirin use, depression, and cognitive impairment in later life: the health in men study. *J Am Geriatr Soc*. 2010;58(5):990–992.

140. Fields C, Drye L, Vaidya V, Lyketsos C, Group AR. Celecoxib or naproxen treatment does not benefit depressive symptoms in persons age 70 and older: findings from a randomized controlled trial. *The American Journal of Geriatric Psychiatry*. 2012;20(6):505–513.

141. Gallagher PJ, Castro V, Fava M, et al. Antidepressant response in patients with major depression exposed to NSAIDs: a pharmacovigilance study. *Am J Psychiatry*. 2012;169(10):1065–1072.

142. Muller N, Schwarz MJ, Dehning S, et al. The cyclooxygenase-2 inhibitor celecoxib has therapeutic effects in major depression: results of a double-blind, randomized, placebo controlled, add-on pilot study to reboxetine. *Mol Psychiatr*. 2006;11(7):680–684.

143. Musil R, Schwarz MJ, Riedel M, et al. Elevated macrophage migration inhibitory factor and decreased transforming growth factor-beta levels in major depression–no influence of celecoxib treatment. *J Affect Disord*. 2011;134(1–3):217–225.

144. Nery FG, Monkul ES, Hatch JP, et al. Celecoxib as an adjunct in the treatment of depressive or mixed episodes of bipolar disorder: a double-blind, randomized, placebo-controlled study. *Hum Psychopharmacol*. 2008; 23(2):87–94.

145. Pasco JA, Jacka FN, Williams LJ, et al. Clinical implications of the cytokine hypothesis of depression: the association between use of statins and aspirin and the risk of major depression. *Psychother Psychosom*. 2010;79(5):323–325.

146. Uher R, Carver S, Power RA, et al. Non-steroidal anti-inflammatory drugs and efficacy of antidepressants in major depressive disorder. *Psychol Med*. 2012:1–9.

147. Warner-Schmidt JL, Vanover KE, Chen EY, Marshall JJ, Greengard P. Antidepressant effects of selective serotonin reuptake inhibitors (SSRIs) are attenuated by antiinflammatory drugs in mice and humans. *Proc Natl Acad Sci U S A*. 2011;108(22):9262–9267.

148. Shelton RC. Does concomitant use of NSAIDs reduce the effectiveness of antidepressants? *Am J Psychiatry*. 2012; 169(10):1012–1015.

149. Muller N. The role of anti-inflammatory treatment in psychiatric disorders. *Psychiatr Danub*. 2013;25(3): 292–298.

150. Fond G, Hamdani N, Kapczinski F, Boukouaci W, Drancourt N, Dargel A, Oliveira J, Le Guen E, Marlinge E, Tamouza R. Effectiveness and tolerance of anti-inflammatory drugs' add-on therapy in major mental disorders: a systematic qualitative review. *Acta Psychiatrica Scandinavica*. 2014;129(3):163–179.

151. Almeida OP, Flicker L, Yeap BB, Alfonso H, McCaul K, Hankey GJ. Aspirin decreases the risk of depression in older men with high plasma homocysteine. *Transl Psychiatry*. 2012;2:e151.

152. Iyengar RL, Gandhi S, Aneja A, et al. NSAIDs are associated with lower depression scores in patients with osteoarthritis. *Am J Med*. 2013;126(11):1017 e1011–1017 e1018.

153. Davis A, Gilhooley M, Agius M. Using non-steroidal anti-inflammatory drugs in the treatment of depression. *Psychiatr Danub*. 2010;22(suppl 1):S49–S52.

154. Maes M. Targeting cyclooxygenase-2 in depression is not a viable therapeutic approach and may even aggravate the pathophysiology underpinning depression. *Metab Brain Dis*. 2012;27(4):405–413.

155. Aid S, Bosetti F. Targeting cyclooxygenases-1 and -2 in neuroinflammation: therapeutic implications. *Biochimie*. 2011;93(1):46–51.

156. Berk M, Dean O, Drexhage H, et al. Aspirin: a review of its neurobiological properties and therapeutic potential for mental illness. *BMC Medicine*. 2013;11:74.

157. Choi SH, Aid S, Choi U, Bosetti F. Cyclooxygenases-1 and -2 differentially modulate leukocyte recruitment into the inflamed brain. *Pharmacogenomics J*. 2010;10(5): 448–457.

158. Eyre HA, Stuart MJ, Baune BT. A phase-specific neuroimmune model of clinical depression. *Prog Neuropsychopharmacol Biol Psychiatry*. 2014;54:265–274.

159. Mendlewicz J, Kriwin P, Oswald P, Souery D, Alboni S, Brunello N. Shortened onset of action of antidepressants in major depression using acetylsalicylic acid augmentation: a pilot open-label study. *Int Clin Psychopharmacol*. 2006;21(4):227–231.

160. lou Camara M, Corrigan F, Jaehne EJ, Jawahar MC, Anscomb H, Baune BT. Effects of centrally administered etanercept on behavior, microglia, and astrocytes in mice following a peripheral immune challenge. *Neuropsychopharmacology*. 2015;40(2):502–512.

161. Monje ML, Toda H, Palmer TD. Inflammatory blockade restores adult hippocampal neurogenesis. *Science*. 2003; 302(5651):1760–1765.

162. Zheng L-S, Kaneko N, Sawamoto K. Minocycline treatment ameliorates interferon-alpha-induced neurogenic defects and depression-like behaviors in mice. *Front Cell Neurosci*. 2015;9.

163. Fischer CW, Eskelund A, Budac DP, et al. Interferon-alpha treatment induces depression-like behaviour accompanied by elevated hippocampal quinolinic acid levels in rats. *Behav Brain Res*. 2015;293:166–172.

164. Tikka T, Fiebich BL, Goldsteins G, Keinänen R, Koistinaho J. Minocycline, a tetracycline derivative, is neuroprotective against excitotoxicity by inhibiting activation and proliferation of microglia. *J Neurosci*. 2001; 21(8):2580–2588.

165. Perneger TV, Whelton PK, Klag MJ. Risk of kidney failure associated with the use of acetaminophen, aspirin, and nonsteroidal antiinflammatory drugs. *N Engl J Med*. 1994;331(25):1675–1679.

166. Rainsford K. Profile and mechanisms of gastrointestinal and other side effects of nonsteroidal anti-inflammatory drugs (NSAIDs). *Am J Med*. 1999; 107(6):27–35.

167. Auriel E, Regev K, Korczyn AD. Nonsteroidal anti-inflammatory drugs exposure and the central nervous system. *Handb Clin Neurol*. 2014;119:577−584.

168. Goshen I, Kreisel T, Ben-Menachem-Zidon O, et al. Brain interleukin-1 mediates chronic stress-induced depression in mice via adrenocortical activation and hippocampal neurogenesis suppression. *Mol Psychiatr*. 2008;13(7): 717−728.

169. Koo JW, Duman RS. Evidence for IL-1 receptor blockade as a therapeutic strategy for the treatment of depression. *Curr Opin Investig Drugs*. 2009;10(7):664−671.

170. Kreisel T, Frank MG, Licht T, et al. Dynamic microglial alterations underlie stress-induced depressive-like behavior and suppressed neurogenesis. *Mol Psychiatr*. 2014;19(6): 699−709.

171. Gleeson M, Bishop NC, Stensel DJ, Lindley MR, Mastana SS, Nimmo MA. The anti-inflammatory effects of exercise: mechanisms and implications for the prevention and treatment of disease. *Nat Rev Immunol*. 2011; 11(9):607−615.

172. Petersen AMW, Pedersen BK. The anti-inflammatory effect of exercise. *J Appl Physiol*. 2005;98(4): 1154−1162.

173. Ernst C, Olson AK, Pinel JP, Lam RW, Christie BR. Antidepressant effects of exercise: evidence for an adult-neurogenesis hypothesis? *J Psychiatry Neurosci*. 2006; 31(2):84.

174. Hoffman-Goetz L, Pedersen BK. Exercise and the immune system: a model of the stress response? *Immunol Today*. 1994;15(8):382−387.

175. Nieman DC, Nehlsen-Cannarella SL. The immune response to exercise. In: *Paper Presented at: Seminars in Hematology*. 1994.

176. Smith J, Telford R, Mason I, Weidemann M. Exercise, training and neutrophil microbicidal activity. *Int J Sports Med*. 1990;11(03):179−187.

177. Nehlsen-Cannarella SL. Cellular responses to moderate and heavy exercise. *Can J Physiol Pharmacol*. 1998;76(5): 485−489.

178. Su K-P, Huang S-Y, Chiu C-C, Shen WW. Omega-3 fatty acids in major depressive disorder: a preliminary double-blind, placebo-controlled trial. *Eur Neuropsychopharmacol*. 2003;13(4):267−271.

179. Grenyer BF, Crowe T, Meyer B, et al. Fish oil supplementation in the treatment of major depression: a randomised double-blind placebo-controlled trial. *Prog Neuro Psychopharmacol Biol Psychiatr*. 2007;31(7):1393−1396.

180. Haroon E, Raison CL, Miller AH. Psychoneuroimmunology meets neuropsychopharmacology: translational implications of the impact of inflammation on behavior. *Neuropsychopharmacology*. 2012;37(1):137−162.

181. Kato TA, Kanba S. Are microglia minding us? Digging up the unconscious mind-brain relationship from a neuropsychoanalytic approach. *Front Hum Neurosci*. 2013;7:13.

CHAPTER 7

Psychiatric Comorbidity in Major Depressive Disorder

JUNGJIN KIM, MD • THOMAS L. SCHWARTZ, MD

INTRODUCTION

Major depressive disorder (MDD) frequently co-occurs with other psychiatric disorders, but these comorbidities are often underrecognized and undertreated because they are either overpowered symptomatically or disguised by MDD symptomatology.[1,2] In comparison to patients with only MDD, patients with co-occurring psychiatric disorders tend to have greater severity of illness and poorer longitudinal courses and outcomes. Additionally, these patients have higher healthcare utilization rates and greater impairment of psychosocial functioning, adding to the overall economic and social burden of MDD. Clinicians are, thus, encouraged to be diligent in screening for these co-occurring disorders as the resultant assessment may influence the clinical outcome narrowly and the public healthcare burden broadly. To that end, this chapter provides a synthesized overview of the epidemiological data of MDD's most frequent comorbidities: anxiety disorders, attention-deficit hyperactivity disorder (ADHD), substance use disorder (SUD), psychotic disorders, and personality disorders. In conclusion, the authors will provide practical assessment and treatment strategies in the management of comorbid MDD and these psychiatric disorders. The goal is to improve the readers' awareness of these co-occurrences and confidence to treat more effectively when these clinical challenges occur in day-to-day practice.

ANXIETY DISORDERS

Anxiety disorders are probably the most frequently encountered comorbid psychiatric conditions when treating patients with MDD. A lifetime prevalence study in the Netherlands ($n = 1783$) has shown that 75% of those with MDD suffered from concomitant anxiety disorder whereas 79% of those with anxiety disorders had MDD.[3] A larger, international study (24 countries,

$n = 74,045$) corroborated this finding: 45.7% of individuals with MDD had a lifetime diagnosis of one or more anxiety disorder.[4]

Twelve-month prevalence studies yield similar results. The National Comorbidity Survey Replication (NCS-R) of nationally representative sample in the United States (US), 65.2% of respondents with 12-month MDD had at least one other disorder and more than half of them (56.5%) were anxiety disorders.[5] Another epidemiological study in the Netherlands ($n = 7076$) showed that the rate of comorbid mood and anxiety disorders is 3.5%, higher than the rate of pure mood disorder (3.1%) but lower than that of having a pure anxiety disorder (7.7%).[6] Of those with mood disorder, 60.5% had comorbid mental health problems with anxiety topping the list at 54.3%. The approximate prevalence of MDD and each of the five anxiety disorders pooled from these epidemiological studies is shown in Table 7.1.

In addition to high rates of co-occurrence, patients with comorbid MDD and anxiety disorders tend to have poorer response to treatment than to the individual disorders.[7] These patients tend to have a more persistent and chronic course of MDD symptoms, greater overall symptom severity, increased functional impairment, and a lower quality of life.[1,7,8] Given the high rate of comorbidity and the associated clinical consequences, a thorough and systematic evaluation is needed at the time of initial psychiatric evaluation. This usually occurs when a psychiatric review of systems (discussed later in this chapter) is conducted.

The Canadian Network for Mood and Anxiety Treatment (CANMAT) task force has published useful guiding principles for managing comorbid psychiatric conditions.[9] These are (1) establishing accurate diagnoses, (2) diligent risk assessment, (3) establishing appropriate treatment settings, (4) addressing chronic disease management, (5) consideration for concurrent or

Major Depressive Disorder. https://doi.org/10.1016/B978-0-323-58131-8.00007-0

TABLE 7.1 Approximate MDD	
MDD + GAD	58%
MDD + PD	55%
MDD + OCD	37%
MDD + SAD	37%
MDD + PTSD	48%

sequential treatment, based on hierarchical assessment, and (6) use of measurement-based care. These general principles are useful when managing not only comorbid MDD and anxiety disorders but also other psychiatric disorders. Some of these skills will be discussed in the latter half of this chapter.

The diagnosis of both MDD and a co-occurring anxiety disorder is based on the DSM-5 criteria for the individual disorders. However, anxiety disorders and MDD have several overlapping symptoms, making the diagnosis at times complex. Common to both diagnoses include the following symptoms: irritability, psychomotor activation, difficulty with concentration, fatigue, and insomnia. What is not typical for anxiety disorders, however, is a pervasive depressed or sad affect, remarkable loss of interest, and a preoccupation with thoughts of death. Specifically interviewing for these later symptoms may be helpful and pivotal during assessment.

It is also important to establish whether the observed anxiety and depressive symptoms are due to MDD with anxious distress (a DSM-5 specifier for MDD) or MDD co-occurring with a premorbid, separate anxiety disorder. Anxiety symptoms in MDD with anxious distress are usually restricted and only occur during depressive episodes and resolve with effective MDD treatment. Presence of a separate anxiety disorder is likely to persist even longer and needs to be treated even when the MDD symptoms remit. The anxious subgroup of patients in the Sequenced Treatment Alternatives to Relieve Depression (STAR*D) trial indeed tended to have lower rates of antidepressant response and remission compared to the nonanxious subgroup.[10]

There are two other clinical and diagnostic conventions to consider if a clinician wishes to determine if a truly comorbid anxiety disorder is present with MDD. If the anxiety symptoms meet DSM-5 criteria and predate MDD, then it is felt to be that two separate disorders exist. In addition, if after a successful MDD treatment remission, anxiety symptoms meeting the DSM-5 criteria continue, then the disorders are considered separate and distinct.

The psychopharmacologic treatment of choice with the broadest coverage for all five anxiety disorders and MDD are the serotonergic antidepressants: selective serotonin reuptake inhibitors (SSRIs) and the selective serotonin-norepinephrine reuptake inhibitors (SNRIs). The agents that have dual approval for both MDD and anxiety disorders by the US Food and Drug Administration (FDA) are laid out in Table 7.2. The agent selection should be guided by patient preference and risk profile and the agent needs to be titrated throughout the effective therapeutic range. For rapid symptom relief for certain anxiety disorders—for example, generalized anxiety disorder (GAD), social anxiety disorder (SAD), or panic disorder (PD)—without a history of substance misuse, an addition of a long-acting benzodiazepine may be considered. Psychotherapy can be combined with pharmacotherapy to optimize outcome. Cognitive-behavioral therapy (CBT), acceptance and commitment therapy (ACT), and psychodynamic therapy are evidence-based treatment options for both MDD and anxiety disorders.[11,12]

ATTENTION-DEFICIT HYPERACTIVITY DISORDER

ADHD is a neurodevelopmental disorder of childhood onset associated with significant cognitive, academic, occupational, and social impairment. Approximately 7% of school-aged children meet the criteria for ADHD.[13] ADHD frequently persists into adulthood: up to 36% of adults with ADHD had been diagnosed with ADHD as children.[14] The adult ADHD prevalence rate is estimated to be 4.4%.[15]

The prevalence of MDD comorbid with ADHD ranges from 9% to 50% across a number of different studies.[15–17] The National Comorbidity Survey (NCS-RS), for instance, reported prevalence rates of MDD in individuals diagnosed with ADHD at 18.6% compared to just 7.8% in those without ADHD.[15] Individuals with comorbid MDD and ADHD are at higher risk, compared to those with ADHD alone, for poorer academic or occupational performance, mental health utilization rates, suicide risk, and social/vocational outcomes.[16–18] Oftentimes, ADHD impairs occupational and interpersonal function, which in turn leads to commensurate financial and social stress that predispose an individual with ADHD to development of MDD. Therefore, a low threshold of suspicion for comorbid depression should exist when managing patients with ADHD.

TABLE 7.2
Pharmacologic Agents That Have FDA Dual Approval for MDD

	MDD	GAD	Panic	OCD	SAD	PTSD
SELECTIVE SEROTONIN REUPTAKE INHIBITORS (SSRIS)						
Fluoxetine	X		X	X		
Sertraline	X		X	X	X	X
Paroxetine	X	X	X	X	X	X
Fluvoxamine				X		
Citalopram	X					
Escitalopram	X	X				
SELECTIVE SEROTONIN-NOREPINEPHRINE REUPTAKE INHIBITORS (SNRIS)						
Venlafaxine	X	X	X		X	
Desvenlafaxine	X					
Duloxetine	X	X				
Levomilnacipran	X					
SSRI-PLUS AGENTS						
Vilazodone	X					
Vortioxetine	X					
TRICYCLIC ANTIDEPRESSANTS (TCAS)						
Imipramine	X					
Amitriptyline	X					
Clomipramine	X			X		
Doxepin	X					
MONOAMINE OXIDASE INHIBITORS (MAOIS)						
Selegiline	X					
Phenelzine	X					
Tranylcypromine	X					

Diagnosing a comorbid depressive episode in an ADHD patient can be complicated by overlapping symptoms—inattention, distractibility, restlessness, or psychomotor activation. In addition, the consequences of untreated ADHD often result in recurrent social stressors, multiple adjustment disorders with resultant disappointments and demoralization that may mimic MDD. However, both the ADHD symptoms and its adverse psychosocial sequelae should dissipate with adequate treatment of ADHD with pharmacotherapy.

Persistent depressed or sad affect and preoccupation with suicidal ideas are not typical in patients with only ADHD and may thus serve as a symptomatic clue to the presence of comorbid MDD. McIntosh et al. (2009)[19] have compiled an expert consensus of practical assessment strategies that start with a 3-question screen

("have you ever been diagnosed with ADHD? Do you have a family history of ADHD? Did you have any difficulty in school – did you daydream or have difficulty paying attention? did you get your homework done on time, were you disruptive?"), followed by a functional impairment screen ("Do you currently have substantial difficulties with forgetfulness, attention, impulsivity or restlessness that are interfering with your relationships or your success at work?"). If answers to both of these are positive, then the clinician is encouraged to refine the diagnosis by completing a full diagnostic interview based on the DSM-5 criteria and then to administer the adult ADHD Self-Report Scale (ASRS). A thorough review of the patient's medical and psychiatric history and collection of data from collateral sources can be of great diagnostic value as well.

TABLE 7.3
Agents With Prominent Noradrenergic Effects That May Be Considered as Off-Label Treatment for ADHD.

SNRIs	Noradrenergic and Specific Serotonergic Antidepressants (NaSSA)	TCAs
Venlafaxine	Mirtazapine	Desipramine
Desvenlafaxine		Nortriptyline
Duloxetine		Protriptyline
Levomilnacipran		Imipramine (Metabolites)
		Amitriptyline (Metabolites)
Norepinephrine dopamine reuptake inhibitor (NDRIs)	**MAOIs**	**Second-generation antipsychotics (SGAs)**
Bupropion XL	Selegiline	Quetiapine
	Isocarboxazid	
	Phenelzine	
	Tranylcypromine	

Once the diagnoses of comorbid ADHD and MDD are both established, a sequential treatment strategy based on a hierarchy of greater clinical importance is often appropriate. In this strategy, the clinician treats the more symptomatically severe or functionally impairing disorder first—that is, if MDD is the most pressing clinical concern, it is treated first and vice versa. If MDD needs to be addressed first, a trial of antidepressant treatment should be started. If effective, the cognitive impairments associated with MDD should improve together with the affective symptoms. Should the patient still have cognitive difficulties despite improvement in mood symptoms, the cognitive symptoms may then be attributed to a comorbid diagnosis i.e. ADHD that subsequently needs to be treated.

When choosing an antidepressant to treat the comorbid ADHD and MDD, the clinician should consider an agent that increases synaptic norepinephrine such as bupropion, (des)venlafaxine, duloxetine, levomilnacipran, and TCAs as these agents work via norepinephrine reuptake inhibition similar to the ADHD-approved atomoxetine.[20,21] Atomoxetine has no known antidepressant effect so it should not be a monotherapy approach. Knowing these antidepressants with prominent noradrenergic effects may be helpful in strategizing off-label treatment for ADHD (Table 7.3). Currently, there are no jointly approved medications for MDD and ADHD as there exists for the MDD-anxiety comorbidity.

If ADHD is deemed more acute, a trial of long-acting stimulants, guided by risk–benefit discussion and patient preference, is often the next step in management. The use of stimulants to treat MDD may be considered as an off-label option, but there are no definitive data that they are effective as an MDD monotherapy. For patients at risk of substance abuse, nonaddictive alternatives such as the FDA-approved NRI atomoxetine or alpha 2 agonists (guanfacine or clonidine) are preferred. Once ADHD symptoms improve with these medications, MDD symptoms should be revisited to assess whether further treatment is needed to gain remission of both disorders.

Whether treating MDD first or ADHD first, it is often helpful to know how long it takes for each therapeutic option to exert its effect. For example, it can take 2–6 weeks for antidepressants to become effective,[22] while a stimulant titration to an effective dose may take a week.[23] Knowing the time course to response may guide the clinician as to which disorder is actually responding to treatment or is most prominent.

SUBSTANCE USE DISORDER

SUD is a serious public health concern that commonly co-occurs with MDD. Several epidemiological data confirm the high frequency of co-occurrence. The Epidemiological Catchment Area (ECA) study ($n = 20,291$) in the 1980's revealed that the rates of co-occurring alcohol use disorder (AUD) and nonalcohol SUD in patients with MDD were 16.5% and 18.0%, respectively.[24] The diagnosis of SUD (either alcohol or drug) almost doubled the risk of having a comorbid MDD when compared to individuals without a history of SUD. The US National Comorbidity Survey (NCS; $n = 5877$) conducted in the 1990s indicated that individuals with MDD were three times more likely to have a 12-month co-occurrence of SUD and twice as more likely to have a lifetime co-occurrence of SUD compared to the general population.[25] The National Study of Alcoholism and Related Conditions (NESARC; $n = 43,093$) conducted in the early 2000s have yielded even higher rates of co-occurrence with MDD: 3.7 times more likely for AUD and 9.0 times more likely for nonalcohol SUD.[26] Putting these results together, the presence of SUD consistently and remarkably increases the risk of MDD and the converse is also true. Similar to ADHD, SUD often remarkably increases interpersonal stress, social estrangement, and financial distress, making MDD more likely to occur.

Regarding different substances of abuse, the lifetime prevalence rates of MDD and AUD (20%–67%), cocaine use disorder (30%–40%), and opioid use disorder (54%) vary.[27] Common across these different substances are that the co-occurrence of MDD and SUD leads to greater symptom burden, higher rates of hospitalization and relapse, delayed recovery, and elevated risk of suicide.[28–32]

Diagnostic refinement regarding these common comorbidities can be made possible through (1) a careful history focusing on the symptom onset chronology of both MDD and SUD and (2) verification of patient history through data from multiple sources (e.g., collateral information from family, physical exam, laboratory tests). Ideally, the patient could be monitored during periods of abstinence from the substance of abuse or during periods of stable affective symptoms for clearer diagnosis. For example, MDD symptoms that follow increases of alcohol daily use or only after a cocaine binge do not strongly support a primary affective disorder but most likely a drug-induced depressive state. To do this, knowing the pharmacokinetics of each drug of abuse is essential (e.g., absorption, half-life, etc.).

Once the diagnosis of MDD and co-occurring SUD is established, treatment should follow. Three models of treatment exist for addressing co-occurring MDD and SUD: sequential, parallel, and integrated.[33] In the sequential treatment, SUD is treated first before targeting the comorbid MDD. In parallel treatment, both disorders are treated simultaneously but by two different clinicians, one for each disorder. For an integrated approach, both disorders are treated by the same clinician/team of clinicians, and there is increasing consensus that integrated treatment most often leads to improved clinical outcomes.[34–36]

Choice of treatment model often depends on available resources, but regardless of the model, the combination of psychosocial intervention and pharmacotherapy is the cornerstone of treatment.[33,37,38] Motivational interviewing (MI),[39] CBT,[40] and Community Reinforcement Approach (CRA)[41] have all shown efficacy for reducing substance misuse and depressive symptoms. Attendance at self-help groups (i.e., Alcoholics Anonymous [AA]) is encouraged and there is some evidence that long-term AA attendance may reduce depressive symptoms.[42]

Regarding pharmacotherapy, adjunctive antidepressant treatment to pharmacotherapy targeting the primary SUD (e.g., buprenorphine, methadone, naltrexone, acamprosate, etc.) may be considered. In several meta-analysis studies, it has been shown that antidepressant treatment may be helpful in improving depressive outcomes in depressed AUD patients but the result was more equivocal for depressed patients with opioid or cocaine use disorder.[43,44] It has been proposed that antidepressant treatment may be effective at reducing substance abuse by reducing depressive symptoms but by themselves may not improve substance abuse outcome independent of affective normalization.[45] Among antidepressants, TCAs, mirtazapine (NaSSA), and venlafaxine (SNRI) have shown more consistent efficacy than SSRIs. SSRI use is discouraged in patients with MDD and co-occurring early-onset, Babor's Type B AUD due to its association with worse clinical outcomes.[46]

PSYCHOTIC DISORDERS

Schizophrenia is a severe and chronic mental disorder that affects 1% of the population. Due in part to a striking resemblance of negative symptoms of schizophrenia—lack of spontaneous speech or movement, psychomotor retardation, blunted affect, lack of volition, and paucity of social interactions—with neurovegetative symptoms in a depressed individual, a comorbid MDD is often missed when treating patients with schizophrenia. It has been suggested that the estimated lifetime prevalence of MDD and schizophrenia is close to 25%,[47,48] which is well above the prevalence of MDD in the general population (17%). Schizophrenic patients are already inherently at higher risk of death by suicide, and when combined with depression, these patients are at even greater risk of self-harm.[49] In addition, a comorbid schizophrenia and MDD is associated with greater symptom severity and duration, higher frequency of psychotic relapse and rehospitalization, SUD, and diminished quality of life.[47,48,50–52] It is therefore important, both clinically and public healthwise, to screen for comorbid MDD when treating schizophrenic patients.

Diagnosing MDD in patients with schizophrenia can be challenging due to a long list of differential diagnoses. A systematic way of serially ruling out these possibilities and the patience to carry out this diagnostic investigation over several follow-ups are helpful. Siris and Bench (2007)[48] have described a useful list of differential diagnoses and steps to sequentially evaluate this. In this strategy, an organic etiology—including depressogenic medical problems, medications, substance misuse issues—is evaluated first, often in collaboration with the primary care physician. Acute psychosocial stressors are also assessed with a close follow-up scheduled. In the follow-up visit, depressive symptoms should have run its course if these were an acute psychological reaction to a proximal psychosocial stressor. Depressive symptoms may also be a marker for early stages of psychotic relapse. Careful screening for covert psychotic symptom emergence, together with antipsychotic adherence evaluation, and, if necessary, dose adjustment, may avert a relapse into a full psychotic decompensation.

If the depressive symptoms were not due to an acute psychological stress reaction or a prodromal psychotic relapse, antipsychotic-induced extrapyramidal side effects need to be ruled out. Parkinsonism with bradykinesia and masked facies may mimic MDD. A trial of anticholinergic agents to target bradykinesia may be warranted. In addition, akathisia may present as MDD with anxious distress. A trial of a benzodiazepine or a β-blocker to target akathisia may confirm or dismiss these clinical possibilities.

If psychotic symptoms are stable but depressive symptoms persist, a careful antipsychotic dose lowering may be required to rule out the possibility of an antipsychotic-induced dysphoria. Antipsychotic-induced dysphoria, commonly known as neuroleptic dysphoria, is a poorly understood phenomenon that is theorized to result from prefrontal dopamine blockade, causing executive dysfunction and increased negative symptoms from inhibited limbic dopamine neuronal pathways.[53] It is equivocal whether a particular antipsychotic is associated with higher or lower incidence of this phenomenon, but using this theory, a lower potency antipsychotic such as quetiapine, iloperidone, clozapine, or olanzapine may theoretically have lower risk of neuroleptic dysphoria.

If the psychotic symptoms are stable but the depressive symptoms persist despite above interventions, an adjunctive antidepressant treatment may be considered. SSRIs are usually given initial consideration, though patient preference and risk–benefit considerations should guide the overall selection process. Of note, SSRIs, particularly fluvoxamine, need to be used cautiously with clozapine as they may raise clozapine levels inappropriately via pharmacodynamic drug–drug interaction.[54] Tricyclic antidepressants may also be considered but their anticholinergic side effects may be additive to those of concurrent antipsychotic treatment.

It should be noted that the evidence base to support the use of adjunctive antidepressant is weak.[55,56]

A meta-analysis of 82 randomized controlled trials (RCTs; $n = 3608$)[50] examining depression scores for a wide range of antidepressants used in schizophrenics with MDD, did however find a statistically significant modest improvement in depressive symptom outcome (number needed to treat [NNT] = 5) similar to the NNT for individuals diagnosed only with MDD.[57] This study was limited by heterogeneity of results, disparate outcome reporting and failure to address multiple confounding factors. Although it is noteworthy that adjunctive antidepressant therapy was safe in combination with antipsychotics in this study, more investigation is needed to establish the efficacy of adjunctive antidepressant treatment for co-occurring schizophrenia and depression. Theoretically, second-generation antipsychotics with known antidepressant effects in MDD/bipolar depression could be preferentially prescribed (e.g., risperidone, olanzapine, quetiapine, aripiprazole, brexpiprazole, lurasidone). Lastly, a concurrent psychosocial intervention, such as CBT for psychosis and vocational rehabilitation, should accompany pharmacotherapy to optimize treatment outcome.[58]

PERSONALITY DISORDERS

Considering the impact of character pathology is important when evaluating patients with MDD. Personality disorders (PDO) are highly prevalent in depressed individuals in both inpatient and outpatient settings. A meta-analysis across 122 studies ($n = 24,867$) observed the rate of at least one PDO concurrent with MDD at 45%.[59] This rate was even higher at 60% for persistent depressive disorder in the same study. The most common PDOs were "cluster C personality disorders" (avoidant, dependent, and obsessive-compulsive) and borderline personality disorder (BPD) as laid out in Table 7.4. The presence of these comorbid personality pathologies, particularly BPD, has been associated with persistent and protracted courses of MDD, higher likelihood of SUD and self-harm behaviors.[60]

A detailed description of the MDD-PDO interplay and diagnostic assessment is outside the scope of this chapter, but the key to assessing comorbid PDO in depressed patients is the presence of longitudinal symptomatology. Symptoms due to personality pathology are often chronic and enduring whereas symptoms of a pure mood disorder are often limited and episodic. It is not uncommon to take several clinical sessions to link together to arrive at the diagnosis of a PDO.

Unfortunately, no medication is remarkably efficacious for PDO per se, but the comorbid depressive episodes may have a better chance of responding to

TABLE 7.4 MDD-PDO Prevalence Rates.[59]	
MDD + Any PDO	**45%**
MDD + Cluster A PDO	**9%**
MDD + Paranoid PDO	7%
MDD + Schizoid PDO	2%
MDD + Schizotypal PDO	3%
MDD + Cluster B PDO	**19%**
MDD + Antisocial PDO	3%
MDD + Borderline PDO	14%
MDD + Histrionic PDO	6%
MDD + Narcissistic PDO	4%
MDD + Cluster C PDO	**30%**
MDD + Avoidant PDO	16%
MDD + Dependent PDO	10%
MDD + Obsessive-compulsive PDO	9%

comorbid psychiatric disorders. To avoid overlooking a comorbidity, the clinician should assess the patient systematically using a psychiatric ROS, much like the way a nonpsychiatric physician would use a medical ROS. It is often helpful to categorize the psychiatric disorders into eight major clusters: (1) depressive disorders, (2) bipolar disorders, (3) psychotic disorders, (4) anxiety disorders, (5) substance use disorders, (6) personality disorders, (7) ADHD and cognitive disorders, and (8) negative body perception disorders (i.e., eating disorders, somatization disorders). The clinician would then interview regarding each of the disorders with screening questions. A positive response to the screening questions should prompt more thorough follow-up questions guided by the full DSM-5 criteria, and if needed, supplementation with pertinent psychometric scales and collateral information from family and friends, to refine the diagnosis. Useful screening questionnaires adapted from Schwartz (2017)[69] are summarized in Table 7.5.

pharmacotherapy with concurrent psychological or psychosocial intervention. Psychosocial treatment is the centerpiece of PDO treatment. Bateman et al. (2015)[61] have described the existing evidence-based psychosocial, psychological and pharmacotherapeutic treatment options for a wide range of PDOs. CBT and psychodynamic therapy have been shown to be effective for "cluster C personality disorders" with reports of medium to large positive effect sizes.[62,63] No randomized controlled trials of medications have been reported for "cluster C personality disorders." For BPD, several psychotherapeutic modalities—dialectical behavioral therapy (DBT),[64] mentalization-based therapy (MBT),[65] transference-focused therapy (TFT),[66] good psychiatric management (GPM),[67] and dynamic deconstructive psychotherapy (DDP)[68]—have an evidence base to support their use, but these treatments vary widely in their accessibility, time commitment, and cost. It is also unclear how these work when PDO and MDD are comorbid. Drug treatment for BPD should be used cautiously and adjunctively added to psychosocial treatments to target specific symptoms, keeping in mind the risk of intentional overdose.

CONDUCTING A GOOD PSYCHIATRIC REVIEW OF SYSTEMS

A good psychiatric review of systems (ROS) can be both useful and critical in identifying patients with

MEASUREMENT-BASED CARE: USE IT!

There are several validated rating scales that can supplement the diagnostic interview. Rating scales are completed by the patient or the provider on paper or electronically at each clinical encounter. The same scale should be used consistently so that the clinician can obtain a baseline and follow the trajectory of the symptoms and impairments longitudinally. Abnormal findings should prompt the clinician to make adjustments to the treatment accordingly. The scales vary widely in their sensitivity, specificity, price, and length. For MDD, the Patient Health Questionnaire (PHQ-9), the Hamilton Rating Scale for Depression (HAM-D), the Montgomery-Asberg Depression Rating Scale (MADRS), the Beck Depression Inventory (BDI), and the Quick Inventory of Depressive Symptomatology (QIDs) are all valid scales.[70,71] For anxiety disorders, Generalized Anxiety Disorder-7 (GAD-7) can be used for GAD, Social Anxiety Questionnaire for Adults (SAQ) or Liebowitz Social Anxiety Scale (LSAS) for SAD, the DSM Severity Measure for Panic Disorder for panic disorder, the PTSD Civilian Checklist (PCL-5) for PTSD, and Obsessive-Compulsive Inventory (OCI-R) or Yale-Brown Obsessive-Compulsive Scale (YBOCS) for OCD.[71] For ADHD, the Adult ADHD Self-Report Scale (ASRS) is validated and widely used.[72] For schizophrenia, the Brief Psychiatric Rating Scale (BPRS), Clinical Global Impression (CGI), and Positive and Negative Syndrome Scale (PANSS) are commonly used.[73] For SUD, Alcohol Use Disorders

TABLE 7.5
Screening Questions for Psychiatric ROS.

DEPRESSIVE DISORDERS

MDD

- In the last 2 weeks, have you been feeling down, depressed, or hopeless?
- In the last 2 weeks, have you had little interest or pleasure in doing things?

PDD

- Have you been feeling sad or low more often than not over two or more years continuously?
- Have you functioned alright despite this?

Premenstrual dysphoric disorder (PMDD)

- Do you typically only get depressed, anxious, or irritable just before and/or during your period?
- Do you completely recover from these symptoms outside of this timeframe?

MDD with a seasonal pattern

- Do you typically function well all year, and then suffer depression only during the winter months?

BIPOLAR DISORDER

- Have there been times lasting at least 4 days when you felt abnormally high, on top of the world, or overly happy?
- What about a period lasting at least 4 days when you needed little sleep but were full of energy and never tired despite not sleeping?

PSYCHOTIC DISORDERS

- In your life, have you ever saw or heard things that others cannot or that did not make sense?
- Have you ever been paranoid or felt people were out to get you, trying to harm you, or following you around?

ANXIETY DISORDERS

- Do you worry, more often than not, continuously about multiple different things for more than 6 months?
- Do you fear being the center of attention or being scrutinized by others where you feel you will be embarrassed? Do you avoid certain places or events because of this?
- Do you have panic attacks where you have a sudden rush of physical symptoms such as feeling sweaty, shaky, jittery, and heart beating fast, for no apparent reason?
- Have you been in a traumatic event like a mugging, assault, natural disaster, car crash, etc., where despite being safe months after, you still had nightmares and recurrent thoughts about the event?
- Do you have repetitive, intrusive thoughts that are distasteful, bothersome, or disturbing that are hard to dismiss? How about repetitive behaviors like hand washing, checking things, etc., that you feel like cannot stop doing?

SUBSTANCE USE DISORDERS

- Do you drink or use drugs at all? Ever?
- Have you ever gotten in trouble in relationships, at work, or legally, because you lost control over the amount you used?

ADHD

- Do you often make careless mistakes at home, work, or school because you are not paying attention?
- Is it hard for you to sit still?
- What problems do these behaviors cause at school, work or home?
- How old were you when you began these behaviors?

COGNITIVE DISORDERS

- Do you find yourself losing things more easily? Have you found it difficult to learn new things late?
- Have you recently noticed any memory problems?

EATING DISORDERS

- How do you feel about your weight? What do you make of your body size and how comfortable are you with yourself in this aspect?

- Do you ever go through short periods of time where you feel compelled to eat tons of food? Have you made yourself throw up after eating?

SOMATIZATION DISORDERS

- In the past several months, have you been persistently bothered by any physical symptoms? How about physical appearance? Or spent a lot of time thinking that you have or will get a serious illness?

Identification Test (AUDIT), and Drug Abuse Screen Test (DAST-10) are helpful and are being increasingly used in primary care settings.[74] Alternatively, a clinician may use a single, longer full DSM inventory such as the Psychiatric Diagnostic Screening Questionnaire (PDSQ).[75] For PDOs, the Standardized Assessment of Personality-Abbreviated Scale (SAPAS), Personality Diagnostic Questionnaire-4 (PDQ-4), and self-report Iowa Personality Disorder Screen (IPDS) are short and useful.[76]

Although the use of measurement-based care has been associated with improved outcomes and shorter time to response and remission,[77] it is important to note that the use of scales should be thought of as a supplement to, and not a replacement for an empathic, responsive, professional diagnostic interview. Judicious and consistent use of these scales allows for a faster, more focused clinical encounters during which the clinician can use the remaining time for rapport-building, informed consent, safety assessment, and use core psychotherapy techniques such as motivational interviewing to improve clinical outcome.

CONCLUDING REMARKS

The co-occurrence of MDD and other psychiatric disorders is quite common. The clinical implications generally amount to greater symptom severity and worsened longitudinal course and poorer outcome. Despite the high frequency of co-occurrence and clinical implications, there is yet limited prospective research aimed at identifying overlapping etiologic commonalities and improving treatment outcome. The joint occurrence of MDD and psychiatric disorders remains an underexplored therapeutic frontier that may offer opportunities for refining disease models and improving clinical outcome in this population with clearly unmet treatment needs.

DISCLOSURE

Authors have no conflicts of interest to disclose.

REFERENCES

1. Johansson R, Carlbring P, Heedman A, Paxling B, Andersson G. Depression, anxiety and their comorbidity in the Swedish general population: point prevalence and the effect on health-related quality of life. *Peer J.* 2013;1: e98.
2. Kessler RC, Chiu WT, Demler O, Merikangas KR, Walters EE. Prevalence, severity, and comorbidity of 12-month DSM-IV disorders in the national comorbidity survey replication. *Arch Gen Psychiatr.* 2005;62(6):617—627.
3. Lamers F, van Oppen P, Comijs HC, et al. Comorbidity patterns of anxiety and depressive disorders in a large cohort study: The Netherlands Study of Depression and Anxiety (NESDA). *J Clin Psychiatry.* 2011;72(3):341—348.
4. Kessler RC, Sampson NA, Berglund P, et al. Anxious and non-anxious major depressive disorder in the World Health Organization World Mental Health Surveys. *Epidemiol Psychiatr Sci.* 2015;24(3):210—226.
5. Kessler RC, Berglund P, Demler O, et al. The epidemiology of major depressive disorder: results from the National Comorbidity Survey Replication (NCS-R). *JAMA.* 2003; 289(23):3095—3105.
6. de Graaf R, Bijl RV, Smit F, Vollebergh WA, Spijker J. Risk factors for 12-month comorbidity of mood, anxiety, and substance use disorders: findings from The Netherlands Mental Health Survey and Incidence Study. *Am J Psychiatry.* 2002;159(4):620—629.
7. Penninx BW, Nolen WA, Lamers F, et al. Two-year course of depressive and anxiety disorders: results from The Netherlands Study of Depression and Anxiety (NESDA). *J Affect Disord.* 2011;133(1—2):76—85.
8. Kessler R, White LA, Birnbaum H, et al. Comparative and interactive effects of depression relative to other health problems on work performance in the workforce of a large employer. *J Occup Environ Med.* 2008;50(7): 809—816.
9. McIntyre RS, Rosenbluth M, Ramasubbu R, et al. Managing medical and psychiatric comorbidity in individuals

with major depressive disorder and bipolar disorder. *Ann Clin Psychiatr.* 2012;24(2):163–169.

10. Fava M, Rush AJ, Alpert JE, et al. Difference in treatment outcome in outpatients with anxious versus nonanxious depression: a STAR*D report. *Am J Psychiatry.* 2008; 165(3):342–351.

11. Arch JJ, Eifert GH, Davies C, Plumb Vilardaga JC, Rose RD, Craske MG. Randomized clinical trial of cognitive behavioral therapy (CBT) versus acceptance and commitment therapy (ACT) for mixed anxiety disorders. *J Consult Clin Psychol.* 2012;80(5):750–765.

12. Fonagy P. The effectiveness of psychodynamic psychotherapies: an update. *World Psychiatry.* 2015;14(2):137–150.

13. Thomas R, Sanders S, Doust J, Beller E, Glasziou P. Prevalence of attention-deficit/hyperactivity disorder: a systematic review and meta-analysis. *Pediatrics.* 2015;135(4): e994–1001.

14. Kessler RC, Adler LA, Barkley R, et al. Patterns and predictors of attention-deficit/hyperactivity disorder persistence into adulthood: results from the national comorbidity survey replication. *Biol Psychiatry.* 2005;57(11):1442–1451.

15. Kessler RC, Adler L, Barkley R, et al. The prevalence and correlates of adult ADHD in the United States: results from the National Comorbidity Survey Replication. *Am J Psychiatry.* 2006;163(4):716–723.

16. Biederman J, Ball SW, Monuteaux MC, et al. New insights into the comorbidity between ADHD and major depression in adolescent and young adult females. *J Am Acad Child Adolesc Psychiatry.* 2008;47(4):426–434.

17. Gjervan B, Torgersen T, Nordahl HM, Rasmussen K. Functional impairment and occupational outcome in adults with ADHD. *J Atten Disord.* 2012;16(7):544–552.

18. Furczyk K, Thome J. Adult ADHD and suicide. *Attention deficit and hyperactivity disorders.* 2014;6(3):153–158.

19. McIntosh D, Kutcher S, Binder C, Levitt A, Fallu A, Rosenbluth M. Adult ADHD and comorbid depression: a consensus-derived diagnostic algorithm for ADHD. *Neuropsychiatr Dis Treat.* 2009;5:137–150.

20. Wilens TE, Spencer TJ, Biederman J, et al. A controlled clinical trial of bupropion for attention deficit hyperactivity disorder in adults. *Am J Psychiatry.* 2001;158(2):282–288.

21. Park P, Caballero J, Omidian H. Use of serotonin norepinephrine reuptake inhibitors in the treatment of attention-deficit hyperactivity disorder in pediatrics. *Ann Pharmacother.* 2014;48(1):86–92.

22. Lam RW. Onset, time course and trajectories of improvement with antidepressants. *Eur Neuropsychopharmacol.* 2012;22(suppl 3):S492–S498.

23. Medori R, Ramos-Quiroga JA, Casas M, et al. A randomized, placebo-controlled trial of three fixed dosages of prolonged-release OROS methylphenidate in adults with attention-deficit/hyperactivity disorder. *Biol Psychiatry.* 2008;63(10):981–989.

24. Regier DA, Farmer ME, Rae DS, et al. Comorbidity of mental disorders with alcohol and other drug abuse. Results from the Epidemiologic Catchment Area (ECA) Study. *JAMA.* 1990;264(19):2511–2518.

25. Kessler RC, Nelson CB, McGonagle KA, Edlund MJ, Frank RG, Leaf PJ. The epidemiology of co-occurring addictive and mental disorders: implications for prevention and service utilization. *Am J Orthopsychiatry.* 1996; 66(1):17–31.

26. Hasin DS, Goodwin RD, Stinson FS, Grant BF. Epidemiology of major depressive disorder: results from the national epidemiologic survey on alcoholism and related conditions. *Arch Gen Psychiatr.* 2005;62(10): 1097–1106.

27. Ross S. Substance abuse and mental illness. In: *The American Psychiatric Publishing Textbook of Substance Abuse Treatment.* American Psychiatric Publishing; 2014.

28. Hser YI, Grella C, Evans E, Huang YC. Utilization and outcomes of mental health services among patients in drug treatment. *J Addict Dis.* 2006;25(1):73–85.

29. Cornelius JR, Salloum IM, Mezzich J, et al. Disproportionate suicidality in patients with comorbid major depression and alcoholism. *Am J Psychiatry.* 1995;152(3): 358–364.

30. Bovasso GB. Cannabis abuse as a risk factor for depressive symptoms. *Am J Psychiatry.* 2001;158(12):2033–2037.

31. Havard A, Teesson M, Darke S, Ross J. Depression among heroin users: 12-Month outcomes from the Australian Treatment Outcome Study (ATOS). *J Subst Abus Treat.* 2006;30(4):355–362.

32. Landheim AS, Bakken K, Vaglum P. Impact of comorbid psychiatric disorders on the outcome of substance abusers: a six year prospective follow-up in two Norwegian counties. *BMC Psychiatry.* 2006;6(1):44.

33. Kim Y, Hack LM, Ahn ES, Kim J. Practical outpatient pharmacotherapy for alcohol use disorder. *Drugs Context.* 2018; 7:212308.

34. Weiss RD, Griffin ML, Kolodziej ME, et al. A randomized trial of integrated group therapy versus group drug counseling for patients with bipolar disorder and substance dependence. *Am J Psychiatry.* 2007;164(1):100–107.

35. Mangrum LF, Spence RT, Lopez M. Integrated versus parallel treatment of co-occurring psychiatric and substance use disorders. *J Subst Abus Treat.* 2006;30(1):79–84.

36. Lydecker KP, Tate SR, Cummins KM, McQuaid J, Granholm E, Brown SA. Clinical outcomes of an integrated treatment for depression and substance use disorders. *Psychol Addict Behav.* 2010;24(3):453–465.

37. Reus VI, Fochtmann LJ, Bukstein O, et al. The American psychiatric association practice guideline for the pharmacological treatment of patients with alcohol use disorder. *Am J Psychiatry.* 2018;175(1):86–90.

38. Murthy P, Chand P. Treatment of dual diagnosis disorders. *Curr Opin Psychiatr.* 2012;25(3):194–200.

39. Satre DD, Leibowitz A, Sterling SA, Lu Y, Travis A, Weisner C. A randomized clinical trial of Motivational Interviewing to reduce alcohol and drug use among patients with depression. *J Consult Clin Psychol.* 2016;84(7): 571–579.

40. Hides L, Samet S, Lubman DI. Cognitive behaviour therapy (CBT) for the treatment of co-occurring depression

and substance use: current evidence and directions for future research. *Drug Alcohol Rev.* 2010;29(5):508−517.

41. Higgins ST, Sigmon SC, Wong CJ, et al. Community reinforcement therapy for cocaine-dependent outpatients. *Arch Gen Psychiatr.* 2003;60(10):1043−1052.

42. Wilcox CE, Pearson MR, Tonigan JS. Effects of long-term AA attendance and spirituality on the course of depressive symptoms in individuals with alcohol use disorder. *Psychol Addict Behav.* 2015;29(2):382−391.

43. Torrens M, Fonseca F, Mateu G, Farre M. Efficacy of antidepressants in substance use disorders with and without comorbid depression. A systematic review and meta-analysis. *Drug Alcohol Depend.* 2005;78(1):1−22.

44. Nunes EV, Levin FR. Treatment of depression in patients with alcohol or other drug dependence: a meta-analysis. *JAMA.* 2004;291(15):1887−1896.

45. Nunes E, Weiss R. Co-occurring addiction and affective disorders. In: *Principles of addiction medicine.* 4. 2009.

46. Dundon W, Lynch KG, Pettinati HM, Lipkin C. Treatment outcomes in type A and B alcohol dependence 6 months after serotonergic pharmacotherapy. *Alcohol Clin Exp Res.* 2004;28(7):1065−1073.

47. Buckley PF, Miller BJ, Lehrer DS, Castle DJ. Psychiatric comorbidities and schizophrenia. *Schizophr Bull.* 2009; 35(2):383−402.

48. Siris SG, Bench C. Depression and schizophrenia. In: Hirsch SR, R WD, eds. *Schizophrenia.* Malden, MA: Blackwell Publishing Company; 2007:142−167.

49. Popovic D, Benabarre A, Crespo JM, et al. Risk factors for suicide in schizophrenia: systematic review and clinical recommendations. *Acta Psychiatr Scand.* 2014;130(6): 418−426.

50. Johnson DA. The significance of depression in the prediction of relapse in chronic schizophrenia. *Br J Psychiatry.* 1988;152:320−323.

51. Mandel MR, Severe JB, Schooler NR, Gelenberg AJ, Mieske M. Development and prediction of postpsychotic depression in neuroleptic-treated schizophrenics. *Arch Gen Psychiatr.* 1982;39(2):197−203.

52. Sim K, Mahendran R, Siris SG, Heckers S, Chong SA. Subjective quality of life in first episode schizophrenia spectrum disorders with comorbid depression. *Psychiatr Res.* 2004;129(2):141−147.

53. Awad AG, Voruganti LN. Neuroleptic dysphoria: revisiting the concept 50 years later. *Acta Psychiatr Scand Suppl.* 2005; (427):6−13.

54. Centorrino F, Baldessarini RJ, Frankenburg FR, Kando J, Volpicelli SA, Flood JG. Serum levels of clozapine and norclozapine in patients treated with selective serotonin reuptake inhibitors. *Am J Psychiatry.* 1996;153(6): 820−822.

55. Buoli M, Serati M, Ciappolino V, Altamura AC. May selective serotonin reuptake inhibitors (SSRIs) provide some benefit for the treatment of schizophrenia? *Expert Opin Pharmacother.* 2016;17(10):1375−1385.

56. Helfer B, Samara MT, Huhn M, et al. Efficacy and safety of antidepressants added to antipsychotics for schizophrenia:

a systematic review and meta-analysis. *Am J Psychiatry.* 2016;173(9):876−886.

57. Gibbons RD, Hur K, Brown CH, Davis JM, Mann JJ. Benefits from antidepressants: synthesis of 6-week patient-level outcomes from double-blind placebo-controlled randomized trials of fluoxetine and venlafaxine. *Arch Gen Psychiatr.* 2012;69(6):572−579.

58. Turner DT, van der Gaag M, Karyotaki E, Cuijpers P. Psychological interventions for psychosis: a meta-analysis of comparative outcome studies. *Am J Psychiatry.* 2014; 171(5):523−538.

59. Friborg O, Martinsen EW, Martinussen M, Kaiser S, Overgard KT, Rosenvinge JH. Comorbidity of personality disorders in mood disorders: a meta-analytic review of 122 studies from 1988 to 2010. *J Affect Disord.* 2014; 152−154:1−11.

60. Yoshimatsu K, Palmer B. Depression in patients with borderline personality disorder. *Harv Rev Psychiatry.* 2014;22(5):266−273.

61. Bateman AW, Gunderson J, Mulder R. Treatment of personality disorder. *Lancet.* 2015;385(9969):735−743.

62. Svartberg M, Stiles TC, Seltzer MH. Randomized, controlled trial of the effectiveness of short-term dynamic psychotherapy and cognitive therapy for cluster C personality disorders. *Am J Psychiatry.* 2004;161(5):810−817.

63. Simon W. Follow-up psychotherapy outcome of patients with dependent, avoidant and obsessive-compulsive personality disorders: a meta-analytic review. *Int J Psychiatry Clin Pract.* 2009;13(2):153−165.

64. van den Bosch LM, Verheul R, Schippers GM, van den Brink W. Dialectical Behavior Therapy of borderline patients with and without substance use problems. Implementation and long-term effects. *Addict Behav.* 2002; 27(6):911−923.

65. Bateman A, Fonagy P. Randomized controlled trial of outpatient mentalization-based treatment versus structured clinical management for borderline personality disorder. *Am J Psychiatry.* 2009;166(12):1355−1364.

66. Clarkin JF, Levy KN, Lenzenweger MF, Kernberg OF. Evaluating three treatments for borderline personality disorder: a multiwave study. *Am J Psychiatry.* 2007;164(6): 922−928.

67. Gunderson J, Masland S, Choi-Kain L. Good psychiatric management: a review. *Curr Opin Psychol.* 2018;21: 127−131.

68. Gregory RJ, DeLucia-Deranja E, Mogle JA. Dynamic deconstructive psychotherapy versus optimized community care for borderline personality disorder co-occurring with alcohol use disorders: a 30-month follow-up. *J Nerv Ment Dis.* 2010;198(4):292−298.

69. Schwartz TL. *Practical Psychopharmacology: Basic to Advanced Principles.* 2017.

70. Furukawa TA. Assessment of mood: guides for clinicians. *J Psychosom Res.* 2010;68(6):581−589.

71. Baer L, Blais MA. *Handbook of Clinical Rating Scales and Assessment in Psychiatry and Mental Health.* New York: Humana; 2012.

72. Kessler RC, Adler L, Ames M, et al. The World Health Organization Adult ADHD Self-Report Scale (ASRS): a short screening scale for use in the general population. *Psychol Med.* 2005;35(2):245–256.

73. Mortimer AM. Symptom rating scales and outcome in schizophrenia. *Br J Psychiatr Suppl.* 2007;50:s7–14.

74. Maisto SA, Carey MP, Carey KB, Gordon CM, Gleason JR. Use of the AUDIT and the DAST-10 to identify alcohol and drug use disorders among adults with a severe and persistent mental illness. *Psychol Assess.* 2000;12(2):186–192.

75. Zimmerman M, Mattia JI. The psychiatric diagnostic screening questionnaire: development, reliability and validity. *Compr Psychiatr.* 2001;42(3):175–189.

76. Germans S, Van Heck GL, Hodiamont PP. Results of the search for personality disorder screening tools: clinical implications. *J Clin Psychiatry.* 2012;73(2):165–173.

77. Guo T, Xiang YT, Xiao L, et al. Measurement-based care versus standard care for major depression: a randomized controlled trial with blind raters. *Am J Psychiatry.* 2015; 172(10):1004–1013.

CHAPTER 8

Pharmacological Treatment of Major Depressive Disorder

JOSHUA D. ROSENBLAT, BSC, MD • ROGER S. MCINTYRE, MD, FRCP(C)

INTRODUCTION

Major depressive disorder (MDD) is the leading cause of disability worldwide, affecting more than 350 million people globally.[1] As such, the effective treatment and prevention of MDD is an international priority. Antidepressants have a strong evidence base for the treatment of MDD, for moderate-to-severe major depressive episodes (MDEs).[2] Psychotherapy (e.g., cognitive behavioral therapy) and brain stimulation (e.g., electroconvulsive therapy [ECT]) are important alternative modalities of treatment; however, they have several limitations, including but not limited, availability, scalability, acceptability, cost, tolerability, and safety. Therefore, pharmacotherapy remains the cornerstone of treatment for MDD in most parts of the world.[3]

Most currently approved antidepressants modulate the monoamine system (e.g., serotonin, norepinephrine, dopamine). Targeting the monoamine system to treat depression was serendipitously discovered through observing antidepressant "side effects" of iproniazid, a monoamine oxidase inhibitor (MAO-I), initially developed for the treatment of tuberculosis (TB) in the early 1950s.[4] Iproniazid was soon after studied specifically for the treatment of depression and found to have significant antidepressant effects in most patients, thus making iproniazid the first effective pharmacological treatment of MDD. This serendipitous discovery lead to the articulation of the monoamine hypothesis of depression, which, on a societal level, also lead to the further development of the biological model of depression.[5] The biological model allowed for depression to be understood as a product of neurobiological changes in the brain and body, rather than solely the result of unresolved psychodynamic tensions of the mind.[6] Indeed, this new biological understanding of depression sparked the investigation of numerous new pharmacological treatments over the past 60 years,

targeting the monoamine system from a variety of angles, yielding the large number of monoaminergic antidepressants currently available today (e.g., tricyclic antidepressants [TCAs], selective serotonin reuptake inhibitors [SSRIs]).[4]

Although the development of monoaminergic antidepressants greatly advanced the field of psychiatry, the sole focus on the monoamine system has also hampered the development of novel antidepressants targeting other systems.[5] Newer "me too" monoaminergic antidepressants have yielded minimal improvements in efficacy, but rather have primarily made improvements in tolerability. Moreover, after decades of drug development, currently available treatments continue to have high rates of treatment resistance, with approximately one-quarter of patients failing to achieve remission after several trials of evidence-based antidepressant monotherapies and augmentation strategies.[7] Replicated evidence has also demonstrated that patients who have achieved remission (i.e., based on depressive symptom severity scores being in the normal range) frequently continue to experience persistent functional and cognitive impairments with poor quality of life being commonly reported.[8,9] As such, there is still a great need to discover new pharmacological treatments for MDD with superior efficacy and disease-modifying effects.

This chapter will focus on pharmacological treatments of MDD. Numerous evidence-based treatments are currently available. In addition, new treatments are currently being investigated that hold promise for improved treatment outcomes. The specific objectives of this chapter are to review evidence-based pharmacological treatments, including recently approved antidepressants, along with promising experimental pharmacological treatments that are likely to be translated into clinical practice in the near future. After reviewing the various drug classes and specific agents,

Major Depressive Disorder. https://doi.org/10.1016/B978-0-323-58131-8.00008-2

the general principles of pharmacological treatment of MDD will be discussed, including principles of initial antidepressant selection and management of treatment-resistant depression (TRD).

CURRENTLY APPROVED PHARMACOLOGICAL TREATMENTS OF DEPRESSION

As shown in Table 8.1, there are numerous different evidence-based antidepressants that are subcategorized into drug classes based on the primary mechanism of action. The main drug classes of antidepressants are SSRIs, selective serotonin and norepinephrine reuptake inhibitors (SNRIs), norepinephrine and dopamine reuptake inhibitors (NDRI), noradrenergic and specific serotonergic agents (NaSSAs), TCAs, MAO-Is, and melatonin modulators (agomelatine). More recently, multimodal serotonin modulator and stimulator (SMS) antidepressants (e.g., vortioxetine and vilazodone) have also been Food and Drug Administration (FDA)-approved, targeting the serotonin transporter (SERT) along with modulating specific serotonin receptors. This section reviews these drug classes and commonly prescribed antidepressants of each class. The classes are discussed in order of discovery to provide a historical context to drug development and to set the stage for a discussion of recently approved antidepressants along with promising experimental treatments.

Monoamine Oxidase Inhibitors

Soon after the observation of the antidepressant effects of iproniazid in TB (1952), MAO-Is became the first effective pharmacological treatment for depression and were highly prescribed from the 1950s to 1970s.[5] Further investigation into the mechanism of action lead to the articulation of the monoamine hypothesis of depression and the identification of specific MAO enzymes, namely, MAO-A and MAO-B, responsible for breaking down serotonin, norepinephrine, and dopamine. The "classic" MAO-Is, such as iproniazid, phenelzine, and tranylcypromine, are nonselective (e.g., inhibiting both MAO-A&B), irreversible inhibitors with potent antidepressant effects, however, also with poor tolerability, significant safety concerns, and problematic drug interactions (e.g., with other drugs, foods, and beverages).[10] The major safety concern with classic MAO-Is is the risk of a fatal hypertensive crisis and serotonin syndrome, as the result of increased levels of serotonin and norepinephrine.[11] This potentially fatal outcome is the product of the strong and irreversible MAO inhibition that would prevent the breakdown of

serotonin and norepinephrine, leading to potentially toxic monoamine levels. On their own, MAO-Is are relatively safe; however, when combined with another substance that increases monoamine levels, a hypertensive crisis could be precipitated.[11] To prevent this outcome, careful attention to coadministered medications (that could also increase monoamine levels) and diet are needed. When taking a nonselective irreversible MAO-I, patients are required to avoid other monoaminergic medications and limit food and beverages containing tyramine (e.g., fermented substances such as aged cheese and alcoholic beverages).[10] With the burden of these precautions and significant safety concerns if not followed adequately, the use of classic MAO-Is significantly decreased in the 1970s with new, safer alternatives emerging. However, phenelzine and tranylcypromine remain effective third-line options (with level 1 evidence for efficacy) for patients that are reliable to follow necessary dietary precautions and have failed to respond to other treatments.[12]

More recently, the use of MAO-Is has been revisited through the development of reversible inhibitors of MAO (RIMAs; e.g., moclobemide) and selective MAO-Is (e.g., selective MAO-B inhibitors such as selegiline). These newer alternatives are at significantly lower risk of precipitating a hypertensive crisis or serotonin syndrome and do not require the same strict dietary precautions. Additionally, efficacy and tolerability of moclobemide is similar to SSRIs.[13]

Tricyclic Antidepressants

Soon after the discovery of the antidepressant effects of MAO-Is (i.e., early 1950s), TCAs emerged as a new class of antidepressants. Imipramine was the first TCA to be FDA-approved for the treatment of MDD in 1959. Imipramine was initially evaluated in the treatment of schizophrenia; however, it did not have significant antipsychotic effects. However, Kuhn (1958) observed that patients with schizophrenia treated with imipramine "commence some activity of their own, again seeking contact with other people, they begin to entertain themselves, take part in the games, become more cheerful and are once again able to laugh … The patients express themselves as feeling much better, fatigue disappears, the feeling of heaviness in the limbs vanish, and the sense of oppression in the chest gives way to a feeling of relief."[14] These observations in the schizophrenia population were the first to suggest an antidepressant effect of TCAs and lead to further study in MDD populations, demonstrating robust antidepressant effects.[15,16] The tolerability of imipramine was also markedly improved compared to MAO-Is.

TABLE 8.1
Evidence-Based Antidepressants.

Generic Name	Half-life (hours)	Initial Dose (mg/days)	Maintenance Dose (mg/days)	Maximum Dose (mg/d)
SSRIS				
Sertraline[a]	<104	25–50	100–200	200
Escitalopram[a]	27–32	5–10	10–20	20
Citalopram[a]	23–45	10	20–40	40
Fluoxetine[a]	10–14 days	10	20–40	80
Paroxetine[a]	3–65	10	20–50	60
Fluvoxamine[a]	9–28	50	100–300	300
SNRIS				
Venlafaxine XR[a]	9–13	37.5	150–225	225
Desvenlafaxine[a]	11	50	50	100
Duloxetine[a]	8–17	30	60–90	120
Levomilnacipran	12–14	20	40–80	120
NDRIS				
Bupropion XL[a]	15–25	150	150–300	300
Bupropion SR	10–30	100	150 (BID)	300
NASSA				
Mirtazapine[a]	20–40	7.5–15	30–45	60
SARI				
Trazodone	4–9	25–50	Hypnotic: 50–150 Antidepressant: 200–500	600
MULTIMODALS/SMS				
Vortioxetine[a]	50–70	5	10–20	20
Vilazodone	20–30	10	40	80
MELATONIN AGONIST				
Agomelatine[a]	2–4	25	25–50	50
RIMA				
Moclobemide	1–3	150	300–600 (split BID/TID)	600
TCA—SECONDARY AMINES				
Desipramine	12–72	25	75–200	300
Nortriptyline	13–88	25	50–150	150
TCA—TERTIARY AMINES				
Amitriptyline	10–46	25	100–200	300
Clomipramine	17–37	25	100–300	300
Imipramine	4–34	25	100–300 (split BID/TID)	300
IRREVERSIBLE MAO-IS				
Phenelzine	1.5–4	15	45–90 (split BID/TID)	90
Tranylcypromine	2–4	10	20–40	40
Seleginine transdermal (selective MAO-B)	2–10	6	6–12	12

[a] First line based on CANMAT 2016 guidelines. Including half-life of active metabolites.[12]

After the approval of imipramine for MDD, numerous other TCAs were developed and approved for the treatment of MDD.[14] There are two major groups of TCAs: secondary amines (e.g., desipramine, nortripty-line) and tertiary amines (e.g., clomipramine, imipra-mine, amitriptyline). The primary mechanism of action of TCAs is similar to SNRIs; however, the class of TCAs is extremely heterogeneous as some TCAs are mostly serotonergic (e.g., clomipramine, imipramine), whereas others are more noradrenergic (e.g., desipramine, nortriptyline) and others exert fairly balanced inhibition of both serotonin and norepinephrine reuptake (e.g., amitriptyline, doxepin).[17] The off-target effects are highly variable as well, leading to dissimilar adverse effect pro-files (e.g., desipramine is often wake promoting whereas amitriptyline and doxepin are very sedating).

For decades, TCAs were by far the most popular an-tidepressant class, with strong antidepressant effects demonstrated in numerous randomized controlled tri-als (RCTs).[15] Currently, TCAs remain one of the most effective treatments of MDD; however, they have been largely replaced by newer classes of antidepressants (e.g., SSRIs) due to improved tolerability and safety.[16] One significant safety concern with TCAs is the narrow therapeutic window and potential lethality in an over-dose.[17] Given the high rates of suicidal ideations in MDD, the potential for lethal overdose with TCAs greatly limit their use. Conversely, with most new anti-depressant classes (e.g., SSRIs, SNRIs, NaSSAs, and SMSs), lethal overdose is extremely unlikely.[18] Never-theless, TCAs remain second line in most MDD treat-ment guidelines, with level-1 evidence for efficacy, and are suitable alternatives for patients who are at low risk of overdose and are failing to respond to mul-tiple first-line treatments (e.g., SSRIs).[12]

Selective Serotonin Reuptake Inhibitors

Soon after the advent of MAO-Is and TCAs, serotonin was identified as a key neurotransmitter mediating the antidepressant and anxiolytic effects of antidepres-sants.[6] As such, SSRIs were developed and remain the most commonly prescribed antidepressants. Fluoxetine was the first SSRI developed, demonstrating robust an-tidepressant efficacy, with improved tolerability and safety compared to earlier treatments (e.g., MAO-Is and TCAs).[19] Fluoxetine has the added benefit of a long half-life, preventing serotonin discontinuation symptoms with missed doses. Fluoxetine also continues to be the most well-studied antidepressant in children and adolescence, making it the treatment of choice in this population.[20]

After the development of fluoxetine, numerous other SSRIs were developed, including paroxetine,

fluvoxamine, sertraline, citalopram, and escitalopram. Notably, while all of these agents were initially classi-fied as SSRIs, there is significant variability in binding affinity to specific monoamine transporters, making the pharmacodynamics of SSRIs highly variable. For example, fluoxetine and paroxetine also have significant norepinephrine reuptake inhibition (NRI), whereas cit-alopram and escitalopram are very specific to serotonin reuptake inhibition (SRI) with negligible effects on norepinephrine transporters. Of the SSRIs, escitalopram has been shown to have the greatest efficacy and tolera-bility, through network meta-analyses and direct anti-depressant comparator studies.[2]

Selective Serotonin and Norepinephrine Reuptake Inhibitors

Soon after the development of SSRIs, the role of norepi-nephrine and dopamine were also identified as impor-tant in the pathophysiology and treatment of MDD.[6] As such, SNRIs were developed in an attempt to improve efficacy while maintaining the improved tolerability profile of SSRIs (as compared to MAO-Is and TCAs). In theory, increased norepinephrine signaling was postulated to improve energy, motivation, and cognitive function. Numerous SNRIs have now been developed (venlafaxine, desvenlafaxine, duloxetine, milnacipran, and levomilnacipran) and remain the second most commonly prescribed class of antidepressants.

Of the SNRIs, venlafaxine has the greatest evidence for efficacy[2]; however, it is notably associated with sig-nificant discontinuation symptoms with missed doses due to the short half-life. Notably, venlafaxine is con-verted by CYP450 2D6 into desvenlafaxine that has greater NRI effects. As such, for patients with decreased CYP450 2D6 activity (either through genetics or a drug–drug interaction), the effects of venlafaxine may be similar to an SSRI. Therefore, desvenlafaxine was developed, as the active metabolite, to provide consis-tent SNRI effects, regardless of CYP450 2D6 activity. Duloxetine is also commonly prescribed, especially for patients with comorbid pain, as duloxetine is also efficacious for neuropathic pain, fibromyalgia and chronic pain.[21] Milnacipran is not currently FDA-approved for MDD, but only for fibromyalgia. Howev-er, the levorotatory enantiomer of milnacipran, levomilnacipran, was recently FDA-approved for MDD in 2013, as the newest SNRI. The relative efficacy of levomilnacipran compared to other SSRIs and SNRIs remains largely unknown due to a lack of head-to-head trials[2]; however, levomilnacipran appears to be particularly effective at improving measures of motiva-tion, energy, and interest, potentially secondarily to the potent NRI effects.[22]

Nonserotonergic Agents—Norepinephrine and Dopamine Reuptake Inhibitors and Norepinephrine Reuptake Inhibitors

As the appreciation of MDD as a biologically heterogeneous disorder grew, and moving away from the initial hypothesis that only serotonin was responsible for the pathophysiology of MDD, newer treatments were developed that did not target serotonin at all. Replicated evidence demonstrated the importance of norepinephrine and dopamine in the pathophysiology of MDD, especially in the domains of motivation, hedonic drive, energy, and cognitive function.[23] Numerous NDRIs and NRIs have been developed primarily for the treatment of attention deficit hyperactivity disorder (ADHD) and narcolepsy with bupropion (NDRI) and reboxetine (NRI) being evaluated as monotherapies specifically for MDD.

Replicated evidence demonstrated strong antidepressant efficacy and excellent tolerability of bupropion.[24] Bupropion was also void of some of the problematic serotonergic adverse effects of earlier antidepressants, showing no sexual side effects, no weight gain, and no serotonin discontinuation symptoms (since serotonin was not affected). Clinical lore suggests that bupropion should not be used first for cases with significant comorbid anxiety (as serotonin is still believed to be the most important monoamine for anxiolytic effects); however, this practice has not been substantiated by robust evidence. Notably, bupropion is also specifically indicated for prevention of seasonal affective disorder, as an aid for smoking cessation and more recently as a weight loss agent when combined with naltrexone.[25,26] Other NDRIs indicated for ADHD, such as methylphenidate, have demonstrated antidepressant effects and are part of augmenting strategies, however, are not approved for MDD and typically should not be used as monotherapy.[27]

Reboxetine (NRI) was initially preliminarily FDA-approved for the treatment of MDD in 1999, however, more recent clinical studies, prompted by the FDA, resulted in a letter of nonapproval due to poor efficacy. Furthermore, numerous meta-analyses have demonstrated reboxetine to be significantly less efficacious compared to all other antidepressants.[2]

Serotonin Antagonists/Reuptake Inhibitors

Numerous studies suggested that 5HT1A was the most important serotonin receptor for SSRIs antidepressant and anxiolytic effects,[28] while 5HT2A/C stimulation was responsible for several unwanted adverse effects, such as sexual dysfunction, insomnia, and treatment emergent anxiety.[29] As such, serotonin antagonists/reuptake inhibitors (SARIs) were developed to target SERT while also antagonizing 5HT2A/C to prevent unwanted adverse effects of increased serotonin, while boosting antidepressant effects. Trazodone and nefazodone were both approved for MDD; however, nefazodone was later withdrawn from the market due to rare liver toxicity. Trazodone is now rarely used as a primary monotherapy for MDD, but more frequently is used as a hypnotic, for patients with or without MDD. At lower dose (25–150 mg oral at night), trazodone primarily antagonizes 5HT2A, alpha-1 and histamine-1 receptors, leading to strong hypnotic effects. Much higher doses (200–600 mg daily) are needed for SRI activity to allow for antidepressant effects; however, at these higher doses, tolerability of trazodone is extremely poor with common treatment discontinuation. As such, trazodone is rarely prescribed as a monotherapy for MDD, but rather as a sleep aid.[30]

Noradrenergic and Specific Serotonin Agents

Although earlier antidepressants primarily targeted increasing monoamine levels through reuptake and monoamine oxidase inhibition, more recent strategies have also targeted specific monoamine receptors in an attempt to further optimize antidepressant benefits while minimizing adverse effects caused by modulation of off-target receptors. Mirtazapine is the only FDA-approved NaSSA for MDD; however, mianserin is another NaSSA approved in Europe. Mirtazapine acts as an alpha-2-antagonist to effectively inhibit the inhibition of release of serotonin and norepinephrine, leading to increased release of serotonin and norepinephrine from the raphe nuclei and locus coeruleus, respectively. Additionally, mirtazapine inhibits 5HT2C/2A/3, which is believed to further mediate antidepressant and anxiolytic effects along with antiemetic effects and increasing appetite. Strong antihistaminergic (H1) effects that are believed to mediate the strong sedating effects of mirtazapine are also observed. As such, mirtazapine serves as a unique antidepressant, which may be of particular benefit for patients with significant insomnia and decreased appetite/weight loss.[31] Similar to bupropion, mirtazapine also has no sexual side effects and is not associated with serotonin discontinuation with missed doses.

New and Emerging Antidepressants

As described, antidepressant drug development has evolved to more specifically target monoamines implicated in MDD pathophysiology while avoiding monoaminergic alterations that may lead to unwanted adverse effects. The numerous antidepressants described earlier provide a large variety of options to alter monoamines through increasing the release (e.g., NaSSAs), decreasing the reuptake (e.g., TCAs, SSRIs, SNRIs, and NDRIs), or decreasing the breakdown (MAO-Is) of serotonin, norepinephrine, and dopamine. These pharmacodynamically diverse agents allow for differential modulation of specific monoamine(s) levels.

The development of these agents certainly moved the field forward to allow for more targeted treatment (i.e., by targeting specific monoamines), however, more recently, the classic monoamine hypothesis has been revisited, with replicated evidence demonstrating that the increase in monoamines in itself does not exert the antidepressant effects, but rather the downstream effects from monoamine receptor signaling is chiefly responsible for mediating both antidepressant and adverse effects.[6] Furthermore, the same neurotransmitter (e.g., serotonin) may have desirable effects when binding to one of its receptors (e.g., antidepressant and anxiolytic effects when serotonin binds to 5HT1A) while having undesirable adverse effects when binding to another receptor (e.g., sexual side effects from serotonin binding to 5HT2A/C). As such, to further improve antidepressant efficacy and tolerability, targeting *specific receptors* was believed to be the next step, rather than trying to further optimize the magnitude and ratio of increased serotonin, norepinephrine, and dopamine.

Multimodal Antidepressants—Serotonin Modulator and Stimulators

The advent of multimodal (SMS) antidepressants was the first attempt at more specifically targeting receptors to achieve greater antidepressant efficacy, tolerability, and safety. These agents are described as "multimodal" as they both directly target specific serotonin receptors while still inhibiting reuptake of serotonin (i.e., SRI activity). The two recently approved SMS antidepressants are vortioxetine and vilazodone. Vilazodone was FDA-approved in 2011 for the treatment of MDD. As the first SMS, vilazodone has SRI activity along with partial agonism of 5HT1A, with negligible effects on other monoamine transporters and receptors. Agonism of 5HT1A has been shown to be an important mediator of the antidepressant and anxiolytic effects or SSRI and SNRIs.[28] As such, in theory, specifically targeting 5HT1A may allow for improved efficacy that may potentially be achieved at lower doses, thus limiting the undesirable off-target effects of greatly increased serotonin levels. Vilazodone has been demonstrated to be efficacious

with good tolerability; however, it has not demonstrated superiority compared to earlier treatments.[2]

Vortioxetine, the second SMS, was FDA-approved in 2013 as a monotherapy for MDD with level-1 evidence for efficacy along with good tolerability and safety.[12] Vortioxetine has SRI and, to a lesser extent, NRI activity. Additionally, vortioxetine is a full agonist of 5HT1A, the receptor shown to mediate the antidepressant and anxiolytic effects of SSRIs, as previously described. Vortioxetine also antagonizes 5HT1D, 5HT3, and 5HT7 and is a partial agonist of 5HT1B. Vortioxetine has been shown to be the only antidepressant to robustly improve cognitive function, which is believed to be mediated via 5HT7 antagonism.[32] Notably, no other antidepressant has been consistently shown to improve cognitive function, even with remission of depressive symptom. In addition to the procognitive benefits, antidepressant efficacy and tolerability of vortioxetine have been found to be superior compared to other antidepressants in head-to-head trials,[2] adding further merit to the further development of multimodal antidepressants.

Novel Experimental Antidepressants

Numerous new treatments are being currently investigated, with the focus shifting away from targeting monoamines to identifying novel targets that might allow for the discovery of potentially disease-modifying treatments and preventative strategies. Several alternate pathways involved in the pathophysiology of MDD have been uncovered including, but not limited to, the following: inflammatory pathways, the oxidative stress pathway, the hypothalamic–pituitary–adrenal axis, the metabolic and bioenergetics system, neurotrophic pathways, the glutamate system, the opioid system, the cholinergic system, and sleep–wake cycle disturbances (e.g., melatonin and orexin systems).[33,34] For each of these systems, several targets have been shown promise and are further discussed in other chapters. Notably, to date (as of 2018), only one agent has been approved as an antidepressant monotherapy for MDD with a primary target that is outside of the monoaminergic system; while not approved in North America, agomelatine, a melatonin receptor agonist, has been approved in Europe and Australia, with numerous studies showing antidepressant efficacy and good tolerability.[2]

Currently, the most promising novel pharmacological treatment for MDD, acting outside of the monoaminergic system, is ketamine, targeting the glutamate system through N-methyl-D-aspartate (NMDA) receptor antagonism (further discussed in Chapter 12).

Ketamine represents a new class of "rapid acting" antidepressants, exerting antidepressant effects within hours of administration.[35] Before its approval, ketamine has already been prescribed off-label for MDD at numerous clinics around the world for the past few years. The evidence for ketamine is primarily when given via the intravenous (IV) route, with most studies only assessing efficacy and tolerability after a single IV dose, showing rapid antidepressant effects, lasting 2–14 days after a single dose with good tolerability.[36] Furthermore, increasing evidence has suggested an antisuicide effect.[37,38] Of note, only two previous treatments have been shown to have antisuicide effects, namely lithium and clozapine.[39]

Numerous concerns around unknown long-term safety, misuse/abuse potential, psychotomimetic effects, feasibility and scalability of ketamine for MDD (given that the treatment is IV) have arisen, leading to the investigation of alternatives targeting the same system (i.e., the glutamate system). An intranasal formulation of esketamine has now been developed with promising results that would allow for home self-administration, along with numerous other experimental agents that target the glutamate system in different ways.[35,40] Although numerous other agents show promise as novel treatments of depression (e.g., antiinflammatories), glutamate receptor modulators, such as ketamine, are likely to be the next major antidepressant drug class.

GENERAL PRINCIPLES TO THE PHARMACOLOGICAL TREATMENT OF MDD

As discussed and shown in Table 8.1, there are numerous FDA-approved pharmacological treatments for MDD. Approval is based on a minimum of two phase III RCTs demonstrating antidepressant efficacy compared to placebo. Clinical trials primarily assess antidepressant efficacy, safety, and tolerability. Other factors, such as symptom profile, cost, local availability, and drug interactions, may also impact selection of treatment. The current section reviews these factors that may guide selection of an antidepressant.

The first step to select the most appropriate pharmacological treatment is conducting a detailed clinical assessment. Of particular importance, with direct management implications, is an evaluation of suicidality, bipolarity, comorbidity (both medical and psychiatric), current medications, allergies, symptom specifiers/dimensions (e.g., mixed features, psychotic features, and anxious distress), and previous treatments (including previous antidepressant trial doses, duration, response, and adverse effects). If the current depressive symptoms are believed to be part of a bipolar disorder, the symptoms should be treated in accordance with evidence-based bipolar guidelines,[41] which are outside of the scope of this chapter. Similarly, if the depressive symptoms are due to another medical condition (e.g., hypothyroidism), then this condition should be treated first, and then the depressive symptoms should be reevaluated.

If a diagnosis of MDD with a current MDE is identified, then evaluating symptom count and severity, along with functional impairment, is essential in determining if pharmacotherapy will be indicated. If the patient is found to have MDD with a current moderate-to-severe MDE, pharmacotherapy is indicated and a discussion with the patient regarding initiation of an evidence-based antidepressant should ensue. If the current MDE is mild, psychoeducation, self-management, and psychological treatments are the preferred treatments. However, in some cases, pharmacotherapy may be indicated for mild depression if there is a strong patient preference, previous response to antidepressants, or lack of response to nonpharmacological interventions.[12]

Before initiating treatment, quantitative baseline measures of depressive symptom severity and functional impairment should be obtained. Once treatment is initiated, the first follow-up visit should be within 2 weeks, with follow-up every 2–4 weeks thereafter until remission is achieved. At each follow-up visit, depressive symptom severity should be reevaluated using validated rating tools (e.g., Quick Inventory of Depressive Symptomatology) as measurement-based care has been repeatedly demonstrated to significantly improve outcomes in the treatment of MDD.[42]

In selecting initial pharmacological treatment, several patient and medication factors should be considered and discussed with the patient to collaboratively select the most appropriate treatment. Important patient factors to consider include patient preference, clinical features and dimensions, comorbid medical and psychiatric conditions and history of response and adverse effects of previous antidepressant trials. Additionally, medication factors including comparative efficacy, tolerability, potential interactions, cost, availability, and simplicity of use should be considered. For the purpose of this chapter, for brevity, the discussion will be focused on a subset of key patient (clinical features and dimensions) and medication factors (comparative efficacy and tolerability).

Comparative Efficacy and Tolerability

After seeing the large list of antidepressants, often the first two questions from patients, clinicians, researchers, and pharmaceutical investors are "which one works best?" and "which one has the least side effects?" These seemingly simple questions are surprisingly difficult to answer as there have been hundreds of RCTs evaluating the efficacy and tolerability of different antidepressants.[2] Furthermore, differences in study design, study populations, placebo response rates, comorbidities, funding sources, and publication bias make it extremely difficult to accurately and reliably answer these two fundamental questions. Ideally, a large clinical trial could be conducted that comparatively evaluates all antidepressants in the same population, however, such a study would likely not be feasible given the large sample size required to be adequately powered. As such, the most reliable method that has been employed to evaluate comparative efficacy and tolerability has been network meta-analyses.

A network meta-analysis pools together both placebo-controlled trials and active-comparator head-to-head studies using a validated mathematical algorithm to determine comparative efficacy and overall tolerability (based on overall dropout rates), even for medications that were never directly compared in a single study. This method has been employed in fields outside of psychiatry for decades; however, in the past decade, it has been adopted in psychiatry and applied to determine comparative efficacy of treatments for numerous psychiatry disorders, including MDD. The initial network meta-analysis for MDD was conducted in 2009 comparing 12 antidepressants[43] and was recently updated by Cipriani et al. (2018) to compare more recently approved treatments, including 21 antidepressants in total.[2]

Cipriani et al. included 522 trials comprising 116,477 participants, finding all antidepressants were more effective than placebo, with odds ratios (ORs) ranging between 2.13 (95% credible interval [CrI] 1.89–2.41) for amitriptyline and 1.37 (95% CrI 1.16–1.63) for reboxetine. For acceptability, only agomelatine (OR 0.84%; 95% CrI 0.72–0.97) and fluoxetine (OR 0.88%; 95% CrI 0.80–0.96) were associated with fewer dropouts than placebo, whereas clomipramine was worse than placebo (OR 1.30%; 95% CrI 1.01–1.68). When results from all trials were pooled, differences in ORs between antidepressants ranged from 1.15 to 1.55 for efficacy and from 0.64 to 0.83 for overall tolerability (as determined by dropout rates), with wide CrIs on most of the comparative analyses. In head-to-head studies, agomelatine, amitriptyline,

escitalopram, mirtazapine, paroxetine, venlafaxine, and vortioxetine were more effective than other antidepressants (range of ORs 1.19–1.96), whereas fluoxetine, fluvoxamine, reboxetine, and trazodone were the least efficacious drugs (0.51–0.84). For tolerability, agomelatine, citalopram, escitalopram, fluoxetine, sertraline, and vortioxetine had the lowest dropout rates compared to other antidepressants (range of ORs 0.43–0.77), whereas amitriptyline, clomipramine, duloxetine, fluvoxamine, reboxetine, trazodone, and venlafaxine had the relatively higher dropout rates compared to other antidepressants (range of ORs 1.30–2.32). The superiority and inferiority data are further summarized in Table 8.2.

Taken together, all antidepressants were found to be more efficacious than placebo with some antidepressants emerging as more efficacious than others in head-to-head trials. Intriguingly, no particular class of antidepressant emerged as the most effective, as head-to-head trials revealed the most effect antidepressants included a TCA (amitriptyline), SSRIs (escitalopram, paroxetine), an SNRIs (venlafaxine), a NaSSAs (mirtazapine), and an SMS (vortioxetine). For tolerability, however, mostly SSRIs (citalopram, escitalopram, fluoxetine, sertraline) along with vortioxetine and agomelatine emerged as having the best tolerability. Only vortioxetine, escitalopram, and agomelatine had evidence to support superiority in both efficacy and overall tolerability. This is a notable different finding compared to the 2009 network meta-analysis that found sertraline and escitalopram were the only agents with superiority in both domains of tolerability and efficacy.[43]

Although a network meta-analysis may clearly provide answers for comparable efficacy, evaluating comparative tolerability is often more complicated as different adverse effects are subjectively more or less tolerable for different patients. Overall, discontinuation rate is a generally accepted proxy of overall tolerability; however, overall discontinuation does not provide information about specific adverse effects. The importance of avoiding specific adverse effects is often variable depending on patient preferences. For example, for a fatigued depressed patient sleeping 14 hours per day, an antidepressant with sedating effects should be avoided; however, in a depressed patient with insomnia, the adverse effect of sedation may be preferable. As such, an appreciation of common adverse effects and the relative frequency of these effects for specific agents should also be discussed and integrated into the process of selecting a suitable antidepressant.

TABLE 8.2
Comparative Efficacy and Tolerability of Antidepressants Based Network Meta-Analysis of Head-To-Head Trials (Original Table Produced Using data From Cipriani et al.[2]).

	Efficacy	Overall tolerability
Superiority	Agomelatine	Agomelatine
	Amitriptyline	Citalopram
	Escitalopram	Escitalopram
	Mirtazapine	Fluoxetine
	Paroxetine	Sertraline
	Vortioxetine	Vortioxetine
	Venlafaxine	
Inferiority	Fluoxetine	Amitriptyline
	Fluvoxamine	Clomipramine
	Reboxetine	Duloxetine
	Trazodone	Fluvoxamine
		Reboxetine
		Trazodone
		Venlafaxine

To further highlight superior agents, in box of agents with superior efficacy, green indicates these agents also had superior tolerability, whereas red indicates evidence for inferior tolerability.

A short list of general adverse effects for antidepressants are summarized in Table 8.3. Many of these adverse effects occur at similar frequencies in various antidepressants; however, there is significant variability in the relative sedating, wake promoting, and sexual adverse effects when comparing antidepressants. Discussing with the patient these differences in adverse effect profiles often plays a role in selecting an antidepressant, as patients often feel strongly about avoiding certain adverse effects (e.g., sexual dysfunction, drowsiness, and weight gain).

As shown in Fig. 8.1, there is particular variability in the effect of antidepressants on wakefulness/sedation with some antidepressants promoting wakefulness (SNRIs, NDRIs, vortioxetine, and some SSRIs), some being sleep—wake neutral (citalopram, escitalopram) and others being very sedating (fluvoxamine, mirtazapine, and trazodone). As such, selecting an antidepressant that fits with the patient's current symptom profile (e.g., hypersomnia with anergia vs. insomnia) may help avoid worsening of depressive symptoms from treatment emergent adverse effects (e.g., worsening insomnia with a wake-promoting antidepressant or vice versa). Additionally, timing of the antidepressant (e.g., in the morning vs. at night) may be tailored to the sedative versus wake-promoting effects of the given antidepressant. Of note, individual patient effects, particularly sedation, are often different than expected so timing of doses may need to be adjusted based on individual patient experiences. For example, agents that are often wake promoting (SNRIs) or sleep—wake neutral might be experienced as having sedating effects for an individual patient and may then be required to be dosed at night.

Similarly, frequency of sexual adverse effects (i.e., decreased libido, anorgasmia, erectile dysfunction) are extremely variable. Data on sexual adverse effects are historically poor as often these effects were not systematically screened for. These effects may be particularly problematic as they are unlikely to resolve with time (in the absence of a change in treatment), patients often do not spontaneously report these effects and clinicians often forget to discuss and ask about these effects. Although the quality of the reported data is poor, previous studies suggest frequency of sexual adverse effects range from being equivalent to placebo to greater than 50% with other antidepressants as shown in Table 8.4.

Patient Factors—Clinical Features and Dimensions

Evaluating and discussing the relative efficacy, tolerability and safety of first-line antidepressants often largely dictate the treatment selection. However, there are additional patient factors to consider that might also impact treatment selection. Certainly cost, availability, and patient preference are important factors to be considered with any pharmacological treatment, regardless of the disorder being treated. Specific to the treatment of MDD is a careful consideration of symptom profile to determine the dimensions (e.g.,

TABLE 8.3
General Adverse Effects Associated With Antidepressants.

Transient adverse effects that typically resolve in first few weeks	Anxiety/Nervousness/ Agitation Gastrointestinal upset (nausea, constipation, diarrhea) Headache Dizziness Sweating Insomnia Vivid dreams
Adverse effects that often persist (sometimes resolve with time)	Dry mouth Appetite/weight changes Drowsiness/fatigue/ somnolence Sexual dysfunction (decreased libido, anorgasmia, erectile dysfunction)
Rare but serious adverse effects	Serotonin syndrome Bleeding risk (mostly upper gastrointestinal bleed when used with NSAIDs) Priapism Hypo/manic induction (if underlying/undiagnosed bipolar disorder)
Age specific effects: over 60:	Prolonged QTc, potentially leading to Torsade de pointes (black box warning for citalopram/escitalopram) Hyponatremia Falls and fractures
Under 24:	Suicidal ideations (black box warning under age 24)

Notably, adverse effects occur at variable frequencies depending on antidepressant.

cognitive dysfunction, sleep disturbance) that are being affected and causing functional impairment, as these dimensions may be important to specifically target.[12] If cognitive dysfunction is prominent and functionally impairing, vortioxetine may be preferable, as the only antidepressant that has demonstrated procognitive effects.[32] If low energy and hypersomnia is present, wake-promoting agents such as SNRIs (Fig. 8.1) may be preferable. Conversely, if insomnia is of particular concern, more sedating antidepressants may be preferable. These factors do not completely dictate treatment selection; however, they may be helpful to consider and discuss with the patient.[12]

Additionally, the identification of clinical features, specifically the presence of mixed, psychotic, or catatonic features or anxious distress would directly impact the evidence-based pharmacological treatment to be selected. If psychotic features are identified, level-1 evidence supports the use of combining an antidepressant with an antipsychotic.[12,44] For catatonic features, benzodiazepines and ECT are the only evidence-based treatments as no antidepressants have been studied.

The "mixed features" specifier was added to the DSM-5 to represent the current understanding of mixed states. Indeed, before the DSM-5, mixed state would automatically denote a diagnosis of bipolar disorder, so by definition, you could not be in a mixed state with unipolar MDD. Currently, however, the DSM-5 allows for mixed features to be present in MDD (i.e., syndromal MDE with subsyndromal symptoms of hypo/mania). Only lurasidone and ziprasidone monotherapy has been studied for MDD with mixed features and have demonstrated efficacy.[45,46] Expert consensus suggests that pharmacological treatment with mood stabilizing properties (e.g., second-generation antipsychotics) is required for MDD with mixed features; however, further study is needed to determine optimal treatment.[47] Additionally, discontinuation of antidepressants and stimulants should be considered when mixed features are present as these agents may be worsening symptoms of hypo/mania.[44]

When anxious distress is present, expert consensus suggests that an antidepressant with demonstrated efficacy for anxiety disorders would be preferable; however, studies have failed to demonstrate a significant difference between SSRIs, SNRIs, and bupropion.[12,44]

APPROACH TO TREATMENT NONRESPONSE AND TREATMENT RESISTANCE

The previous sections mostly describe the selection and initiation of antidepressant monotherapy. This section will discuss pharmacological management strategies when the first antidepressant trials are inadequately effective and/or poorly tolerated. The same basic principles discussed in the previous sections of considering both patient and medication factors apply to selecting treatments for TRD (broadly defined as inadequate response to two adequate antidepressant trials).

Before considering switching or adjunctive treatment strategies, the adequacy of the current trial should be determined. At least 2–4 weeks of treatment at an adequate dose is required before determining nonresponse. If no response (<25% symptom score reduction)

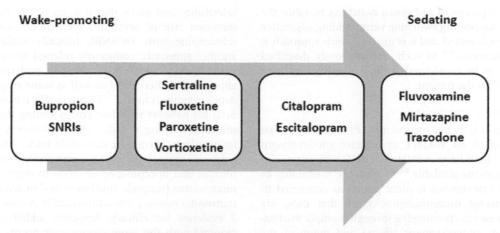

FIG. 8.1 Sleep–wake effects of commonly prescribed antidepressants.

TABLE 8.4
Frequency of Treatment Emergent Sexual Adverse Effects (i.e., Decreased Libido, Anorgasmia, Erectile Dysfunction) With Commonly Prescribed Antidepressants (Based on Product Monographs).

Frequency of Treatment Emergent Sexual Dysfunction	Antidepressants
>40%	Fluoxetine Fluvoxamine Paroxetine Sertraline
15%–40%	Citalopram Duloxetine Escitalopram Venlafaxine
<15%	Bupropion Mirtazapine Moclobemide Vortioxetine Vilazodone Levomilnacipran

or only a partial response (25%–50% reduction) is observed, the dose should be further optimized and given another 2–4 weeks to observe for an improved response.[12] Additionally, adherence should be evaluated, as the serum antidepressant levels may be subtherapeutic if numerous doses are being missed on a regular basis, leading to nonresponse. Throughout treatment, whenever inadequate response is observed, a reevaluation of the initial diagnosis and formulation is also prudent as this reevaluation may greatly alter treatment. For example, if the current MDE is found to be part of a bipolar disorder, the treatment approach would need to be completely changed, due to the known inefficacy and risks of antidepressants in bipolar depression. Similarly, if current symptoms are formulated to be more in keeping with a personality disorder, psychotherapeutic interventions may be required to achieve symptomatic improvements.

If the first adequate trial (adequate dose for adequate duration with a first-line antidepressant with >80% adherence) is found to have no response, switching to another first-line antidepressant with evidence for superiority (e.g., escitalopram, vortioxetine, and venlafaxine) should be considered. Specific dose titration schedules for safely switching antidepressants can be found at switchrx.ca as some switches require special considerations, such as a washout period when switching to a classic MAO-I (e.g., need greater than five half-lives of current SSRI/SNRI of washout period before starting MAO-I) or from an MAO-I (e.g., need 2-week washout period before starting a new antidepressant to allow new MAO enzymes to be synthesized).

If there is nonresponse to a second adequate antidepressant trial, both switching or adding an adjunctive treatment should be considered. Switching may be preferable if the current antidepressant is poorly tolerated, found to have zero benefit or if the patient prefers to switch rather than add. Adding an adjunctive medication may be preferable when there have been two or more previous antidepressant trials, there is a partial response (>25% improvement) to the current antidepressant, the current treatment is well tolerated, or if the patient prefers to add versus switching. Notably, the evidence supporting switching versus adding adjunctive treatments is mixed and it is unclear which approach is more efficacious.[48] As such, the previously described factors may be considered while discussing treatment options with the patient.

Adjunctive Treatments

Numerous adjunctive treatments (i.e., medications that are added in an attempt to increase antidepressant response) have been evaluated in RCTs with many efficacious options available.[48–50] Notably, tolerability of adjunctive treatments is often poorer as compared to antidepressant monotherapies, given that there are now adverse effects emerging through multiple medications (e.g., polypharmacy effects) and many of the adjunctive treatments (e.g., antipsychotics) may have problematic adverse effects that are significantly less common with most antidepressants (e.g., metabolic effects, extrapyramidal effects [EPS]).[51] Nevertheless, adjunctive treatments are still often merited when patients remain symptomatic and functionally impaired even with optimization of antidepressant monotherapy. Evidence-based adjunctive treatments include (1) antipsychotics, (2) antidepressants (e.g., combining two antidepressants), (3) lithium, (4) stimulants, (5) triiodothyronine (T3), and (6) ketamine (experimental, not yet approved), each to be discussed in turn.

Of the adjunctive options, second-generation antipsychotics (SGAs) have the strongest evidence for efficacy.[50] Specifically, aripiprazole, quetiapine, risperidone, brexpiprazole, and olanzapine have all demonstrated level-1 evidence for efficacy as adjunctive treatments for TRD.[12] Although efficacious, there are significant safety/tolerability concerns with regards to metabolic adverse effects (e.g., weight gain, hypercholesterolemia, and insulin resistance) with some of these agents; specifically, olanzapine and quetiapine have been associated with significant weight gain.[51] Brexpiprazole and aripiprazole are relatively weight neutral; however, all SGAs carry the risk of metabolic effects.[52] For risperidone, given the strong dopamine-2 (D2) receptor blockade, there are also concerns of hyperprolactinemia and EPS. Also of note, as shown in Table 8.5, doses of SGAs are significantly lower when being used for MDD, as compared to antipsychotic dose ranges. Although prescribed at lower doses, SGA guideline-concordant metabolic monitoring is still indicated.[53,54]

Combining two antidepressants is another adjunctive option; however, more recent studies have questioned the relative efficacy of this approach.[50] The addition of bupropion has level-2 evidence for

tolerability and given that it is an NDRI, there is no increased risk of serotonin syndrome.[12] Combining mirtazapine with an SNRI, typically venlafaxine, is another approach, commonly referred to as "Californian Rocket Fuel" with level-2 evidence.[12] This approach has theoretical as well as some empirical evidence to support its use.[55] Theoretically, it may be beneficial for patients with low energy during the day and difficulty sleeping at night. The SNRI may have stimulating effects during the day while mirtazapine would help with sleep, with both synergistically increasing serotonin and norepinephrine levels through dissimilar mechanisms (reuptake inhibition and increased neurotransmitter release). The addition of TCAs also has level-2 evidence for efficacy; however, added caution is required with the more serotonergic agents (e.g., clomipramine) increasing the risk of serotonin syndrome when used with SSRIs/SNRIs.[12] Additional concerns about QTc prolongation are present, as TCAs along with some SSRIs (e.g., escitalopram, citalopram) may cause QTc prolongation.[56] Other antidepressants may be combined with less evidence; however, MAO-Is should not be combined with other monoaminergic agents due to the significant risk of serotonin syndrome.

Lithium was historically one of the primary adjunctive treatments for MDD; however, it is used considerably less frequently given the increased number of other adjunctive options. Similar to bipolar disorder, lithium should be dosed to therapeutic serum levels. Lithium has level-2 evidence for efficacy as an adjunctive treatment of MDD.[12] Lithium has the added benefit of having robust antisuicide effects[39]; whereas, all other psychotropics (with the exception of clozapine and possibly ketamine) have failed to demonstrate antisuicide effects. Although lithium is often well tolerated with good efficacy, several notable adverse effects should be considered including the risk of lithium toxicity, thyroid dysfunction, renal dysfunction, treatment emergent tremor, leukocytosis, arrhythmias, electrolyte changes, and metabolic effects.[57–59] Regular monitoring of serum levels and for treatment emergent adverse effects (e.g., hypothyroidism, renal dysfunction) is also required, along with special caution when prescribing agents that may alter levels or effect kidney function, such as diuretics and antiinflammatories.[59]

Level-2 evidence supports T3 as an adjunctive treatment.[60] Effects are usually seen within the first 2 weeks at 25–50 mcg daily. If no effects are observed after 1 month of 50 mcg daily, T3 may be discontinued.[12]

Wake-promoting agents and stimulants have also been shown to be efficacious adjunctive treatments with level 2–3 evidence for efficacy, depending on the

TABLE 8.5
Recommendations for Adjunctive Medications for Nonresponse or Partial Response to an Antidepressant.

Recommendation	Adjunctive Agent	Level of Evidence	Dosing
First line	Aripiprazole	Level 1	2–15 mg
	Quetiapine	Level 1	150–300 mg
	Risperidone	Level 1	1–3 mg
Second line	Brexpiprazole[a]	Level 1	1–3 mg
	Bupropion	Level 2	150–300 mg
	Lithium	Level 2	600–1200 mg (therapeutic serum levels)
	Mirtazapine/mianserin	Level 2	30–60 mg
	Modafinil	Level 2	100–400 mg
	Olanzapine	Level 1	2.5–10 mg
	Triiodothyronine	Level 2	25–50 mcg
Third line	Other antidepressants	Level 3	Various
	Other stimulants (methylphenidate, lisdexamfetamine, etc.)	Level 3	Various
	TCAs (e.g., desipramine)	Level 2	Various
	Ziprasidone	Level 3	20–80 mg bid
Experimental	Ketamine	Level 1	0.5 mg/kg, single intravenous dose[b]
Not recommended	Pindolol	Level 1 (lack of efficacy)	Not applicable

TCA, tricyclic antidepressant.
[a] Newly approved since the 2009 Canadian Network for Mood and Anxiety Treatments (CANMAT) guidelines.
[b] For acute treatment.
With permission from 2016 CANMAT MDD guidelines.[12]

agent.[27] These agents are typically selected to target low energy/fatigue and would usually be avoided when insomnia or significant anxiety is present. These agents may be especially helpful for patients with comorbid medical conditions that may be contributing to fatigue.[61,62] It is often difficult to differentiate if fatigue is a result of the medical illness versus the depression; however, stimulants have evidence for antidepressant and energizing effects in both scenarios.[61,62] Modafinil has the strongest evidence for efficacy with good tolerability as an adjunctive agent.[61,63] Short-acting methylphenidate also has replicated evidence for antidepressant effects.[27,64] Stimulants are typically well tolerated with the main adverse effects of concern being treatment emergent anxiety, agitation, insomnia, decreased appetite, and cardiac effects.

As discussed previously, ketamine is a promising new "rapid-acting" antidepressant that is currently being used experimentally and off-label for TRD. American and Canadian guidelines recommend that ketamine use be restricted to academic centers of excellence, while recognizing ketamine as an important treatment option for TRD.[12,65] Notably Janssen has been developing intranasal esketamine (i.e., the S-enantiomer of ketamine that binds more strongly with NMDA), which will likely have FDA approval for MDD in the near future and might increase the availability of usage.[40] Concerns of poorly understood long-term adverse effects and abuse potential are still being evaluated.[65] It is also unknown how "rapid-acting" antidepressants may alter patient expectations, with patients preferring to be prescribed ketamine rather than more well-studied antidepressants, given the lag time to effect. Indeed, most mood disorder experts contend that ketamine will play an important role in the treatment of depression; however, it should not be used first line, but rather reserved for more severe and treatment refractory cases.[65] Ketamine and other glutamate modulators are further discussed in Chapter 12.

Although outside of the scope of this chapter, the addition of physical activity, psychotherapy, and brain stimulation (e.g., ECT) may be considered at any point while treating TRD. These options are often limited based on cost, availability, and feasibility; however, they are very efficacious options, especially when used in combination with adequate pharmacotherapy.

New and Emerging Treatment Approaches

As in other fields of medicine, psychiatry is investigating ways to make treatments more personalized or "precision-based."[66] Current treatment algorithms, as described previously, rely mostly on a trial-and-error approach, which can often greatly delay the identification of the most effective treatment (or combination of treatments). As such, numerous investigators are trying to identify reliable ways to predict what patient factors will predict response to specific treatments. Factors considered include, but are not limited to, demographics, symptom profile, family history, pharmacogenomics, epigenetics, environmental factors, neuroimaging, and serum biomarkers.[66–68] Several studies have also applied machine-learning algorithms to integrate factors from numerous domains (e.g., integrating symptom profile with neuroimaging and genetic testing) to more accurately predict who will respond to what treatment.[69,70]

Currently, these predictive models are promising, but have yet to robustly demonstrate clinical utility. For example, numerous commercial pharmacogenomics tests are currently being marketed as having the ability to provide personalized guidance for antidepressant selection based on testing genes involved in antidepressant pharmacodynamics and pharmacokinetics.[71] Although results have been promising, RCTs have failed to demonstrate clinical utility, as pharmacogenomic-guided antidepressant selection failed to improve treatment efficacy (i.e., treatment efficacy was the same for participants who received trial-and-error treatment as usual as compared to participants with pharmacogenomic-guided treatment).[71] Treatments based on symptom profile or neuroimaging findings have similarly failed to robustly demonstrate improved efficacy. Taken together, there is significant interest and promise in more personalized treatments with numerous large studies underway; however, the field of precision medicine in psychiatry is still greatly lagging behind other fields, such as oncology (e.g., treatments are specific for cancer type based on biopsy results) and infectious disease specialties (e.g., antimicrobials prescribed based on specific cultures and sensitives).

CONCLUSION

Pharmacotherapy remains the cornerstone of treatment for moderate-to-severe depression. Numerous efficacious and well-tolerated antidepressants are currently available. More recently approved antidepressants have modest improvements in efficacy and significant improvements in tolerability and safety, as compared to older antidepressants. Considering both patient and medication factors can guide treatment selection; however, treatment is still largely based on trial and error. Currently available treatments are associated with unacceptably high rates of treatment nonresponse, meriting the discovery of new treatments with novel targets acting outside of the monoamine system. Experimental treatments for MDD are exploring novel pathways implicated in the pathophysiology of MDD (e.g., glutamate, inflammation, oxidative stress). Among these new treatments, glutamate receptor modulators, such as ketamine, show the most promise, demonstrating robust and rapid antidepressant effects. The quest for precision medicine in the treatment of MDD is also currently underway, which may lead to predictive models that would allow for early remission and recovery through selecting the optimal treatment at the beginning of MDD management, rather than identifying it eventually through the trial-and-error method.

COMPETING INTERESTS

JDR and YL have no competing interests to declare. RSM has received research grant support from Lundbeck, JanssenOrtho, Shire, Purdue, AstraZeneca, Pfizer, Otsuka, Allergan, Stanley Medical Research Institute (SMRI); speaker/consultation fees from Lundbeck, Pfizer, AstraZeneca, Elli-Lilly, JanssenOrtho, Purdue, Johnson & Johnson, Moksha8, Sunovion, Mitsubishi, Takeda, Forest, Otsuka, Bristol-Myers Squibb, and Shire.

REFERENCES

1. WHO. *Depression Fact Sheet*. 2017.
2. Cipriani A, Furukawa TA, Salanti G, et al. Comparative efficacy and acceptability of 21 antidepressant drugs for the acute treatment of adults with major depressive disorder: a systematic review and network meta-analysis. *The Lancet*. 2018;0(0). https://doi.org/10.1016/S0140-6736(17)32802-7.
3. Hasin DS, Sarvet AL, Meyers JL, et al. Epidemiology of adult DSM-5 major depressive disorder and its specifiers in the United States. *JAMA Psychiatry*. February 2018. https://doi.org/10.1001/jamapsychiatry.2017.4602.
4. Lopez-Munoz F, Alamo C. Monoaminergic neurotransmission: the history of the discovery of antidepressants from 1950s until today. *Curr Pharm Des*. 2009;15:1563–1586.
5. Hillhouse TM, Porter JH. A brief history of the development of antidepressant drugs: from monoamines to glutamate. *Exp Clin Psychopharmacol*. 2015;23(1):1–21. https://doi.org/10.1037/a0038550.

6. Hirschfeld RM. History and evolution of the monoamine hypothesis of depression. *J Clin Psychiatry*. 2000;61(suppl 6):4–6.

7. Gaynes BN, Warden D, Trivedi MH, Wisniewski SR, Fava M, Rush AJ. What did STAR*D teach us? Results from a large-scale, practical, clinical trial for patients with depression. *Psychiatr Serv*. 2009;60:1439–1445. https://doi.org/10.1176/appi.ps.60.11.1439.

8. IsHak WW, Greenberg JM, Balayan K, et al. Quality of life: the ultimate outcome measure of interventions in major depressive disorder. *Harv Rev Psychiatry*. 2011;19(5):229–239. https://doi.org/10.3109/10673229.2011.614099.

9. Hasselbalch BJ, Knorr U, Hasselbalch SG, Gade A, Kessing LV. Cognitive deficits in the remitted state of unipolar depressive disorder. *Neuropsychology*. 2012;26:642–651. https://doi.org/10.1037/a0029301.

10. Flockhart DA. Dietary restrictions and drug interactions with monoamine oxidase inhibitors: an update. *J Clin Psychiatry*. 2012;73(suppl 1):17–24. https://doi.org/10.4088/JCP.11096su1c.03.

11. Stahl SM, Felker A. Monoamine oxidase inhibitors: a modern guide to an unrequited class of antidepressants. *CNS Spectr*. 2008;13(10):855–870.

12. Kennedy SH, Lam RW, McIntyre RS, et al. Canadian network for mood and anxiety treatments (CANMAT) 2016 clinical guidelines for the management of adults with major depressive disorder: section 3. Pharmacological treatments. *Can J Psychiatry*. 2016;61:540–560. https://doi.org/10.1177/0706743716659417.

13. Papakostas GI, Fava M. A metaanalysis of clinical trials comparing moclobemide with selective serotonin reuptake inhibitors for the treatment of major depressive disorder. *Can J Psychiatry Rev Can Psychiatr*. 2006;51(12):783–790. https://doi.org/10.1177/070674370605101208.

14. Pletscher A. The discovery of antidepressants: a winding path. *Experientia*. 1991;47(1):4–8.

15. Anderson IM. Selective serotonin reuptake inhibitors versus tricyclic antidepressants: a meta-analysis of efficacy and tolerability. *J Affect Disord*. 2000;58(1):19–36. https://doi.org/10.1016/S0165-0327(99)00092-0.

16. Arroll B, Macgillivray S, Ogston S, et al. Efficacy and tolerability of tricyclic antidepressants and SSRIs compared with placebo for treatment of depression in primary care: a meta-analysis. *Ann Fam Med*. 2005;3(5):449–456. https://doi.org/10.1370/afm.349.

17. Gillman PK. Tricyclic antidepressant pharmacology and therapeutic drug interactions updated. *Br J Pharmacol*. 2007;151(6):737–748. https://doi.org/10.1038/sj.bjp.0707253.

18. Barbey JT, Roose SP. SSRI safety in overdose. *J Clin Psychiatry*. 1998;59(suppl 15):42–48.

19. Anderson IM, Tomenson BM. The efficacy of selective serotonin re-uptake inhibitors in depression: a meta-analysis of studies against tricyclic antidepressants. *J Psychopharmacol (Oxf)*. 1994;8(4):238–249. https://doi.org/10.1177/026988119400800407.

20. Cipriani A, Zhou X, Del Giovane C, et al. Comparative efficacy and tolerability of antidepressants for major depressive disorder in children and adolescents: a network meta-analysis. *The Lancet*. 2016;388(10047):881–890. https://doi.org/10.1016/S0140-6736(16)30385-3.

21. Raskin J, Wiltse CG, Siegal A, et al. Efficacy of duloxetine on cognition, depression, and pain in elderly patients with major depressive disorder: an 8-week, double-blind, placebo-controlled trial. *Am J Psychiatry*. 2007;164:900–909. https://doi.org/10.1176/appi.ajp.164.6.900.

22. Ragguett R-M, Yim SJ, Ho PT, McIntyre RS. Efficacy of levomilnacipran extended release in treating major depressive disorder. *Expert Opin Pharmacother*. 2017;18(18):2017–2024. https://doi.org/10.1080/14656566.2017.1410540.

23. Lambert G, Johansson M, Ågren H, Friberg P. Reduced brain norepinephrine and dopamine release in treatment-refractory depressive illness: evidence in support of the catecholamine hypothesis of mood disorders. *Arch Gen Psychiatry*. 2000;57(8):787–793. https://doi.org/10.1001/archpsyc.57.8.787.

24. Moreira R. The efficacy and tolerability of bupropion in the treatment of major depressive disorder. *Clin Drug Investig*. 2011;31(suppl 1):5–17. https://doi.org/10.2165/1159616-s0-000000000-00000.

25. McElroy SL, Guerdjikova AI, Kim DD, et al. Naltrexone/Bupropion combination therapy in overweight or obese patients with major depressive disorder: results of a pilot study. *Prim Care Companion CNS Disord*. 2013;15. https://doi.org/10.4088/PCC.12m01494.

26. Wilkes S. Bupropion. *Drugs Today Barc Spain 1998*. 2006;42(10):671–681.

27. McIntyre RS, Lee Y, Zhou AJ, et al. The efficacy of psychostimulants in major depressive episodes: a systematic review and meta-analysis. *J Clin Psychopharmacol*. 2017;37(4):412–418. https://doi.org/10.1097/JCP.0000000000000723.

28. Hjorth S, Bengtsson HJ, Kullberg A, Carlzon D, Peilot H, Auerbach SB. Serotonin autoreceptor function and antidepressant drug action. *J Psychopharmacol (Oxf)*. 2000;14(2):177–185. https://doi.org/10.1177/026988110001400204.

29. Celada P, Puig MV, Amargós-Bosch M, Adell A, Artigas F. The therapeutic role of 5-HT1A and 5-HT2A receptors in depression. *J Psychiatry Neurosci*. 2004;29(4):252–265.

30. James SP, Mendelson WB. The use of trazodone as a hypnotic: a critical review. *J Clin Psychiatry*. 2004;65(6):752–755.

31. Anttila SAK, Leinonen EVJ. A review of the pharmacological and clinical profile of mirtazapine. *CNS Drug Rev*. 2001;7(3):249–264. https://doi.org/10.1111/j.1527-3458.2001.tb00198.x.

32. Rosenblat JD, Kakar R, McIntyre RS. The cognitive effects of antidepressants in major depressive disorder: a systematic review and meta-analysis of randomized clinical trials. *Int J Neuropsychopharmacol*. 2015;19(2). https://doi.org/10.1093/ijnp/pyv082.

33. Rosenblat JD, McIntyre RS, Alves GS, Fountoulakis KN, Carvalho AF. Beyond monoamines-novel targets for treatment-resistant depression: a comprehensive review. *Curr Neuropharmacol*. 2015;13(5):636–655.

34. Alamo C, Lopez-Munoz F. New antidepressant drugs: beyond monoaminergic mechanisms. *Curr Pharm Des.* 2009;15:1559–1562.

35. Caddy C, Amit BH, McCloud TL, et al. Ketamine and other glutamate receptor modulators for depression in adults. *Cochrane Database Syst Rev.* 2015:CD011612. https://doi.org/10.1002/14651858.CD011612.pub2.

36. Coyle CM, Laws KR. The use of ketamine as an antidepressant: a systematic review and meta-analysis. *Hum Psychopharmacol.* 2015;30:152–163. https://doi.org/10.1002/hup.2475.

37. Ballard ED, Ionescu DF, Vande Voort JL, et al. Improvement in suicidal ideation after ketamine infusion: relationship to reductions in depression and anxiety. *J Psychiatr Res.* 2014;58:161–166. https://doi.org/10.1016/j.jpsychires.2014.07.027.

38. Wilkinson ST, Ballard ED, Bloch MH, et al. The effect of a single dose of intravenous ketamine on suicidal ideation: a systematic review and individual participant data meta-analysis. *Am J Psychiatry.* 2018;175(2):150–158. https://doi.org/10.1176/appi.ajp.2017.17040472.

39. Cipriani A, Hawton K, Stockton S, Geddes JR. Lithium in the prevention of suicide in mood disorders: updated systematic review and meta-analysis. *BMJ.* 2013;346:f3646. https://doi.org/10.1136/bmj.f3646.

40. Daly E, Singh J, Fedgchin M. Intranasal esketamine in treatment-resistant depression, a dose response study: double blind and open label extension data. In: *Presented at the: The 54th Annual Meeting of the American College of Neuropsychopharmacology.* 2015.

41. Yatham LN, Kennedy SH, Parikh SV, et al. Canadian Network for Mood and Anxiety Treatments (CANMAT) and International Society for Bipolar Disorders (ISBD) collaborative update of CANMAT guidelines for the management of patients with bipolar disorder: update 2013. *Bipolar Disord.* 2013;15:1–44. https://doi.org/10.1111/bdi.12025.

42. Fortney JC, Unutzer J, Wrenn G, et al. A tipping point for measurement-based care. *Psychiatr Serv.* 2017;68: 179–188. https://doi.org/10.1176/appi.ps.201500439.

43. Cipriani A, Furukawa TA, Salanti G, et al. Comparative efficacy and acceptability of 12 new-generation antidepressants: a multiple-treatments meta-analysis. *Lancet.* 2009; 373:746–758. https://doi.org/10.1016/S0140-6736(09)60046-5.

44. McIntyre RS. *Florida Best Practice Psychotherapeutic Medication Guidelines for Adults.* 2015.

45. Suppes T, Silva R, Cucchiaro J, et al. Lurasidone for the treatment of major depressive disorder with mixed features: a randomized, double-blind, placebo-controlled study. *Am J Psychiatry.* 2016;173:400–407. https://doi.org/10.1176/appi.ajp.2015.15060770.

46. Patkar A, Gilmer W, Pae CU, et al. A 6 week randomized double-blind placebo-controlled trial of ziprasidone for the acute depressive mixed state. *PLoS One.* 2012;7: e34757. https://doi.org/10.1371/journal.pone.0034757.

47. Stahl SM, Morrissette DA, Faedda G, et al. Guidelines for the recognition and management of mixed depression. *CNS Spectr.* 2017;22:203–219. https://doi.org/10.1017/S1092852917000165.

48. Connolly KR, Thase ME. If at first you don't succeed: a review of the evidence for antidepressant augmentation, combination and switching strategies. *Drugs.* 2011;71: 43–64. https://doi.org/10.2165/11587620-000000000-00000.

49. Papakostas GI, Shelton RC, Smith J, Fava M. Augmentation of antidepressants with atypical antipsychotic medications for treatment-resistant major depressive disorder: a meta-analysis. *J Clin Psychiatry.* 2007;68: 826–831.

50. Zhou X, Ravindran AV, Qin B, et al. Comparative efficacy, acceptability, and tolerability of augmentation agents in treatment-resistant depression: systematic review and network meta-analysis. *J Clin Psychiatry.* 2015;76(4): e487–498. https://doi.org/10.4088/JCP.14r09204.

51. Himmerich H, Minkwitz J, Kirkby KC. Weight gain and metabolic changes during treatment with antipsychotics and antidepressants. *Endocr Metab Immune Disord - Drug Targets.* 2015;15:252–260.

52. Bak M, Fransen A, Janssen J, van Os J, Drukker M. Almost all antipsychotics result in weight gain: a meta-analysis. *PLoS One.* 2014;9:e94112. https://doi.org/10.1371/journal.pone.0094112.

53. Mitchell AJ, Delaffon V, Vancampfort D, Correll CU, De Hert M. Guideline concordant monitoring of metabolic risk in people treated with antipsychotic medication: systematic review and meta-analysis of screening practices. *Psychol Med.* 2012;42:125–147. https://doi.org/10.1017/S003329171100105X.

54. Simon V, van Winkel R, De Hert M. Are weight gain and metabolic side effects of atypical antipsychotics dose dependent? A literature review. *J Clin Psychiatry.* 2009;70: 1041–1050.

55. Carpenter LL, Yasmin S, Price LH. A double-blind, placebo-controlled study of antidepressant augmentation with mirtazapine. *Biol Psychiatry.* 2002;51:183–188. pii: S0006322301012628.

56. Beach SR, Celano CM, Noseworthy PA, Januzzi JL, Huffman JC. QTc prolongation, torsades de pointes, and psychotropic medications. *Psychosomatics.* 2013;54(1): 1–13. https://doi.org/10.1016/j.psym.2012.11.001.

57. Bauer M, Dopfmer S. Lithium augmentation in treatment-resistant depression: meta-analysis of placebo-controlled studies. *J Clin Psychopharmacol.* 1999;19:427–434.

58. Garland EJ, Remick RA, Zis AP. Weight gain with antidepressants and lithium. *J Clin Psychopharmacol.* 1988;8: 323–330.

59. McKnight RF, Adida M, Budge K, Stockton S, Goodwin GM, Geddes JR. Lithium toxicity profile: a systematic review and meta-analysis. *Lancet.* 2012;379: 721–728. https://doi.org/10.1016/S0140-6736(11)61516-X.

60. Aronson R, Offman HJ, Joffe RT, Naylor CD. Triiodothyronine augmentation in the treatment of refractory depression. A meta-analysis. *Arch Gen Psychiatry.* 1996;53: 842–848.

61. DeBattista C, Doghramji K, Menza MA, Rosenthal MH, Fieve RR. Adjunct modafinil for the short-term treatment of fatigue and sleepiness in patients with major depressive disorder: a preliminary double-blind, placebo-controlled study. *J Clin Psychiatry.* 2003;64:1057—1064.

62. Ng CG, Boks MP, Roes KC, et al. Rapid response to methylphenidate as an add-on therapy to mirtazapine in the treatment of major depressive disorder in terminally ill cancer patients: a four-week, randomized, double-blinded, placebo-controlled study. *Eur Neuropsychopharmacol.* 2014;24:491—498. https://doi.org/10.1016/j.euroneuro.2014.01.016.

63. Fava M, Thase ME, DeBattista C, Doghramji K, Arora S, Hughes RJ. Modafinil augmentation of selective serotonin reuptake inhibitor therapy in MDD partial responders with persistent fatigue and sleepiness. *Ann Clin Psychiatry.* 2007;19:153—159. https://doi.org/10.1080/10401230701464858.

64. Lavretsky H, Reinlieb M, St Cyr N, Siddarth P, Ercoli LM, Senturk D. Citalopram, methylphenidate, or their combination in geriatric depression: a randomized, double-blind, placebo-controlled trial. *Am J Psychiatry.* February 2015. https://doi.org/10.1176/appi.ajp.2014.14070889. appiajp.201414070889.

65. Sanacora G, Frye MA, McDonald W, et al. A consensus statement on the use of ketamine in the treatment of mood disorders. *JAMA Psychiatry.* 2017;74:399—405. https://doi.org/10.1001/jamapsychiatry.2017.0080.

66. Insel TR. The NIMH research domain criteria (RDoC) project: precision medicine for psychiatry. *Am J Psychiatry.* 2014;171(4):395—397. https://doi.org/10.1176/appi.ajp.2014.14020138.

67. Uher R, Perlis RH, Henigsberg N, et al. Depression symptom dimensions as predictors of antidepressant treatment outcome: replicable evidence for interest-activity symptoms. *Psychol Med.* 2012;42:967—980. https://doi.org/10.1017/S0033291711001905.

68. Kautzky A, Dold M, Bartova L, et al. Refining prediction in treatment-resistant depression: results of machine learning analyses in the TRD III sample. *J Clin Psychiatry.* 2017;79(1). https://doi.org/10.4088/JCP.16m11385.

69. Etkin A, Patenaude B, Song YJC, et al. A cognitive-emotional biomarker for predicting remission with antidepressant medications: a report from the iSPOT-D trial. *Neuropsychopharmacol Off Publ Am Coll Neuropsychopharmacol.* 2015;40(6):1332—1342. https://doi.org/10.1038/npp.2014.333.

70. Patel MJ, Andreescu C, Price JC, Edelman KL, Reynolds CF, Aizenstein HJ. Machine learning approaches for integrating clinical and imaging features in late-life depression classification and response prediction. *Int J Geriatr Psychiatry.* 2015;30(10):1056—1067. https://doi.org/10.1002/gps.4262.

71. Rosenblat JD, Lee Y, McIntyre RS. Does pharmacogenomic testing improve clinical outcomes for major depressive disorder? A systematic review of clinical trials and cost-effectiveness studies. *J Clin Psychiatry.* 2017;78:720—729. https://doi.org/10.4088/JCP.15r10583.

CHAPTER 9

Neurocircuitry-Based Treatments for Major Depressive Disorder

PETER GIACOBBE, MD, MSC, FRCPC • KARIM MITHANI, M.ENG •
VENKAT BHAT, MD, MSC, FRCPC, DABPN • YING MENG, MD

INTRODUCTION

Originating in the 1930s, electroconvulsive therapy was the first bonafide treatment available for those with mood disorders, predating the advent of antidepressant medications. In recent years, there has been a renaissance in the interest in brain stimulation as a treatment for refractory psychiatric illness due to multiple converging factors. The fact that more than one in three patients with major depressive disorder (MDD) receive inadequate symptom relief from evidence-based medication and psychotherapy has led to the fervent exploration of other therapeutic modalities for the treatment of this disorder. Furthermore, in the last 2 decades, there has been continued development of neurocircuitry models of the brain, leading to hypothesis-driven direct-to-brain interventional approaches to the treatment of MDD.[1] Additionally, advances in technology have provided multiple means of modulating activity in key structures in the brain.[2] This chapter will outline the existing evidence base for a variety of neuromodulatory approaches, including repetitive transcranial magnetic stimulation (rTMS), electroconvulsive therapy (ECT) and magnetic seizure therapy (MST), deep brain stimulation (DBS), vagus nerve stimulation (VNS), and magnetic resonance imaging (MRI)-guided focused ultrasound (FUS). For further information about transcranial direct current stimulation (tDCS), please refer to.[3]

REPETITIVE TRANSCRANIAL MAGNETIC STIMULATION

In the late 20th century, several scientific teams were exploring the use of magnetic fields to alter electrical signals in the brain. Applying Faraday's Law, Anthony Barker and his colleagues developed the first transcranial magnetic brain stimulator in 1985, which delivered single pulses, used predominantly for diagnostic and research purposes.[4] The therapeutic utility of these devices to deliver repeated trains of magnetic pulses to stimulate the brain for therapeutic reasons began in earnest in the 1990s.[5] The observed benefits of this rTMS on depressive disorders led to the rapid development, investigation, and dissemination of the technology, culminating in the approval of rTMS for MDD by Health Canada in 2002, and by the United States Food and Drug Administration (FDA) in 2008.[6]

rTMS allows for noninvasive modulation of discrete neural structures in a spatially and frequency-dependent manner. High frequency rTMS ($> 10Hz$) has generally excitatory effects, whereas low frequency rTMS ($1Hz$) produces inhibitory effects. Intermediate frequencies produce variable interindividual effects. During the procedure, plastic-encased wire coils are placed on the patient's scalp. Electrical currents are then passed through these coils, generating a changing magnetic field that can penetrate the skin and skull with virtually no resistance. As per Faraday's law of induction, this varying magnetic field in turn produces an electrical current inside the brain, altering the activity of neuronal structures. Using this principle of physics, rTMS can reliably generate electrical changes in targeted areas of the brain.

In contrast to other neuromodulation techniques, rTMS is relatively noninvasive. Compared to convulsive therapies such as ECT and MST, rTMS does not require anesthesia or patient sedation in a hospital setting and does not involve inducing seizures. Nor does it involve the implantation of devices or the creation of ablative lesions, as with DBS, VNS, and FUS. As a result, rTMS may be provided by a psychiatric provider in a wider variety of clinical settings, including both in hospitals and in private offices.

Dozens of randomized controlled trials (RCTs) and meta-analyses have investigated the efficacy of rTMS in treating treatment-resistant depression (TRD).[7,8,9,10,11] In general, these studies have found clinically relevant improvements in depression scores with rTMS compared to sham stimulation, with small-to-medium effect sizes. One of the current factors preventing limiting more widespread delivery of this treatment is the intensity of the treatment protocols. Conventional rTMS protocols require that a patient come into the clinic to receive daily treatments, 5 days a week for 4–6 weeks, for a total of 20–30 sessions.[6] Much research in underway to streamline the delivery of rTMS to maximize its accessibility to patients with MDD.

There appears to be no difference between high frequency of left dorsolateral prefrontal cortex (DLPFC) and low frequency of right DLPFC in terms of antidepressant efficacy, with both forms of rTMS demonstrating response rates in the 40%–55% range and remission rates in the 25%–35% range.[11] The long-term effects of this treatment are unclear; however, RCTs with longer follow-up phases (e.g., 8–16 weeks) tend to have lower effect sizes compared to those with shorter follow-ups (e.g., 1–4 weeks).[9] Most rTMS protocols appear to be less effective than ECT in treating major depression, although they may be better tolerated by patients.[12] The most commonly reported side effect of rTMS is scalp pain, which occurs in 35%–40% of individuals. Other adverse effects include transient headaches after stimulation, mania or hypomania, sleep disturbances, or—in less than 0.01% of cases—seizure.[6] No neurocognitive effects have been noted, and in fact there is some evidence to suggest that rTMS may impart some cognitive benefits.[13]

Several different targets, techniques, and protocols for rTMS have been developed, with variable efficacy in treating TRD. The most common target is the DLPFC, a bilaterally paired structure involved in mediating working memory, decision making, and other executive functions. Hypoactivity in the DLPFC is associated with major depression in functional neuroimaging studies, and rTMS-mediated excitation of this region has shown beneficial effects in TRD.[14] Alternative targets include the dorsomedial prefrontal cortex (DMPFC), frontopolar cortex, ventromedial prefrontal cortex, and ventrolateral prefrontal cortex that have shown promise in uncontrolled case series and await verification in sham-controlled studies.

rTMS is dosed relative to the minimum amount of energy reliably producing a motor reaction, typically of the thumb, when the coil is placed over the motor cortex. This is referred to as motor threshold (MT). The highest tolerable dose of energy is delivered to the DLPFC, typically up to 115%–120% of the MT in high frequency protocols. Other variables that affect rTMS efficacy include length and dosing of treatment regimen, frequency of treatment sessions, unilateral versus bilateral stimulation, targeting techniques, coil type, and stimulation parameters.[15] The frequency of stimulation during an rTMS treatment session can vary across protocols. Presently, the 10 Hz left DLPFC protocol, which takes approximately 37.5 minutes, has the most supporting evidence for the treatment of TRD.[15] A newer form of rTMS called intermittent theta burst stimulation (iTBS), which is a form of patterned stimulation that is excitatory and mimics physiological theta rhythms. A 3-min high frequency iTBS protocol delivered to the left DLPFC at 120% MT has been recently shown to be noninferior to the 10 Hz protocol, leading to its approval by the FDA as an intervention for MDD.[16] Given that one of the major drawbacks to rTMS is the extensive time commitment required this innovation has the potential to dramatically improve patient acceptability of rTMS. Research has explored neuroimaging predictors of treatment response to rTMS, with promising results identifying a biotype responsive to DMPFC rTMS and selecting cortical regions with the maximal anticorrelation in functional connectivity to the subgenual cingulate cortex as a predictor of response to high frequency DLPFC rTMS[17,18]

In summary, rTMS is an established noninvasive neuromodulation technique for MDD, which offers the promise of an incredible degree of flexibility in selecting the neuroanatomical target and personalizing the brain stimulation parameters delivered. The antidepressant effects of rTMS may be equivalent to or superior to pharmacological add-on strategies for those with TRD, but less robust than those of ECT. However, its noninvasive nature, excellent safety profile, and minimal associated side effects make rTMS an appealing initial brain stimulation management option for those with TRD. Future research will continue to clarify the optimal rTMS protocols for individuals with different symptoms clusters of MDD.

CONVULSIVE THERAPIES (ELECTROCONVULSIVE THERAPY AND MAGNETIC SEIZURE THERAPY)

Convulsive treatments are therapeutic procedures that entail an induction of a seizure under general anesthesia. ECT applies an electrical stimulus to the scalp, whereas MST uses a coil that generates a strong magnetic field that is able to cross the skull and soft tissue unimpeded, to reach the brain to elicit a generalized seizure. ECT as a somatic therapy has a long history extending into the first half of the 20th century. Over time, electrically induced seizures under anesthesia and muscle relaxation have supplanted "unmodified" forms of ECT. ECT has demonstrated efficacy in the treatment of many psychiatric disorders, with depressive disorders being the most common treatment indication.[19] MST is a newer form of convulsive treatment that represents a continuation of the trend toward more focal brain stimulation that began with unilateral ECT. MST is being studied as an alternative to ECT, with the promise of maintaining the efficacy of ECT but reducing its associated cognitive side effects. Seizures induced by convulsive treatments are considered to have antidepressant effects through mechanisms including neuroplasticity, neurogenesis, changes in functional connectivity, altered levels of neurotransmitters such as GABA, and neurotrophic factors such as brain-derived neurotropic factor.[20] All convulsive treatments elicit seizures under general anesthesia with assisted ventilation and EEG monitoring and application of a muscle relaxant.

Among established antidepressant treatments, ECT is associated with the fastest onset of clinical effects. The median number of treatments to achieve an antidepressant response, resolution of suicidal ideation and remission of symptoms, is 3, 4 and 7, respectively.[21,22] A typical frequency of ECT during an index course of treatment is 2–3 times per week. More than three treatments per week are not recommended due to significantly higher frequency of cognitive side effects.[23] A course of ECT may yield an antidepressant response in the 50%–80% range, with lower response rates in those higher degrees of prior treatment resistance. Positive prognostic features to ECT in those with MDD, include older age, greater severity of illness, presence of psychosis, and the absence of personality disorders.[24] A meta-analysis of patient-reported quality of life revealed that ECT was associated with large and very large effect size improvements in both mental and physical health confirms that ECT plays a vital role in the treatment of the most severely ill patients with MDD.[25]

ECT has been recommended as a first-line choice in MDD in certain clinical scenarios, such as acute suicidal ideation, psychotic features, TRD, catatonic features, prior favorable response to ECT, rapidly deteriorating physical status, and patient preference.[26] Although ECT has no absolute contraindications, relative contraindications include conditions such as recent cerebral hemorrhage and class 4 or 5 anesthesia risk. MST delivery has followed the ECT schedule (2–3 times per week, index course of 12 treatments), but the

optimal delivery parameters for MST are current topics of investigation. ECT is generally considered to produce superior antidepressant effects than rTMS, with no differences in global cognitive performance as measured by the Mini-Mental State Examination (MMSE).

However, in head-to-head studies, ECT patients had more immediate impairments in visual memory and verbal fluency compared to rTMS.[27] The limited studies comparing MST to sham stimulation suggest response and remission rates similar to those obtained with acute ECT[28] and MST is currently considered an investigational treatment pending positive results in pivotal trials.[26]

Modern ECT entails detailed medical, laboratory, and anesthesia evaluation with appropriate risk–benefit considerations and obtention of informed consent before ECT. ECT is extremely safe, with a procedural mortality rate estimated to be less than 1 death per 98,000 treatments, similar to that of general anesthesia.[29] Transient adverse effects such as headaches (45%), muscle soreness (20%), and nausea (up to 25%) can occur and can be managed symptomatically.[2] Cognitive impairment is the most concerning adverse effect for patients and family members. Transient post-procedural disorientation can occur secondary to postictal confusion and effects of general anesthesia. Anterograde amnesia usually disappears within weeks to months following acute course of ECT and retrograde amnesia as demonstrated by objective tests of autobiographical memory typically does not persist 6 months post-ECT.[30] However, subjective retrograde amnesia is often reported, with self-reports of cognitive dysfunction correlating strongly with persistent depressive symptoms. Clinical factors, including older age, preexisting cognitive impairment, and use of bitemporal ECT, have been associated with greater cognitive impairment.[31]

Lithium use during ECT may increase risk of cognitive side effects, whereas anticonvulsants and benzodiazepines could raise the seizure threshold and decrease seizure efficacy. MST through focal stimulation appears to have lower rates of headaches and muscle aches than ECT, with lower associated rates of anterograde/retrograde anesthesia and reduced reorientation time.[28] There is no evidence of brain damage with ECT; in fact, meta-analyses have indicated that hippocampal volume increases following ECT, suggestive that ECT is a neurorestorative treatment.[32]

Having a seizure is necessary but not sufficient to trigger an antidepressant effect, and doses above seizure threshold (ST) are required. The treatment parameters for ECT include electrode position, electrical intensity, and pulse width. Dose titration techniques have included stimulus dosing, preselected dose, and EEG-based dosing, with stimulus dosing being the most commonly employed method. Bitemporal (BT), bifrontal (BF), or right unilateral (RUL) are the most common electrode placements and have similar efficacy but may affect specific cognitive domains differently.[33] BT and BF ECT is dosed at 1.5—2.0 times ST and RUL at 6—8 times ST. There has been an evolution from sine wave to brief pulse ECT (pulse width>0.5 msec), and ultrabrief (pulse width <0.5 msec) may be associated with less short-term cognitive impairment and specifically the loss of autobiographical memory.[34]

In modern era studies, 51.1% of patients successfully treated with ECT will experience a relapse of their condition within 12 months, with most relapses (37.7%, 95% CI = 30.7%—45.2%) occurring within the first 6 months.[35] Meta-analyses have revealed a trend toward increased post-ECT relapse rates in the 21st century versus the 1960s, which has been attributed to the higher degree of refractory illness seen in those referred for ECT now compared to the past.[35] Expert opinion recommends that some form of post-ECT prophylaxis is required after every successful course of ECT. Evidence-based methods to reduce relapse post-ECT include the use of medications (the combinations of nortriptyline and lithium or venlafaxine and lithium), or maintenance of ECT at a gradually diminishing frequency.[36,37] Recently, the Prolonging Remission in Depressed Elderly (PRIDE) Study, reported a 16% relapse rate over 24 weeks, when venlafaxine and lithium (0.4—0.6 mEq/L), together with weekly ECT for the first 4 weeks, followed by ECT as indicated ("rescue ECT") was provided.[38]

Although ECT continues to be considered the "gold standard" in terms of acute antidepressant effects, there remain numerous opportunities for optimization. This includes developing comparative evidence for delivery parameters (electrode placements, anesthetic agents, stimulus waveform, and dosing), pharmacological augmentation of ECT with existing and novel antidepressant agents, and development of "closed loop" ECT delivery with feedback-driven stimulation. MST may represent the evolution of ECT toward more focal stimulation with less delivery of electricity. Finally, deeper insights into the neural circuitry underlying depression would offer potential biomarkers to predict treatment response and to personalize convulsive treatment parameters to the individual patient.

SURGICAL APPROACHES TO TRD

For individuals with TRD for whom noninvasive and convulsive neuromodulation approaches are ineffective, neurocircuitry-based surgical approaches may be considered. These include implantable device-related approaches such as DBS, VNS, or alternatively an incisionless neuroablative procedure, MRI-guided FUS. Current treatment guidelines consider surgical approaches to TRD as third line or experimental options[26] and should only be offered in specialized centers following a thorough presurgical screening process.

Deep Brain Stimulation

DBS involves directly modulating the activity of discrete neuronal structures or networks via electrodes implanted in the brain, which provide continuous stimulation. An implantable pulse generator, often described as a "pacemaker," is implanted under the clavicle and connected to intracranial electrodes via subcutaneous wires. The electrodes can be precisely targeted through MRI guidance to specific structures in the brain and the stimulation finely calibrated, to achieve the desired effects. DBS has a long history in functional neurosurgery for various indications, most prominently movement disorders, with burgeoning research exploring its efficacy in treating refractory psychiatric disorders, such as treatment-resistant major depressive disorder (TRD).[39]

Different from other types of ablative psychiatric neurosurgeries, DBS offers a relatively less invasive, adjustable, and reversible way to alter the activity of neuronal networks. Advances in structural and functional brain imaging have dramatically improved the accuracy of neurosurgical procedures, including DBS. For example, electrode targeting is augmented by MRI techniques such as diffusion tensor imaging.[40] Postoperative imaging of DBS patients, however, is a controversial topic; although MRI is typically an indispensable method for assessing certain surgical complications, such as hemorrhage or brain shift, its use is limited by concerns about safety and accuracy in these patients. The mechanism of action of DBS is not fully understood, and likely varies by target and indication. Theories of DBS effects include neuronal excitation, neuronal inhibition, a combination of excitation and inhibition, and/or cellular and molecular changes.[41]

In 2005, a seminal pilot study of DBS of the subgenual cingulate white matter revealed acute and sustained improvements in depressive symptoms in four out of six patients with TRD.[42] Many targets for TRD

DBS have been investigated with variable degrees of effectiveness, including subcallosal cingulate gyrus, nucleus accumbens, anterior limb of the internal capsule, caudate nucleus, medial forebrain bundle, lateral habenular complex, inferior thalamic peduncle, and subthalamic nucleus.[42a]

The antidepressant effects of DBS remain controversial, with small observational studies and controlled trials reporting variable results.[43] To date, eight controlled clinical trials have investigated DBS for TRD, six of which were double-blinded RCTs, and two were single-blinded sham-controlled trials. In general, these studies found an improvement in depressive symptoms with deep brain stimulation, albeit with variable efficacy and side-effect profiles depending—in part—on the neuronal target. Modest sample sizes, heterogeneous surgical targets and techniques, and restricted clinical trial designs likely all contribute to this variability, making it difficult to define consistent, practicable guidelines.

A meta-analysis of these controlled trials found odds ratios of "treatment response," defined as a HAMD-17 score of less than eight or a 50% or greater reduction in depression scores, to be between 4.85 and 8.34 depending on the target.[44] The total odds ratio of DBS for TRD was 5.50. The most effective target was the medial forebrain bundle, followed by the subcallosal cingulate and the internal/ventral capsule. Notably, the apparently beneficial effects of DBS were no longer significant when the meta-analysis was restricted only to parallel-group studies, as opposed to crossover designs.

In the same meta-analysis, the most commonly reported adverse events included device-related discomfort, infection, pain around the incision, headache, agitation/restlessness, and hypomania.[44] Notably, the sham stimulation phases of these controlled trials frequently precipitated increased depression or anxiety, as well as suicidal ideation and attempts, providing indirect support for the salutary effects of active stimulation. As always, patients should be fully informed of the numerous risks associated with the procedure, including surgical complications, device-related adverse effects, and the potential for worsening their symptoms.

Importantly, the effects of DBS on long-term functional outcomes and quality of life have not been systematically investigated. This is important because clinical ratings of depressive symptoms do not necessarily correspond to a normalization of perceived quality of life or functioning for many patients with MDD.[25]

In summary, DBS may offer a promising treatment option for patients with debilitating, refractory major depression. Nevertheless, its effectiveness for this indication is inconsistent and still under investigation. The mechanism of action, optimal target, and ideal candidates for DBS are still unclear, and require large, controlled clinical trials to be better delineated. The risks posed by DBS, including those of the surgery and potential return of symptoms with cessation of stimulation, should be thoroughly discussed with patients and carefully balanced with potential benefits.

Vagus Nerve Stimulation

VNS is a device-based therapy that involves the surgical insertion of an implantable pulse generator below the skin of the chest, which is connected to an electrode that stimulates the left vagus nerve in the neck. Among the cranial nerves, vagus nerve is the 10th cranial nerve and the left vagus nerve predominantly comprises afferent nerve fibers that convey impulses to the brain from the periphery.

The rationale for VNS as an antidepressant treatment emerged from evidence of mood improvement in VNS-implanted epilepsy patients, benefits of anticonvulsant therapies for mood stabilization, as well as preclinical literature.[45] VNS is thought to provide electrical stimulation to the nucleus tractus solitarius, which has widely distributed neuronal connections to limbic and cortical regions of the brain and is thus able to impact multiple regions of the brain.[46] VNS was approved initially as an adjunctive therapy for epilepsy in 1997 by the US FDA, and in 2005 as an adjunctive treatment in the long-term management of TRD. The CANMAT neurostimulation guidelines recommend it as a third-line acute treatment with level-3 evidence for efficacy.[26]

The optimal treatment parameters for VNS have not been definitively established. One open-label RCT of VNS compared high (1.25–1.5 mA, 250 ms), medium (0.5–1.0 mA, 250 ms), or low (0.25 mA current, 130 ms pulse width) electrical outputs, and better improvement in depressive symptoms were associated with higher electrical charges.[47] Furthermore, reduction in suicide attempts and more sustained antidepressant responses were predominantly noted in the medium- and high stimulation groups.

VNS may be associated with modest acute antidepressant effects. At 12 weeks, no significant differences in efficacy between active and sham VNS were established in the only RCT conducted to date, although a meta-analysis of open-label studies suggested a response rate of 31.8%.[48] The antidepressant effects of VNS accumulate over time with one study estimating median time to response at 9 months[49] and long-term naturalistic trials with up to 5 years follow-up suggest that enhanced antidepressant effects may further accrue over time with VNS, compared to treatment as usual.[50] In addition, VNS plus treatment as usual (TAU) compared to TAU alone found significantly higher odds ratios (ORs) for response (OR, 3.19) and remission (OR, 4.99) but the absolute response rates were low.[51] VNS has been approved by the FDA for the treatment of adult patients with a major depressive episode who failed to respond to four or more adequate antidepressant treatments, for the adjunct long-term treatment of chronic or recurrent depression.

During long-term treatment with VNS, diminishing rates of adverse events and improving tolerability over time has been reported by patients. After 1 year of VNS for TRD, increased cough (26.4%), pain (28.4%), dyspnea (30.1%), and voice alteration (69.3%) are the most commonly reported adverse effects.[47a] Turning off the stimulation can immediately restore the voice and reduce cough as these are direct effects of VNS stimulation. Treatment-emergent hypomania or mania (2.7%) and suicide or attempted suicide (4.6%) are the main reported serious adverse psychiatric events[47]; however, VNS may increase long-term survival for those with TRD, as lower all-cause mortality rate and suicide has been noted with adjunctive VNS, compared to TAU alone.[52]

Future directions for VNS include alternative means of stimulating the nerve, obviating the need for a surgery. Positive results from a sham-controlled trial of transcutaneous VNS delivering electrical impulses to the afferent auricular branch of the vagus nerve may also represent a promising advance.[53] Of note, there are similarities between the VNS and the DBS literature with accrued evidence for positive clinical effects of long-term stimulation beyond the 6-month durations of double-blind treatment trials. This suggests that alternative trial designs other than short-term comparisons with an active versus sham arm may be needed to capture the full clinical and neurobiological effects of this modality.

MRI-Guided Focused Ultrasound

MRI-guided FUS is an emerging technology for noninvasive therapeutic ablation of brain tissue and nonlesional neuromodulation. Ultrasound refers to high-frequency mechanical vibrations produced by transducers. Although commonly used as a diagnostic tool in medicine, ultrasound may also have a variety of neurobiologic effects, depending on a variety of biophysical parameters. With advances in phased array technology, image guidance, and stereotactic frames, precise transcranial delivery of ultrasound is achievable.[54] The clinician can adjust the energy delivery in

real time in response to the tissue changes detected by MR and MR thermometry to create an anatomically circumscribed ablative lesion. Focused ultrasound is therefore considered to be incisionless neurosurgical intervention.

FUS for neuroablation has established human safety data, stemming from numerous clinical trials of thalamotomy for movement disorders such as essential tremor, Parkinson's disease, and dystonia, as well as pain disorders.[55] Investigations of FUS for medically refractory obsessive-compulsive disorder (OCD) with bilateral anterior capsulotomy have also been reported.[56] The study found gradual improvement in Y-BOCS scores in four patients with OCD and comorbid MDD by 33% at 6 months. Symptoms of depression as measured by the HAMD were reduced by 61.1% at 6 months, without any adverse effects or changes on neuropsychological test scores[57]

FUS neuroablation of the anterior limb of the internal capsule (ALIC) for patients with TRD is currently the target of several ongoing investigations (NCT02348411, NCT02685488). The ALIC consists of a dense set of white matter tracts that connect numerous cortical and subcortical regions, such as the prefrontal cortex, anterior cingulate cortex, hippocampus, amygdala, and thalamus.[58] Imaging studies in human subjects and animal studies have found these targets, part of the cortico-striato-thalamo-cortical model to be implicated in depressive symptoms and other mood disorders. To date, the ALIC target has been used in a single case report of the FUS procedure for TRD.[57] Baseline HAMD of 26 decreased to 8 as early as 1 week, and remained at 7 at 12 months. Although this result seems promising, it requires replication in larger scale studies.

FUS employed at lower intensities than those resulting in thermal ablation can focally and reversibly alter brain activity, although this form of neuromodulation for the treatment of depression remains unexplored. An alternative effect of low-intensity FUS in combination with intravenously injected microbubbles is increased blood-brain barrier (BBB) permeability in the target area. FUS-induced opening of the BBB in the hippocampus was found to have antidepressant effects in one study with rodent forced-swim test model.[61] The mechanism of these effects is unclear, but may be associated with the robust increase in neurogenesis after BBB modulation by FUS. Alterations in neurotrophic factors and neural plasticity, as well as FUS-aided therapeutic delivery, are also areas of investigation.

Overall, FUS for TRD is investigational. Compared to other stereotactic techniques such as radiofrequency ablation and stereotactic radiosurgery, the FUS does not require open surgery or use ionizing radiation and is potentially safer due to the spatial precision and control offered by this image-guided technology. Additionally, it offers the prospect of aiding in the delivery of molecules and/or the temporary disruption of the BBB in anatomically focused manner under MRI-guided FUS. The therapeutic effects of FUS for mood disorders remain to be explored.

CONCLUSION

As the conceptualization of MDD is moving beyond a strict neurotransmitter doctrine to one of a circuit disorder,[59] there has been a rapid expansion in the evidence base for neuromodulation strategies to help those with TRD. This growth has led to the interest in "Interventional Psychiatry" as a subspecialty within our field, which utilizes technologies to identify dysfunctional brain circuitry underlying psychiatric disorders and apply direct-to-brain techniques to modulate that circuitry.[60]

Multiple brain stimulation methods now exist, each with different neurophysiological mechanisms and kinetics of response. Noninvasive stimulation in the form of rTMS has been recommended as a first-line choice for those that have failed to respond to at least one adequate antidepressant medication. ECT has the quickest onset of antidepressant effects, while implantable device-related stimulation (VNS and DBS) appear to have delayed but sustained effects. We await positive results from sham-controlled trials to evaluate the safety and efficacy of the novel techniques of MST and FUS in the treatment of MDD. Future research should prioritize the identification of biomarkers of response and the exploration of when is the optimal point in the disease course for each neuromodulation technique to be provided. This would allow more precise patient selection to maximize clinical and functional outcomes.

REFERENCES

1. Giacobbe P, Mayberg HS, Lozano AM. Treatment resistant depression as a failure of brain homeostatic mechanisms: implications for deep brain stimulation. *Exp Neurol.* 2009; 219:44−52.
2. Lipsman N, Sankar T, Downar J, Kennedy SH, Lozano AM, Giacobbe P. Neuromodulation for treatment-refractory major depressive disorder. *Can Med Assoc J.* 2014;186: 33−39.
3. Brunoni AR, Moffa AH, Fregni F, et al. Transcranial direct current stimulation for acute major depressive episodes: meta-analysis of individual patient data. *Br J Psychiatry.* 2016;208:522−531.
4. Barker AT, Jalinous R, Freeston IL. Non-invasive magnetic stimulation of human motor cortex. *Lancet.* 1985;1(8437): 1106−1107.
5. Kolbinger HM, Höflich G, Hufnagel A, Müller H-J, Kasper S. Transcranial magnetic stimulation (TMS) in the treatment of major depression — a pilot study. *Hum Psychopharmacol Clin Exp.* 1995;10(4):305−310.
6. Downar J, Blumberger DM, Daskalakis ZJ. Repetitive transcranial magnetic stimulation: an emerging treatment for medication-resistant depression. *Can Med Assoc J.* 2016; 188:1175−1177.
7. Berlim MT, van den Eynde F, Tovar-Perdomo S, Daskalakis ZJ. Response, remission and drop-out rates following high-frequency repetitive transcranial magnetic stimulation (rTMS) for treating major depression: a systematic review and meta-analysis of randomized, double-blind and sham-controlled trials. *Psychol Med.* 2014;44:225−239.
8. Kedzior KK, Gellersen HM, Brachetti AK, Berlim MT. Deep transcranial magnetic stimulation (DTMS) in the treatment of major depression: an exploratory systematic review and meta-analysis. *J Affect Disord.* 2015a;187:73−83.
9. Kedzior KK, Reitz SK, Azorina V, Loo C. Durability of the antidepressant effect of the high-frequency repetitive transcranial magnetic stimulation (rTMS) in the absence of maintenance treatment in major depression: a systematic review and meta-analysis of 16 double-blind, randomized, sham-controlled trials. *Depress Anxiety.* 2015b;32: 193−203.
10. Liu B, Zhang Y, Zhang L, Li L. Repetitive transcranial magnetic stimulation as an augmentative strategy for treatment-resistant depression, a meta-analysis of randomized, double-blind and sham-controlled study. *BMC Psychiatry.* 2014;14:342. https://doi.org/10.1186/s12888-014-0342-4.
11. Brunoni AR, Chaimani A, Moffa AH, et al. Repetitive transcranial magnetic stimulation for the acute treatment of major depressive episodes: a systematic review with network meta-analysis. *JAMA Psychiatry.* 2017;74: 143−152.
12. Chen J, Zhao L, Liu Y, Fan S, Xie P. Comparative efficacy and acceptability of electroconvulsive therapy versus repetitive transcranial magnetic stimulation for major depression: a systematic review and multiple-treatments meta-analysis. *Behav Brain Res.* 2017;320:30−36.
13. Martin DM, McClintock SM, Forster JJ, Lo TY, Loo CK. Cognitive enhancing effects of rTMS administered to the prefrontal cortex in patients with depression: a systematic review and meta-analysis of individual task effects. *Depress Anxiety.* 2017;34:1029−1039.
14. Downar J, Daskalakis ZJ. New targets for rTMS in depression: a review of convergent evidence. *Brain Stimul.* 2013; 6:231−240.
15. Health Quality Ontario. Repetitive transcranial magnetic stimulation for treatment-resistant depression: a systematic review and meta-analysis of randomized controlled trials. *Ont Health Technol Assess Ser.* 2016;16(5):1−66. http://www.ncbi.nlm.nih.gov/pubmed/27099642.

16. Blumberger DM, Vila-Rodriguez F, Thorpe KE, et al. Effectiveness of theta burst versus high-frequency repetitive transcranial magnetic stimulation in patients with depression (THREE-D): a randomised non-inferiority trial. *Lancet.* 2018;391(10131):1683−1692.

17. Drysdale AT, Grosenick L, Downar J, et al. Resting-state connectivity biomarkers define neurophysiological subtypes of depression. *Nat Med.* 2017;23:28−38.

18. Weigand A, Horn A, Caballero R, et al. Prospective validation that subgenual connectivity predicts antidepressant efficacy of transcranial magnetic stimulation sites. *Biol Psychiatry.* 2018;84:28−37.

19. Mankad MV, Beyer JL, Weiner RD, Krystal A. *Clinical Manual of Electroconvulsive Therapy.* American Psychiatric Pub; 2010.

20. Brunoni AR, Baeken C, Machado-Vieira R, Gattaz WF, Vanderhasselt M-A. BDNF blood levels after electroconvulsive therapy in patients with mood disorders: a systematic review and meta-analysis. *World J Biol Psychiatr.* 2014;15:411−418.

21. Husain MM, Rush AJ, Fink M, et al. Speed of response and remission in major depressive disorder with acute electroconvulsive therapy (ECT): a Consortium for Research in ECT (CORE) report. *J Clin Psychiatry.* 2004;65:485−491.

22. Kellner CH, Fink M, Knapp R, et al. Relief of expressed suicidal intent by ECT: a consortium for research in ECT study. *Am J Psychiatry.* 2005;162:977−982.

23. Charlson F, Siskind D, Doi SA, McCallum E, Broome A, Lie DC. ECT efficacy and treatment course: a systematic review and meta-analysis of twice vs thrice weekly schedules. *J Affect Disord.* 2012;138:1−8.

24. Nordenskjöld A, von Knorring L, Engström I. Predictors of the short-term responder rate of Electroconvulsive therapy in depressive disorders–a population based study. *BMC Psychiatry.* 2012;12:115. https://doi.org/10.1186/1471-244X-12-115.

25. Giacobbe P, Rakita U, Penner-Goeke K, et al. Improvements in health-related quality of life with electroconvulsive therapy: a meta-analysis. *J ECT.* 2018;34:87−94.

26. Milev RV, Giacobbe P, Kennedy SH, et al. Canadian network for mood and anxiety treatments (CANMAT) 2016 clinical guidelines for the management of adults with major depressive disorder: section 4. Neurostimulation treatments. *Can J Psychiatr.* 2016;61:561−575.

27. Ren J, Li H, Palaniyappan L, et al. Repetitive transcranial magnetic stimulation versus electroconvulsive therapy for major depression: a systematic review and meta-analysis. *Prog Neuro-Psychopharmacol Biol Psychiatry.* 2014;51:181−189.

28. Kayser S, Bewernick BH, Matusch A, Hurlemann R, Soehle M, Schlaepfer TE. Magnetic seizure therapy in treatment-resistant depression: clinical, neuropsychological and metabolic effects. *Psychol Med.* 2015;45:1073−1092.

29. Østergaard SD, Bolwig TG, Petrides G. No causal association between electroconvulsive therapy and death: a summary of a report from the Danish Health and Medicines Authority covering 99,728 treatments. *J ECT.* 2014;30:263−264.

30. Semkovska M, McLoughlin DM. Objective cognitive performance associated with electroconvulsive therapy for depression: a systematic review and meta-analysis. *Biol Psychiatry.* 2010;68:568−577.

31. Kumar S, et al. Systematic review of cognitive effects of electroconvulsive therapy in late-life depression. *Am J Geriatr Psychiatry.* 2016;24:547−565.

32. Wilkinson ST, Sanacora G, Bloch MH. Hippocampal volume changes following electroconvulsive therapy: a systematic review and meta-analysis. *Biol Psychiatry Cogn Neurosci Neuroimaging.* 2017;2(4):327−335.

33. Dunne RA, McLoughlin DM. Systematic review and meta-analysis of bifrontal electroconvulsive therapy versus bilateral and unilateral electroconvulsive therapy in depression. *World J Biol Psychiatr.* 2012;13:248−258.

34. Verwijk E, et al. Neurocognitive effects after brief pulse and ultrabrief pulse unilateral electroconvulsive therapy for major depression: a review. *J Affect Disord.* 2012;140:233−243.

35. Jelovac A, Kolshus E, McLoughlin DM. Relapse following successful electroconvulsive therapy for major depression: a meta-analysis. *Neuropsychopharmacology.* 2013;38:2467−2474.

36. Prudic J, Haskett RF, McCall WV, et al. Pharmacological strategies in the prevention of relapse after electroconvulsive therapy. *J ECT.* 2013;29:3−12.

37. Kellner CH, Knapp RG, Petrides G, et al. Continuation electroconvulsive therapy vs pharmacotherapy for relapse prevention in major depression: a multisite study from the Consortium for Research in Electroconvulsive Therapy (CORE). *Arch Gen Psychiatr.* 2006;63:1337−1344.

38. Kellner CH, Husain MM, Knapp RG, et al. A novel strategy for continuation ECT in geriatric depression: phase 2 of the PRIDE study. *Am J Psychiatry.* 2016;173:1110−1118.

39. Lozano AM, Lipsman N, Bergman H, et al. Deep brain stimulation: current challenges and future directions. *Nat Rev Neurol.* 2019;15:148−160.

40. Rodrigues NB, Mithani K, Meng Y, Lipsman N, Hamani C. The emerging role of tractography in deep brain stimulation: basic principles and current applications. *Brain Sci.* 2018;8(2). https://doi.org/10.3390/brainsci8020023.

41. Lozano AM, Lipsman N. Probing and regulating dysfunctional circuits using deep brain stimulation. *Neuron.* 2013;77:406−424.

42. Mayberg HS, Lozano AM, Voon V, et al. Deep brain stimulation for treatment-resistant depression. *Neuron.* 2005;45:651−660.

42a. Dandekar MP, Fenoy AJ, Carvalho AF, Soares JC, Quevedo J. Deep brain stimulation for treatment-resistant depression: an integrative review of preclinical and clinical findings and translational implications. *Mol Psychiatry.* 2018;23(5):1094−1112.

43. Dougherty DD. Deep brain stimulation: clinical applications. *Psychiatr Clin.* 2018;41:385−394. https://doi.org/10.1016/j.psc.2018.04.004.

44. Kisely S, Li A, Warren N, Siskind D. A systematic review and meta-analysis of deep brain stimulation for depression. *Depress Anxiety*. 2018;35:468—480.

45. George MS, Sackeim HA, Rush AJ, et al. Vagus nerve stimulation: a new tool for brain research and therapy. *Biol Psychiatry*. 2000;47:287—295.

46. Nemeroff CB, Mayberg HS, Krahl SE, et al. VNS therapy in treatment-resistant depression: clinical evidence and putative neurobiological mechanisms. *Neuropsychopharmacology*. 2006;31:1345—1355.

47. Aaronson ST, et al. Vagus nerve stimulation therapy randomized to different amounts of electrical charge for treatment-resistant depression: acute and chronic effects. *Brain stimulation*. 2013;6:631—640.

47a. Berry SM, Broglio K, Bunker M, Jayewardene A, Olin B, Rush AJ. A patient-level meta-analysis of studies evaluating vagus nerve stimulation therapy for treatment-resistant depression. *Med Devices (Auckl)*. 2013;6:17—35.

48. Martin J, Martin-Sanchez E. Systematic review and meta-analysis of vagus nerve stimulation in the treatment of depression: variable results based on study designs. *Eur Psychiatry*. 2012;27:147—155.

49. Schlaepfer T, et al. Vagus nerve stimulation for depression: efficacy and safety in a European study. *Psychol Med*. 2008; 38:651—661.

50. Aaronson ST, et al. A 5-year observational study of patients with treatment-resistant depression treated with vagus nerve stimulation or treatment as usual: comparison of response, remission, and suicidality. *Am J Psychiatry*. 2017;174:640—648.

51. Berry SM, Broglio K, Bunker M, Jayewardene A, Olin B, Rush AJ. A patient-level meta-analysis of studies evaluating vagus nerve stimulation therapy for treatment-resistant depression. *Med Devices (Auckl)*. 2013;6:17—35.

52. Olin B, Jayewardene AK, Bunker M, Moreno F. Mortality and suicide risk in treatment-resistant depression: an observational study of the long-term impact of intervention. *PLoS One*. 2012;7:e48002.

53. Rong P, et al. Effect of transcutaneous auricular vagus nerve stimulation on major depressive disorder. A non-randomized controlled pilot study. *J Affect Disord*. 2016; 195:172—179.

54. Hynynen K, Jones RM. Image-guided ultrasound phased arrays are a disruptive technology for non-invasive therapy. *Phys Med Biol*. 2016;61:R206.

55. Meng Y, et al. Current and emerging brain applications of MR-guided focused ultrasound. *J. Ther. Ultrasound*. 2017;5:26.

56. Jung HH, et al. Bilateral thermal capsulotomy with MR-guided focused ultrasound for patients with treatment-refractory obsessive-compulsive disorder: a proof-of-concept study. *Mol Psychiatr*. 2015;20:1205—1211.

57. Kim SJ, Roh D, Jung HH, Chang WS, Kim CH, Chang JW. A study of novel bilateral thermal capsulotomy with focused ultrasound for treatment-refractory obsessive-compulsive disorder: 2-year follow-up. *J Psychiatry Neurosci*. 2018;43(5):327—337.

58. Safadi Z, Grisot G, Jbabdi S, et al. Functional segmentation of the anterior limb of the internal capsule: linking white matter abnormalities to specific connections. *J Neurosci*. 2018;38:2106—2117.

59. Gordon JA. On being a circuit psychiatrist. *Nat Neurosci*. 2016;19:1385—1386.

60. Williams NR, Taylor JJ, Kerns S, Short EB, Kantor EM, George MS. Interventional psychiatry: why now? *J Clin Psychiatry*. 2014;75:895—897.

61. Mooney SJ, Shah K, Yeung S, Burgess A, Aubert I, Hynynen K. Focused Ultrasound-Induced Neurogenesis Requires an Increase in Blood-Brain Barrier Permeability, 26. 2016;11(7): e0159892.

CHAPTER 10

Pharmacological and Nonpharmacological Treatment Effects on Functional Outcomes in Major Depressive Disorder

TRACY L. GREER, BA, MS, PHD, MSCS • JEETHU K. JOSEPH, BS

INTRODUCTION

In 1962, Drs. J.D. Stoeckle and G.E. Davidson published a case series in the *Journal of the American Medical Association* describing "functional depression" in four depressed individuals,[1] indicated by disturbances in three main areas: (1) bodily feelings, characterized by reduced well-being and somatic symptoms, (2) difficulties in intrapersonal relationships associated with reduced self-esteem and helplessness, and (3) difficulties in interpersonal relationships, associated with symptoms such as irritability and withdrawal. In the next decade, Weissman and colleagues studied the phenomenology and treatment of social functioning in depressions.[2,3] Several years later, Wells et al.[4] reported on the impact of depression on function and well-being based on results from the large-scale Medical Outcomes Study, revealing that depression impairs physical, social, and health functioning to a similar or greater extent than do many other chronic diseases, including hypertension, diabetes, coronary artery disease, angina, arthritis, back problems, lung problems, and gastrointestinal disorders. Furthermore, among these chronic diseases, depression was associated with the poorest perceived health and social function.[4] Since that time, consistent and expanding evidence has shown that depression is associated with a myriad of functional impairments that affect every area of life—including family, social, and occupational function—and decreased overall well-being and quality of life.

Functional impairments can persist, even in the presence of symptomatic remission of depressive symptoms. Thus, patients, providers, and researchers alike are keen to identify treatment approaches that will fully ameliorate functional impairments associated with depression. Indeed, there has been clinical and research evidence demonstrating a variety of improvements associated with pharmacological, behavioral, and lifestyle treatments for depression, as well as neuromodulatory treatment approaches. Furthermore, the field has begun to appreciate the need for targeted treatments that directly improve function, along with other aspects of depression, such as cognitive impairments, that are associated with functional impairment in depression. This chapter will summarize the current state of the field regarding a variety of treatments for depression and their impact on function, as well as highlight further needs to help improve the functioning of depressed individuals.

HOW IS FUNCTION IMPAIRED IN MDD?

Psychosocial function and quality of life are significantly impacted by depression across several life domains, such as interpersonal relationships, physical health, and performance in daily activities, within a variety of settings, including the home, workplace, and/or school, and social contexts.[5,6] A potential hindrance to our detailed understanding of how function is impacted by depression is the myriad of terms that are used interchangeably to describe functioning (e.g., function, functioning, psychosocial functioning, social functioning, quality of life, health-related quality of life, life enjoyment, and satisfaction), and the wealth of potential assessment tools that are utilized to measure it (see Greer et al., 2010[7] or Lam et al., 2011[8] for review). These assessments sometimes focus on general

Major Depressive Disorder. https://doi.org/10.1016/B978-0-323-58131-8.00010-0

functioning within many areas of life, whereas others focus on specific areas (e.g., work, social); they can also be differentiated by their assessment of how one perceives their ability to function versus perceived quality of life and/or satisfaction in various areas. Most are self-reported assessments, but there are some measures that are performance-based and/or administered by a clinician.

Several studies have been conducted to evaluate how function is impaired in depression. For example, IsHak and colleagues[9] evaluated quality of life and function in a naturalistic study of depression in 319 outpatients presenting for treatment. Quality of life was assessed with the Quality of Life Enjoyment and Satisfaction Scale (Q-LES-Q) and the average score in this moderately depressed sample was 39.8%, compared to the community norm average of 78.3%—a value greater than 2 standard deviations below the community norm. Significant impairments were also observed on functional measures, including the Global Assessment of Functioning (GAF), the Sheehan Disability Scale (SDS), the Work and Social Adjustment Scale, and the Endicott Work Productivity Scale. Although higher depressive symptomatology was associated with more impaired quality of life, depressive symptomatology was associated with 48.1% of the variance in Q-LES-Q scores, suggesting it is an important contributor, but that other factors also impact quality of life.[9] The GAF and SDS contributed approximately 30% of the variance on the Q-LES-Q, illustrating the important relationship between functioning and quality of life.

Miller et al.[5] examined a wide variety of functional impairments in a randomized, controlled trial comparing sertraline and imipramine in individuals with chronic major depressive disorder. At baseline, chronic depression was associated with poor or very poor overall functioning in 75% of the sample ($n = 638$) and poor to very poor life satisfaction in 65% of the sample, as measured by the LIFE. Furthermore, average scores on assessments of social and interpersonal functioning were 2 SD higher than community norms, indicating significant functional impairment.

To evaluate the most meaningful impact on function from the patient's perspective, Lam et al.,[10] asked depressed patients to rate how specific symptoms and medication side effects interfered with work function. Patients perceived fatigue and low energy, insomnia, concentration and memory problems, anxiety, and irritability the factors that most interfered with work functioning. Medication side effects, such as sedation,

headache, insomnia, and agitation/anxiety, were also rated as interfering. Some of these same symptoms have been noted to be influential in functioning in general, and may mediate functional outcomes.[11]

Depression is also associated with higher health services utilization worldwide.[12] Major depressive disorder (MDD) has maintained its status as one of the leading chronic diseases associated with disability and has recently advanced to the leading cause according to the World Health Organization (WHO).[13] The effect of depression on functional outcomes is compounded by the presence of comorbid chronic diseases and/or psychiatric disorders.[14,15] Importantly, depressed patients stress the importance of function in their assessment of wellness.[16] The consistent evidence demonstrating that functional impairment is a significant and pervasive consequence of depression and the importance of function to patients with depression underscores the need for evaluation of functional outcomes in the context of treatment of depression.

With respect to depressive symptomatology, there is a negative correlation between depressive symptoms and functioning, with higher depressive symptom severity associated with reduced functioning.[17,18] However, even subthreshold depressive symptoms can impair functioning to levels that are distinct from healthy individuals with no chronic conditions. Furthermore, functional impairments appear to persist, at least to some degree, throughout the long-term course of depression.[19] Clinical characteristics such as age of onset of MDD and number of comorbid medical conditions, and demographic characteristics such as race (African American), ethnicity (Hispanic), marital status (divorced or separated), employment status (unemployed), education level (lower education level), insurance status (having public health insurance), and income level (lower monthly household income) was independently associated with reduced health-related quality of life in depressed individuals, suggesting that individuals with these characteristics may face additional functional burden.[17,18]

TREATMENT EFFECTS ON FUNCTIONAL OUTCOMES IN MDD

Hirshfeld and colleagues[6] note that it is often functional impairments and disrupted quality of life that prompt individuals to seek care for depressive disorders. The impact of a variety of different antidepressant treatments has been investigated in depression, with realized improvements in psychosocial functioning and quality of life.[20–22] Despite these encouraging results, functional impairments frequently persist[20] and remain elevated in comparison to nondepressed individuals,[5] even in the presence of reduced overall depressive symptoms.

The question of what treatments are best at yielding functional improvements in depression has yet to be answered. This may be due in part to the variability seen with respect to the optimal treatment choice for reducing depressive symptoms, which speaks to the heterogeneity of the disease. Furthermore, the wide variety of assessments and lack of a gold standard to assess functioning complicates the synthesis of data to understand the impact of treatments on functioning.[6] Nevertheless, the importance of functioning to patients and the fact that depressive symptoms can be resolved while functional dysfunction sustains necessitates investigation into the best approaches for resolving functional impairments associated with depression. Historically, functional outcomes have been underutilized in research on treatment efficacy of antidepressant treatments, particularly as primary outcomes,[6,8] but there have been promising increases in utilization of these outcomes in recent years that have yielded investigation of a wide variety of treatment approaches. Table 10.1 displays some key evidence linking various treatment approaches to functional outcomes.

Pharmacological Treatments

Some of the earlier treatment efficacy trials examined the impact of less currently utilized antidepressant medications including tricyclics and monoamine oxidase inhibitors (MAOIs). In a study comparing the MAOI phenelzine, the tricyclic imipramine, and placebo,[23] improvements in functioning were associated more with treatment response rather than treatment type. A later open-label study of desipramine treatment[24] found similar differentiation of social function improvement based on achievement of symptom response. Kocsis and colleagues[25] compared imipramine to placebo and found it to be superior with respect to improvements in social function at treatment end, as well as at long-term follow-up,[26] and also observed that functional improvements correlated with symptomatic improvements. These studies shared a short treatment duration period (6 weeks) and most had a small sample size, which may limit the generalizability of results. However, they were consistent in the observations that functional improvements tended to align with symptomatic improvements.

Selective serotonin reuptake inhibitors (SSRIs) remain one of the most commonly utilized antidepressants, and they have also shown to be beneficial for functional outcomes. Quality of life and functioning was examined in 2280 individuals from the large, multicenter Sequenced Treatment Alternatives to Relieve Depression (STAR*D) study, 106 of whom were 65 years of age or older. The $\geq$65 age group had less functional impairment on all functional measures at baseline, with the exception of physical quality of life (as measured by the SF-12 Physical Component Subscale [PCS] score). All ages demonstrated significant functional improvements (change scores from baseline to exit) and a significantly increased number of participants within the normal range of assessment scores following citalopram monotherapy, with the exception of the SF-12 PCS score in the 65 or older age group (which did not show a significant improvement). Kocsis et al.[21] compared the effects of sertraline to placebo on functional outcomes in chronic depression, and showed a significant benefit of sertraline on multiple functional outcomes. Importantly, relapse eliminated functional gains that were achieved in the acute phase trial. Similarly, Heiligenstein and colleagues[27] found that fluoxetine, when compared to placebo, conferred significant improvements in health-related quality of life, as measured by the SF-36, particularly on the mental health scales, role limitations due to emotional problems, bodily pain, and physical functioning. Thus, several trials evaluating depressed persons across a wide age range and with various SSRIs show that this antidepressant class yields improvements within a variety of functional domains.

Pharmacological agents that affect the noradrenergic system (namely, serotonin and norepinephrine reuptake inhibitors [SNRIs] and noradrenergic reuptake inhibitors [NARIs]) also have been shown to improve functional outcomes. A series of five studies[28] examining the SNRI, levomilnacipran, showed greater improvements on overall scores of the SDS, as well as all subscales (work/school, family life, and social life) in those treated with levomilnacipran compared to placebo. Data from the Prevention of Recurrent Episodes of Depression with Venlafaxine ER for Two Years (PREVENT) study showed that venlafaxine ER, also an SNRI, benefited psychosocial outcomes when used as a maintenance treatment (1–2 years),[29] and that maintenance treatment with venlafaxine ER significantly increased the probability of remaining well once normal function was achieved.

Some evidence that pharmacological agents preferentially affecting the noradrenergic system (i.e., NARIs, particularly reboxetine) may yield greater functional improvements than serotonergic agents such as SSRIs.[30–32] Functional outcomes in depressed

TABLE 10.1
Studies Assessing Functional Outcomes Following Antidepressant Treatment.

PHARMACOLOGICAL

SSRI

Author/Date	Sample Characteristics (n, Diagnostic Info, Ages)	Treatment (Duration, Type)	Depression Severity Measures	Functional Outcome Measures	Synopsis of Results	Limitations/Considerations
Kocsis et al. (2002)[21]	$n = 635$; chronic major depression, women mean age 41.6, double depression mean age 24.7, onset of dysthymia mean age 16.2	12-week; 16-week follow-up; then randomized to 18-month maintenance therapy or placebo. Sertraline hydrochloride ($n = 77$); placebo ($n = 84$)	HAM-D$_{24}$, CGI	SAS-SR, SF-36, LIFE	Patients taking sertraline, rather than the placebo, had higher psychosocial functioning. For patients in remission, short-term treatment had higher levels of psychosocial functioning. Results also showed that any psychosocial gain, regardless of treatment, was lost if depression reoccurred.	Relies on subjective measures. Significant degree of attrition.
Steiner et al. (2017)[62]	$n = 2,280$, MDD, ages 18+	Postanalyses of sequenced Treatment alternatives to relieve Depression (STAR*D) study, citalopram monotherapy (fixed-flexible dosing schedule	QIDS-SR	WSAS, Q-LES-Q, SF-12	Significant improvements (medium-large effect sizes) in all ages across depressive symptom severity, functioning, and quality of life (with the exception of SF-12 PCS) measures; remitters had larger quality of life and functional improvements.	Not placebo-controlled; small proportion of older adults.
Miller et al. (1998)[5]	$n = 635$, MDD, mean age 41.1 years	12 weeks; comparison of sertraline and imipramine	SCID, HAM-D, CGI, MADRS, CDRS, BDI$_{21}$	LIFE, SAS-SR, SF-36, Q-LES-Q	Depressed patients who had severely impaired psychosocial functioning, had significant improvement after treatment with sertraline or imipramine.	Reported psychosocial functioning could potentially be biased by the patient's mood state. Patients and interviewers not blinded to the idea that patients were receiving active treatment medication or blind to the time of assessment.
Heiligenstein et al. (1995)[27]	$n = 532$, MDD, ages 60+	6 weeks; fluoxetine (20 mg/day) ($n = 261$) Placebo ($n = 271$)	HAM-D$_{17}$	SF-36	Average increases in functional domain scores were significantly greater in fluoxetine versus placebo for physical functioning (3.2 vs. 0.3), bodily pain (7.1 vs. 2.9), role limitations emotional (16.3 vs. 7.3) and mental health (12.5 vs. 7.2).	Short treatment exposure (6 weeks) and low dose of medication (20 mg fluoxetine).

SNRI/NARI

Study	Sample	Measures	Outcome measure	Results	Notes
Dubini et al. (1997)[30]	$n = 302$, MDE, ages 18–65	8 weeks; placebo ($n = 99$), fluoxetine (SSRI; $n = 100$), reboxetine (NARI; $n = 103$)	HAM-D, CGI, MADRS	SASS	Both treatment groups yielded greater improvements in social functioning than placebo; reboxetine yielded greater and more improvements on individual items than placebo.	Results show that their hypotheses about the specific involvement of noradrenaline in sustaining drive are supported; however, this is contrary to past research and needs to be further explored.
Massana et al. (1999)[31]	$n = 139$, MDD, ages unknown	8 weeks; reboxetine ($n = 63$), fluoxetine ($n = 76$)	HAM-D; CGI, MADRS	SASS	Mean social functioning score, baseline to endpoint in all participants: Reboxetine: 27.3–35.7 Fluoxetine: 27.9–35.1 Subanalysis of severely depressed patients showed reboxetine as more efficacious than fluoxetine and more effective for social functioning in remitted patients.	Results show that reboxetine performed better than fluoxetine; however, an additional comparison arm should be considered to determine if it is the best SNRI for social functioning.
Sambunaris et al. (2014)[28]	Pooled postanalysis of three studies, $n = 2,659$, MDD, ages 18–80	8–10 weeks; two fixed dose studies (40, 80, and 120 mg/day; 40 and 80 mg/day) and three flexible-dose studies (two between 40 and 120 mg/day and one between 75 and 100 mg/day)	MADRS, CGI-S, HAM-D$_{17}$	SDS	Both SDS and MADRS were significantly reduced in the levomilnacipran ER group compared to those in placebo group in 4 out of 5 of the trials included in the pooled analysis—in the fifth study, both outcomes were numerically improved with levomilnacipran ER compared to placebo, but not statistically significant; the overall pooled analysis of these trials resulted in a significantly greater improvement SDS score and each subscale (work/school, family life, social life) in the levomilnacipran ER group compared to placebo.	Post hoc, retrospective analyses; stringent eligibility criteria that may not be generalizable; lack of active comparator; lack of correction for multiple analyses.
Watanabe et al. (2017)[63]	Post hoc analysis; $n = 821$, recurrent MDD, ages 18+	10-week acute phase; (venlafaxine $n = 781$), 6-month continuation phase (venlafaxine $n = 282$), and two consecutive 1-year maintenance phases. (Phase a venlafaxine $n = 65$; placebo $n = 69$) (phase B venlafaxine $n = 15$; placebo $n = 18$)	HAM-D	SAS-SR, LES, Q-LES-Q, SF-36	Patients treated with venlafaxine ER versus placebo had a significantly higher probability of remaining well.	389 patients were excluded from this analysis due to no adequate response if greater than 225 mg/day. Small sample size in maintenance phase B therefore not included in this analysis.

Continued

TABLE 10.1

Studies Assessing Functional Outcomes Following Antidepressant Treatment.—cont'd

Author/Date	Sample Characteristics (n, Diagnostic Info, Ages)	Treatment (Duration, Type)	Depression Severity Measures	Functional Outcome Measures	Synopsis of Results	Limitations/Considerations
Trivedi et al. (2010)[29]	n = 258, adult outpatients with MDD; ages 18+	2 years; response or remission following 6-month treatment with venlafaxine ER was randomized to: Venlafaxine ER (n = 129) or placebo (n = 129). Patients who were not randomized to venlafaxine recurrence during year 1 were randomized to venlafaxine ER (n = 43) or placebo (n = 40) for year 2	HAM-D$_{17}$	Q-LES-Q, LES-S, SAS-SR, SF-36, LIFE	Psychosocial functioning was better in patients receiving venlafaxine ER.	Chronic MD and TRD patients excluded. Adverse events (discontinuation-related) could have compromised the treatment blind. Long-term specialist care was a financial incentive for compliance in treatment.
Multimodal						
Chokka et al. (2018)[35]	n = 196, MDD, ages 18–65	26 sites, 52 weeks; vortioxetine (10–20 mg/day) treatment Independent of study; Vortioxetine as first treatment (n = 97); vortioxetine as a switch (n = 99)	QIDS-SR, CGI-S, CGI-I	PDQ-20, WLQ, WHODAS 2.0, WPAI, SDS, GAD-7, DSST	Significant correlation between PDQ-D-20 and WLQ productivity loss scores (r = 0.634; P < .001). Improvement in work productivity associated with improvement in cognitive dysfunction.	Open-label, no control group.
MAOIs						
Stewart et al. (1988)[23]	n = 189; nonmelancholic depression (DSM-III diagnosis of major depression [n = 101], dysthymic disorder [n = 46] or double depression [n = 40]); ages 18–65	6 weeks; phenelzine (n = 36), imipramine (n = 47), placebo (n = 48)	HRSD$_{21}$ (baseline only), CGI-I	SAS	Baseline HSRD score correlated significantly with SAS score (r = 0.37, P = .000); mean social functioning score baseline to endpoint: Phenelzine − 2.0, Imipramine − 2.2, Placebo − 2.4 P < 0.1T; treatment responders showed significantly greater improvements in functioning, regardless of treatment type.	Chronicity established by chart review based on ordinal scale of 1 = mostly well, 2 = depressed about half the time, 3 = depressed most of the time, and 4 = virtually always depressed; short treatment duration precludes evaluation of whether longer treatment duration and/or higher medication doses may differentiate from placebo.

Tricyclics

Kocsis et al. (1988)[25]	$n = 41$; dysthymic disorder (DSM-III); ages 18+	6 weeks; imipramine 50 mg ($n = 11$), placebo ($n = 13$)	HAM-D$_{24}$, GAS	SAS-SR	Mean social functioning score baseline to endpoint: Imipramine – 2.6–2.0, Placebo – 2.5–2.6 ($P < .5$); Improvement in self-rated SAS was correlated with improvement in depressive symptoms and global severity of illness.	Small sample size and short treatment duration. Distinctive sample but few patients achieved level of adjustment comparable to published norms.
Friedman et al. (1995)[24]	$n = 118$, patients with Dysthymia, mean age 37 (10)	10 weeks; desipramine ($n = 74$)	HAM-D$_{24}$, GAS, CDRS	SAS-SR	Mean social functioning score baseline to endpoint: Responders: 2.4–2.0 Nonresponders: 2.6–2.4 P value < 0.0001 Responders to desipramine showed greater improvement in overall social functioning and improvement in leisure time.	Incomplete data for the nonresponder group increases type II error. No control/comparator group.

BEHAVIORAL

Cognitive Therapy

Hirschfeld et al. (2002)[20]	n-662; chronic MDD, double depression, or recurrent MDD with incomplete interepisode recovery (DSM-IV); mean age = 43 years	12 weeks; CBASP, nefazodone (300–600 mg/day), or combination	HAM-D$_{24}$	SAS-SR, EWPS, SF-36, LIFE	Impairment was significantly worse in this study population versus the community sample. Psychosocial functioning improved throughout the study for all patients. Combined nefazodone and CBASP treatment had significantly higher improvement in psychosocial functioning compared to single treatment.	Patients not blinded to treatment type and there was no control group. All functioning measures were self-report.
Matsunaga et al. (2010)[37]	$n = 43$, MDD (DSM-IV) and met criteria for TRD; mean age = 41.3 (9.2)	12 weeks; CBT added to stable medication;	HRSD	GAF, SF-36, DAS, ATQ-r	Patients improved on all measures of psychosocial functioning, and mood symptom. CBT + medication have a positive effect on social functioning and depressive symptoms.	No control group, improvement in social functioning could be related to natural factors, not clear if medication or CBT is the active factor for improvement. Most of the TRD participants in this study were less severely depressed than other TRD populations.

Continued

TABLE 10.1

Studies Assessing Functional Outcomes Following Antidepressant Treatment.—cont'd

Author/Date	Sample Characteristics (n, Diagnostic Info, Ages)	Treatment (Duration, Type)	Depression Severity Measures	Functional Outcome Measures	Synopsis of Results	Limitations/Considerations
Dunn et al. (2012)[36]	$N = 523$; recurrent MDD (DSM-IV); ages 18–70	12–14 weeks of acute phase cognitive therapy (16 –20 sessions); responders randomized to the following: Continuation phase cognitive therapy (12 –14 weeks), fluoxetine or pill placebo	HAM-D, BDI[21], IDS-SR	SAS-SR, RIFT	Large decreases in psychosocial function after acute phase CT ($d = 1.24$); depressive symptoms improved more quickly and to a greater extent than psychological functioning. Improvement in functioning predicted later improvement in symptoms.	Limit in generalizability (sample demographics and specificity of treatment). Retrospective use of RIFT. Limited degree to replication in a clinical setting. Did not include a control group (therefore could not control for external factors).
Exercise						
Greer et al. (2016)[54]	$n = 126$, patients with MDD and moderate or higher depressive symptoms who partially responded to an SSRI antidepressant treatment, ages 18–70	12 weeks; exercise augmentation; randomized to high (16 kilocalories per kilogram of weight per week [KKW]) ($n = 64$) or low dose (4KKW) exercise ($n = 62$) plus maintained prestudy SSRI	IDS-C[30], HRSD[17], IDS-SR[30]	SF-36, SAS-SR, WSAS, Q-LES-Q, SWLS	Significant improvement in several functional outcomes, with some additional benefits with HD augmentation.	No inactive control group; results could be due to exercise augmentation or external factors. Homogeneous sample population that reduces generalizability.
Yoga						
Uebelacker et al. (2017)[47]	$n = 122$, patients with elevated depression symptoms and antidepressant medication use, ages 18+	10 week acute, 3 and 6 month follow-up; patients randomized to weekly yoga classes ($n = 63$) or health education classes (Healthy Living Workshop (HLW) ($n = 59$)	SCID, QIDS, PHQ-9	SF-20; 2 subscales from the WHODAS 2.0: The "getting along with people" and "life activities" subscale; IPAQ	When adjusting for baseline values, participants in the yoga group had increased general health perceptions, and social, work, and role functioning compared to participants in HLW.	Predominantly female and white/ non-Latino sample population, reduces generalizability. Patients were also not blind to treatment assignment.

NEUROMODULATORY TREATMENTS

TMS

Solvason et al. (2014)[57]	$n = 301$, TRD patients not on medication, ages unknown	6-week acute phase, patients randomized to TMS ($N = 155$) or sham TMS ($N = 146$); partial responders then followed in a 24-week durability phase ($N = 120$)	HAM-D$_{17}$, HAM-D$_{24}$, MADRS	SF-36; Q-LES-Q	For active TMS patients, there was a significant improvement in self-reports of functional status.	Important to consider if the QOL benefit observed is actually clinically significant. This study used standardized effect sizes that are rarely reported for measures of QOL.

ECT

McCall et al. (2018)[56]	$n = 120$, MDD patients, ages 60+	6 months; randomized to the following arms: PHARM (medication only; $n = 59$) or STABLE + PHARM (ECT in combination with medication; $n = 61$)	HRSD$_{24}$	SF-36	Patients who received ECT had better health-related quality of life on all dimensions of the SF-36.	Homogeneous sample population. Study only looked at prevention of depressive relapse so cannot make conclusions on acute antidepressant effects. No clinician reports; therefore, all data rely on patient self-report.

ATQ-R, automatic thought questionnaire-revised; *BDI*, beck depression inventory; *CDRS*, cornell dysthymia rating scale; *CGI*, clinical global impressions; *DAS*, dysfunctional attitudes scale; *DSST*, cigit symbol substitution test; *EWPS*, endicott work productivity scale; *GAD*, generalized anxiety disorder; *GAF*, global assessment of functioning; *GAS*, global assessment scale; *HAM-D*, Hamilton depression rating scale; *HRSD*, Hamilton rating scale for depression; *IDS*, inventory of depressive symptomatology; *IPAQ*, international physical activity questionnaire; *KKW*, kilocalories per kilogram per week; *LD*, low dose; *LES*, life enjoyment scale; *LIFE*, longitudinal interval follow-up evaluation; *MDD*, major depressive disorder; *MADRS*, montgomery asberg depression rating scale; *PDQ*, perceived deficits questionnaire; *PHD*, high dose; *PHQ*, patient health questionnaire; *QIDS-SR*, quick inventory of depressive symptomatology; *Q-LES-Q*, quality of life enjoyment and satisfaction questionna re; *RIFT*, range of impaired functioning tool; *SAS*, social adjustment scale; *SASS*, social adaptation self-evaluation scale; *SCID*, structured clinical interview for dsm; *SDS*, Sheehan disability scale; *SF*, short form health survey; *SSRI*, selective serotonin reuptake inhibitor; *SWLS*, satisfaction with life scale; *WHODAS 2.0*, World Health Organization disability assessment schedule 2.0; *WLQ*, work limitations questionnaire; *WPAI*, work productivity and activity impairment; *WSAS*, work and social adjustment scale.

individuals treated with reboxetine compared to those treated with fluoxetine or placebo showed meaningful improvements in both functional and depression outcomes with both treatments.[30] However, reboxetine showed greater improvements across a wider range of specific functional areas. The advantage of reboxetine compared to fluoxetine has also been observed in remitted severely depressed patients.[31] The data supporting the potential advantage associated with noradrenergic agents in comparison to those specifically influencing the serotonergic system for functioning, and particularly social functioning, showed promise in potentially identifying targeted treatments for functional impairments[32–34]; however, additional research in this area appears to have stagnated and remains limited to these few initial examinations.

Newer agents, such as the multimodal antidepressant, vortioxetine, are being assessed for their impact on functional outcomes[35] and suggest improvements in functional areas, as well as associated symptoms, such as cognition. Additional investigations on antidepressants with atypical and/or novel mechanisms of action are warranted.

Psychotherapy

A variety of cognitive and behavioral therapies have been examined with respect to their impact on functional outcomes. Hirshfeld and colleagues[20] compared the Cognitive Behavioral Analysis System of Psychotherapy (CBASP) to nefazodone or their combination and examined work, social, health, and overall functional outcomes. The primary aim of their investigation was to evaluate whether functional changes were independent of those observed for symptomatic outcomes. Of note, CBASP focuses on interpersonal interactions, and thus may be expected to have a direct impact on functional outcomes. The findings indicate that combination therapy was superior to either treatment alone with respect to all functional outcomes. Specifically, when controlling for depressive symptomatology, combination CBASP and nefazodone yielded significantly greater improvements on overall functioning, work functioning and social functioning compared to nefazodone alone, and significantly greater improvements in social functioning compared to CBASP alone. Additional findings noted in this study that have been very informative with respect to our understanding of how functional changes compare to changes in depressive symptoms include the slower pace at which functional improvements were realized, the fact that psychosocial impairments were still present at study end despite noted improvements, and the fact that there

is some independence between functional and symptomatic changes.

Dunn and colleagues[36] examined functional outcomes associated with 16–20 sessions of cognitive therapy provided over 12–14 weeks, and noted significant improvements in both depressive symptoms and psychosocial function. Similar to Hirshfeld et al.,[20] depressive symptoms improved more robustly and more quickly than did psychosocial function. The impact of cognitive therapy has also been investigated as an augmentation. Matsunga et al.[37] examined the addition of group cognitive behavioral therapy (CBT) to augment medication in patients with treatment resistant depression and showed that those who completed treatment realized benefits in all areas assessed, including depressive symptoms, psychosocial functioning, and dysfunctional cognitions, and that these improvements were sustained at the 12-month follow-up.

Lifestyle Interventions

Several lifestyle interventions, including mindfulness techniques, yoga, and exercise, significantly reduce symptoms of depression, as well as related symptoms such as anxiety.[38–41] Although functional improvements have been observed in association with these interventions, studies are few, and many are focused more on quality of life, rather than function per se. Additionally, many are focused the use of these interventions in other disease states in which function is assessed alongside depressive symptomatology. Nevertheless, these data can be extrapolated to support the use of these interventions in major depressive disorders, although greater research studies are clearly needed in this area.

For example, mindfulness has been used in nondistressed couples to boost relationship functioning.[42] In a study by Carson and colleagues (2004), couples were randomized to a mindfulness-based relationship enhancement condition or wait-list control. Couples in the intervention group saw improvements in both individual well-being and relationship functioning across a wide range of measures, including daily relationship happiness, relationship stress, stress coping efficacy, and overall stress.[42] The authors hypothesized that joint participation in exciting self-expansion activities (that facilitate greater awareness of others outside the self), greater acceptance of others, and relaxation may be potential mechanisms by which the intervention positively affects relationship functioning,[43] although a mediational analysis found the joint participation in the activity to be the only significant variable associated with relationship functioning. Although these data could suggest a similar pattern in couples that include a depressed partner, it would be important to test this, as there may be stressors in the relationship that may alter the pattern of results. In the STAR*D study, being single, separated or divorced was associated with worse health-related quality of life, suggesting a positive impact of being married, cohabitating, or in a committed relationship. The potential positive effect of mindfulness-based interventions could be beneficial to relationship function and quality in depressed individuals and married/cohabitating partners, and could be explored as a way to enhance relationship function and quality of life in those who are experiencing dysfunction.

Yoga has also been associated with improvements in function and quality of life in many chronic diseases and conditions and is frequently practiced with the purpose of improving general wellness and quality of life.[44] However, there are differences between how broadly functional improvements are realized across conditions, with many studies in cancer, for example, showing wide-sweeping functional and quality of life improvements,[45] compared to those focused on individuals with low back pain studies, which show functional improvements that are more specific to back pain disability and little to no impact on general quality of life.[46] Uebelacker and colleagues (2017)[47] compared a 10-week hatha yoga program to health education classes on symptom severity and functional outcomes in depressed individuals who had not shown adequate response to their current treatment regimen (antidepressant medication and/or psychotherapy). Although they did not find significant reduction in depressive symptoms at 10 weeks (the primary outcome), they did show both reduction in depressive symptoms over the follow-up period (6 months), as well as significant improvements in perception of general health, and social and role functioning.

Similar to yoga, exercise has been associated with functional improvements in healthy individuals,[48,49] as well as in individuals with other disorders.[50,51] Exercise has also demonstrated specific benefit to functional and psychosocial outcomes in individuals with depression, including both adolescents[52] and adults.[53,54] Most studies have been small in size, and almost all examine exercise as an augmentation strategy to usual treatment. In a recent meta-analysis, Schuch and colleagues (2016)[53] concluded that exercise significantly improves physical and psychological functioning, and overall quality of life, but does not significantly improve social functioning. Data from the TReatment with Exercise Augmentation for Depression (TREAD) were examined with respect to a wide variety of functional outcomes, including health-related quality of life, work and social functioning, and satisfaction with life. TREAD enrolled 122 partial responders to SSRI who were randomized to either high- (16 kcal/kg of weight/week [KKW]) or low-dose (4-KKW) exercise for 12 weeks.[54] Significant improvements were achieved over the 12-week period in all functional domains assessed, including social functioning, with many participants achieving normalized functioning by study end. Of note, there were minimal between-group differences, suggesting that even low doses of exercise can improve functioning.

Sylvia and colleagues recently piloted an integrative lifestyle intervention, Nutrition Exercise and Wellness Treatment (NEW Tx), in individuals with bipolar disorder.[55] The NEW Tx intervention is CBT-based, and includes psychoeducation and goal-setting to increase exercise and improve nutrition and overall wellness. They compared individuals randomized to the intervention with those in a treatment as usual wait-list control group on measures of mood and functioning. Decreases in depressed mood and illness severity were found over the 20-week intervention period, but only the function measures showed significant improvements. This is an important area of further exploration, as both major depressive disorder and bipolar disorder are associated with medical comorbidities such as obesity and cardiovascular disease. Novel, integrative lifestyle interventions such as NEW Tx may provide a meaningful way to reduce symptoms associated with multiple physical and mental health issues that will improve overall health and functioning.

Neuromodulatory Treatments

Neuromodulatory treatments are employed mostly in individuals with treatment resistant depression, who are likely to have more pronounced functional impairments, due to increased severity and longer course of disease. Furthermore, symptoms known to be highly associated with functioning, such as cognition, are often a concern of individuals who may be prescribed neuromodulatory treatments, particularly electroconvulsive therapy (ECT), and thus identifying how these treatments affect functioning is critical. Fortunately, ECT has been shown to improve a variety of functional outcomes, particularly in combination with medication,[56] although functional assessments were limited to health-related quality of life. Other neuromodulatory treatments, including transcranial magnetic stimulation (TMS), have also been associated with improved functioning.[57]

TABLE 10.2
Synthesis of Associations Between Various Antidepressant Treatments and Functional Outcomes.

Treatment	TYPE OF FUNCTIONING					
	Family	Social	School/Occupational	Activities of Daily Living (ADL)/General/Disability	Quality of Life (QOL)	Satisfaction with Life
PHARMACOLOGICAL						
Selective Serotonin reuptake inhibitors (SSRIs)		Kocsis et al. (2002)[21] Miller et al. (1998)[5]		Heiligenstein et al. (1995)[27]	Steiner et al. (2017)[62]	
Serotonin norepinephrine reuptake inhibitors (SNRIs)	Sambunaris et al. (2014)[28]	Dubini et al. (1997)[30] Sambunaris et al. (2014)[28] Trivedi et al. (2010)[29]		Sambunaris et al. (2014)[28] Watanabe et al. (2017)[63]		
Multimodal			Chokka et al. (2018)[35] Lam et al. (2012)[10]		Saragoussi et al. (2018)[11]	
Monoamine oxidase inhibitors (MAOIs)		Stewart et al. (1988)[23]				
Tricyclics		Kocsis et al. (1988)[25]			Friedman et al. (1995)[24]	
Augmentation		Greer et al. (2010)[7]			Massana et al. (1999)[31]	
BEHAVIORAL						
Cognitive behavioral Therapy (CBT)					Matsunaga et al. (2010)[37]	
Other cognitive Therapy		Dunn et al. (2012)[36]				
Exercise					Greer et al. (2016)[54]	
Yoga		Uebelacker et al. (2017)[47]				
Behavioral activation						
NEUROMODULATORY TREATMENTS						
Transcranial magnetic Stimulation (TMS)					Solvason et al. (2014)[57]	
Electroconvulsive Therapy (ECT)					McCall et al. (2018)[56]	

Strength of evidence based on primary outcome, number of studies examined, and adequate sample size/design.

Trajectory of Functional Improvements during Treatment

Psychosocial improvements tend to lag behind improvement in depressive symptoms. Importantly, a series of recent studies show that psychosocial improvements can be realized early in the course of treatment and that when those are accomplished early, they can be predictive of and associated with better symptomatic outcomes. Data examined from the Combining Medications to Enhance Depression Outcomes (CO-MED), study, in which 665 patients nonpsychotic chronic or recurrent depression were randomized to escitalopram plus placebo (SSRI monotherapy), sustained-release bupropion plus escitalopram (bupropion combination), or 3) extended-release venlafaxine plus mirtazapine (venlafaxine combination), showed that early functional improvement could be attained early in the course of treatment (i.e., 4–6 weeks). Importantly, these early improvements were achieved in quality of life,[58] psychosocial function,[59] and daily activity level,[60] and they positively impacted clinical course, as observed via increased odds of remission at the end of the acute phase of treatment, even after controlling for change in depression severity. Forero[61] observed similar predictive value of early functional improvements, as did Dunn et al.,[36] with cognitive therapy, suggesting that this general effect may be meaningful regardless of treatment type.

CURRENT LIMITATIONS IN THE FIELD AND FUTURE DIRECTIONS

It is promising that functional impairments are improved by a wide variety of pharmacological and nonpharmacological interventions. However, evaluations of functioning as both a clinical and research outcome in depression remain predominantly limited to being sparsely and inconsistently evaluated, and frequently included in clinical trials only as a secondary outcome rather than a primary measure of treatment efficacy. The importance of functional outcomes to patients and the established negative impact of incomplete functional recovery on the long-term course of illness necessitates that we focus significant attention to these important outcomes and redefine our definition of recovery and wellness in depression to include resolution of functional impairment as determined by both patient and clinician.

It is certainly positive that a wide variety of treatments have been associated with improvement in a

wide variety of functional outcomes (see Table 10.2). Equally important are the increasing observations that, despite previous data indicating that functional improvements tend to lag behind improvements in depressive symptoms, functional improvements can indeed be achieved early in the course of treatment, and these early improvements are associated with better long-term outcomes. Treatment approaches should incorporate earlier attention to functional outcomes to improve patient outcomes and promote functional recovery.

Unfortunately, it remains true that many functional impairments do remain despite symptomatic improvement, and these symptoms are associated with poorer quality of life and higher likelihood of relapse. As with depressive symptoms, there is no universal treatment that appears to be effective in resolving functional impairments for all depressed individuals. The variability inherent in the measurements, treatments, and sample characteristics of existing research in this area speak to the need for continued focus on evaluation of functional outcomes in depression to allow for a better understanding of treatment effects. In addition, increasing our attention to related symptoms, such as cognition, that are known to influence functional outcomes, is extremely important. Treatment approaches that specifically target improved functioning, and related symptoms, are imperative, and we should continue to explore potential novel treatments.

REFERENCES

1. Stoeckle JD, Davidson GE. Bodily complaints and other symptoms of depressive reaction. Diagnosis and significance in a medical clinic. *Jama*. 1962;180:134–139.
2. Weissman MM, Klerman GL, Paykel ES, Prusoff B, Hanson B. Treatment effects on the social adjustment of depressed patients. *Arch Gen Psychiatr*. 1974;30(6):771–778.
3. Weissman MM, Bothwell S. Assessment of social adjustment by patient self-report. *Arch Gen Psychiatr*. 1976;33(9):1111–1115.
4. Wells KB, Stewart A, Hays RD, et al. The functioning and well-being of depressed patients. Results from the Medical Outcomes Study. *Jama*. 1989;262(7):914–919.
5. Miller IW, Keitner GI, Schatzberg AF, et al. The treatment of chronic depression, part 3: psychosocial functioning before and after treatment with sertraline or imipramine. *J Clin Psychiatry*. 1998;59(11):608–619.
6. Hirschfeld RM, Montgomery SA, Keller MB, et al. Social functioning in depression: a review. *J Clin Psychiatry*. 2000;61(4):268–275.

7. Greer TL, Kurian BT, Trivedi MH. Defining and measuring functional recovery from depression. *CNS Drugs.* 2010; 24(4):267–284.

8. Lam RW, Filteau MJ, Milev R. Clinical effectiveness: the importance of psychosocial functioning outcomes. *J Affect Disord.* 2011;132(suppl 1):S9–s13.

9. Ishak WW, Balayan K, Bresee C, et al. A descriptive analysis of quality of life using patient-reported measures in major depressive disorder in a naturalistic outpatient setting. *Qual Life Res.* 2013;22(3):585–596.

10. Lam RW, Michalak EE, Bond DJ, Tam EM, Axler A, Yatham LN. Which depressive symptoms and medication side effects are perceived by patients as interfering most with occupational functioning? *Depression Res Treatment.* 2012;2012:630206.

11. Saragoussi D, Christensen MC, Hammer-Helmich L, Rive B, Touya M, Haro JM. Long-term follow-up on health-related quality of life in major depressive disorder: a 2-year European cohort study. *Neuropsychiatric Dis Treatment.* 2018;14:1339–1350.

12. Herrman H, Patrick DL, Diehr P, et al. Longitudinal investigation of depression outcomes in primary care in six countries: the LIDO study. Functional status, health service use and treatment of people with depressive symptoms. *Psychol Med.* 2002;32(5):889–902.

13. Organization WH. *Depression*; 2018. http://www.who.int/news-room/fact-sheets/detail/depression.

14. Moussavi S, Chatterji S, Verdes E, Tandon A, Patel V, Ustun B. Depression, chronic diseases, and decrements in health: results from the World Health Surveys. *Lancet.* 2007;370(9590):851–858.

15. Druss BG, Hwang I, Petukhova M, Sampson NA, Wang PS, Kessler RC. Impairment in role functioning in mental and chronic medical disorders in the United States: results from the National Comorbidity Survey Replication. *Mol Psychiatr.* 2009;14(7):728–737.

16. Zimmerman M, McGlinchey JB, Posternak MA, Friedman M, Attiullah N, Boerescu D. How should remission from depression be defined? The depressed patient's perspective. *Am J Psychiatry.* 2006;163(1): 148–150.

17. Trivedi MH, Rush AJ, Wisniewski SR, et al. Factors associated with health-related quality of life among outpatients with major depressive disorder: a STAR*D report. *J Clin Psychiatry.* 2006;67(2):185–195.

18. Daly EJ, Trivedi MH, Wisniewski SR, et al. Health-related quality of life in depression: a STAR*D report. *Ann Clin Psychiatr.* 2010;22(1):43–55.

19. Judd LL, Schettler PJ, Solomon DA, et al. Psychosocial disability and work role function compared across the long-term course of bipolar I, bipolar II and unipolar major depressive disorders. *J Affect Disord.* 2008;108(1–2): 49–58.

20. Hirschfeld RM, Dunner DL, Keitner G, et al. Does psychosocial functioning improve independent of depressive symptoms? A comparison of nefazodone, psychotherapy, and their combination. *Biol Psychiatry.* 2002;51(2): 123–133.

21. Kocsis JH, Schatzberg A, Rush AJ, et al. Psychosocial outcomes following long-term, double-blind treatment of chronic depression with sertraline vs placebo. *Arch Gen Psychiatr.* 2002;59(8):723–728.

22. Papakostas GI, Petersen T, Denninger JW, et al. Psychosocial functioning during the treatment of major depressive disorder with fluoxetine. *J Clin Psychopharmacol.* 2004; 24(5):507–511.

23. Stewart JW, Quitkin FM, McGrath PJ, et al. Social functioning in chronic depression: effect of 6 weeks of antidepressant treatment. *Psychiatr Res.* 1988;25(2):213–222.

24. Friedman RA, Markowitz JC, Parides M, Kocsis JH. Acute response of social functioning in dysthymic patients with desipramine. *J Affect Disord.* 1995;34(2):85–88.

25. Kocsis JH, Frances AJ, Voss C, Mason BJ, Mann JJ, Sweeney J. Imipramine and social-vocational adjustment in chronic depression. *Am J Psychiatry.* 1988;145(8): 997–999.

26. Kocsis JH, Sutton BM, Frances AJ. Long-term follow-up of chronic depression treated with imipramine. *J Clin Psychiatry.* 1991;52(2):56–59.

27. Heiligenstein JH, Ware Jr JE, Beusterien KM, Roback PJ, Andrejasich C, Tollefson GD. Acute effects of fluoxetine versus placebo on functional health and well-being in late-life depression. *Int Psychogeriatr.* 1995;7(suppl): 125–137.

28. Sambunaris A, Gommoll C, Chen C, Greenberg WM. Efficacy of levomilnacipran extended-release in improving functional impairment associated with major depressive disorder: pooled analyses of five double-blind, placebo-controlled trials. *Int Clin Psychopharmacol.* 2014;29(4): 197–205.

29. Trivedi MH, Dunner DL, Kornstein SG, et al. Psychosocial outcomes in patients with recurrent major depressive disorder during 2 years of maintenance treatment with venlafaxine extended release. *J Affect Disord.* 2010;126(3): 420–429.

30. Dubini A, Bosc M, Polin V. Do noradrenaline and serotonin differentially affect social motivation and behaviour? *Eur Neuropsychopharmacol.* 1997;7(suppl 1):S49–S55. discussion S71-43.

31. Massana J, Moller HJ, Burrows GD, Montenegro RM. Reboxetine: a double-blind comparison with fluoxetine in major depressive disorder. *Int Clin Psychopharmacol.* 1999;14(2):73–80.

32. Bosc M. Assessment of social functioning in depression. *Compr Psychiatry.* 2000;41(1):63–69.

33. Keller M. Role of serotonin and noradrenaline in social dysfunction: a review of data on reboxetine and the Social Adaptation Self-evaluation Scale (SASS). *Gen Hosp Psychiatry.* 2001;23(1):15–19.

34. Briley M, Moret C. Improvement of social adaptation in depression with serotonin and norepinephrine reuptake inhibitors. *Neuropsychiatric Dis Treatment.* 2010;6: 647–655.

35. Chokka P, Bougie J, Rampakakis E, Proulx J. Assessment in Work Productivity and the Relationship with Cognitive Symptoms (AtWoRC): primary analysis from a

Canadian open-label study of vortioxetine in patients with major depressive disorder (MDD). *CNS Spectrums*. 2018: 1–10.

36. Dunn TW, Vittengl JR, Clark LA, Carmody T, Thase ME, Jarrett RB. Change in psychosocial functioning and depressive symptoms during acute-phase cognitive therapy for depression. *Psychol Med*. 2012;42(2): 317–326.

37. Matsunaga M, Okamoto Y, Suzuki S, et al. Psychosocial functioning in patients with Treatment-Resistant Depression after group cognitive behavioral therapy. *BMC Psychiatry*. 2010;10:22.

38. Cooney GM, Dwan K, Greig CA, et al. Exercise for depression. *Cochrane Database Syst Rev*. 2013;(9):Cd004366.

39. Trivedi MH, Greer TL, Church TS, et al. Exercise as an augmentation treatment for nonremitted major depressive disorder: a randomized, parallel dose comparison. *J Clin Psychiatry*. 2011;72(5):677–684.

40. Cramer H, Lauche R, Langhorst J, Dobos G. Yoga for depression: a systematic review and meta-analysis. *Depress Anxiety*. 2013;30(11):1068–1083.

41. Hofmann SG, Gomez AF. Mindfulness-based interventions for anxiety and depression. *Psychiatr Clin*. 2017; 40(4):739–749.

42. Carson JW, Carson MK, Gil MK, Baucom DH. Mindfulness-based relationship enhancement. *Behav Ther*. 2004;35(3):471–494.

43. Carson JW, Carson KM, Gil KM, Baucom DH. Self-expansion as a mediator of relationship improvements in a mindfulness intervention. *J Marital Fam Ther*. 2007; 33(4):517–528.

44. Cramer H, Ward L, Steel A, Lauche R, Dobos G, Zhang Y. Prevalence, patterns, and predictors of yoga use: results of a U.S. Nationally representative survey. *Am J Prev Med*. 2016;50(2):230–235.

45. Buffart LM, van Uffelen JG, Riphagen II , et al. Physical and psychosocial benefits of yoga in cancer patients and survivors, a systematic review and meta-analysis of randomized controlled trials. *BMC Cancer*. 2012;12:559.

46. Cramer H, Lauche R, Haller H, Dobos G. A systematic review and meta-analysis of yoga for low back pain. *Clin J Pain*. 2013;29(5):450–460.

47. Uebelacker LA, Tremont G, Gillette LT, et al. Adjunctive yoga v. health education for persistent major depression: a randomized controlled trial. *Psychol Med*. 2017;47(12): 2130–2142.

48. Kruger J, Bowles HR, Jones DA, Ainsworth BE, Kohl 3rd HW. Health-related quality of life, BMI and physical activity among US adults (>/=18 years): national physical activity and weight loss Survey, 2002. *Int J Obes*. 2007;31(2):321–327.

49. Vuillemin A, Boini S, Bertrais S, et al. Leisure time physical activity and health-related quality of life. *Prev Med*. 2005; 41(2):562–569.

50. Schwandt M, Harris JE, Thomas S, Keightley M, Snaiderman A, Colantonio A. Feasibility and effect of aerobic exercise for lowering depressive symptoms among individuals with traumatic brain injury: a pilot study. *J Head Trauma Rehabil*. 2012;27(2):99–103.

51. Sweegers MG, Altenburg TM, Chinapaw MJ, et al. Which exercise prescriptions improve quality of life and physical function in patients with cancer during and following treatment? A systematic review and meta-analysis of randomised controlled trials. *Br J Sports Med*. 2018;52(8): 505–513.

52. Hughes CW, Barnes S, Barnes C, Defina LF, Nakonezny P, Emslie GJ. Depressed Adolescents Treated with Exercise (DATE): a pilot randomized controlled trial to test feasibility and establish preliminary effect sizes. *Mental Health Phys Activity*. 2013;6(2).

53. Schuch FB, Vancampfort D, Rosenbaum S, Richards J, Ward PB, Stubbs B. Exercise improves physical and psychological quality of life in people with depression: a meta-analysis including the evaluation of control group response. *Psychiatr Res*. 2016;241:47–54.

54. Greer TL, Trombello JM, Rethorst CD, et al. Improvements in psychosocial functioning and health-related quality of life following exercise augmentation in patients with treatment response but nonremitted major depressive disorder: results from the tread study. *Depress Anxiety*. 2016;33(9): 870–881.

55. Sylvia LG, Pegg SL, Dufour SC, et al. Pilot study of a lifestyle intervention for bipolar disorder: nutrition exercise wellness treatment (NEW Tx). *J Affect Disord*. 2019;250: 278–283.

56. McCall WV, Lisanby SH, Rosenquist PB, et al. Effects of continuation electroconvulsive therapy on quality of life in elderly depressed patients: a randomized clinical trial. *J Psychiatr Res*. 2018;97:65–69.

57. Solvason HB, Husain M, Fitzgerald PB, et al. Improvement in quality of life with left prefrontal transcranial magnetic stimulation in patients with pharmacoresistant major depression: acute and six month outcomes. *Brain Stimulation*. 2014;7(2):219–225.

58. Jha MK, Greer TL, Grannemann BD, Carmody T, Rush AJ, Trivedi MH. Early normalization of Quality of Life predicts later remission in depression: findings from the CO-MED trial. *J Affect Disord*. 2016;206:17–22.

59. Jha MK, Minhajuddin A, Greer TL, Carmody T, Rush AJ, Trivedi MH. Early improvement in psychosocial function predicts longer-term symptomatic remission in depressed patients. *PLoS One*. 2016;11(12):e0167901.

60. Jha MK, Teer RB, Minhajuddin A, Greer TL, Rush AJ, Trivedi MH. Daily activity level improvement with antidepressant medications predicts long-term clinical outcomes in outpatients with major depressive disorder. *Neuropsychiatric Dis Treatment*. 2017;13: 803–813.

61. Forero CG, Olariu E, Alvarez P, et al. Change in functioning outcomes as a predictor of the course of depression: a 12-month longitudinal study. *Qual Life Res*. 2018; 27(8):2045–2056.

62. Steiner AJ, Recacho J, Vanle B, et al. Quality of life, functioning, and depressive symptom severity in older adults with major depressive disorder treated with citalopram in the STAR*D study. *J Clin Psychiatry.* 2017;78(7):897–903.

63. Watanabe K, Thase ME, Kikuchi T, et al. Long-term function and psychosocial outcomes with venlafaxine extended release 75-225 mg/day versus placebo in the PREVENT study. *Int Clin Psychopharmacol.* 2017;32(5): 271–280.

CHAPTER 11

Internet-Based/Technology-Based Interventions in Major Depressive Disorder

ARVIND RAJAGOPALAN, MBBS • ROGER CHUN MAN HO, MD, MRCPSYCH, FRCPC

INTRODUCTION

Major depressive disorder (MDD), or depression, is one of the most prevalent psychiatric conditions with the aggregate point, 1-year, and lifetime prevalence of depression calculated prevalences of 12.9%, 7.2%, and 10.8%, respectively.[1] Internet-based and technology-based interventions include computer-based and web-based interventions, text messaging, interactive voice recognition, smartphone apps, and emerging technologies.[2] Such interventions allow collection of clinical data from separate and remote locations in real time.[3] Internet-based and technology-based interventions help patients with chronic diseases to maintain remission[4] and provide individually tailored support with privacy.[5] Internet-based and technology-based interventions play a key role in the management of MDD, which is a chronic disorder, and patients want to receive intervention with privacy.

GLOBAL IMPACT OF MOBILE TECHNOLOGY AND THE INTERNET IN HEALTHCARE

With the advent of smartphone technology, access to the internet and technology-based interventions is higher than it has ever been. In 2016, an estimated 46.1% of the world's population had access to the internet, with mobile and tablet-based internet usage exceeding desktop usage that year.[6,7] It is estimated that for every person in the world, there are at least three mobile phones on the market.[8] The prevalence and accessibility of such technology has made it possible for its use in delivering healthcare and medical interventions, otherwise known as "Digital Medicine."[9] The vast potential of digital platforms in obtaining real-time data from individual patients, therefore making health monitoring easier and more cost-effective, has positioned digital medicine as a burgeoning industry, generating increasing commercial interest. In 2014 alone, companies operating in digital healthcare generated as much revenue as in the previous 3 years combined. Although the question remains as to whether commercialization of digital health technologies would lead to truly healthcare-based interventions, or simply consumer-oriented products aimed at generating revenue, it is undeniable that internet and smartphone-based medical interventions are poised to revolutionize medical management.[9]

The Role of Internet and Technology-Based Interventions in Medicine

The accessibility of mobile technology and the internet has made the use of these technologies in medical management advantageous. A large number of healthcare-based smartphone applications exist on the market, around 40,000 as estimated in 2012.[10,11]

Patient education

A survey of 1000 patients in 2002 found that more than half (53.5%) of them made use of the internet for obtaining medical information.[12] Increasingly, healthcare service providers are making use of the internet to deliver qualified medical information to consumers all over the world.[13] With the capacity to store large volumes of information, technology such as smartphone applications and the internet is able to act as a source of easily accessible information for patients, which removes the need to seek a direct medical consultation to obtain this information. For example, the m.CARAT© mobile application was developed to provide patients with asthma and allergic rhinitis with information on their condition.[14] Patients are able to

Major Depressive Disorder. https://doi.org/10.1016/B978-0-323-58131-8.00011-2

receive up-to-date news and information to allow them to effectively monitor themselves. Although there is a risk that patients may access information from nonqualified sources, governing bodies worldwide are developing guidelines to ensure that medical information available on mobile applications and the internet are evaluated for accuracy and quality. For example, the American Medical Association has developed guidelines for website content, while self-certification models and rating scales have been proposed to ensure quality of medical smartphone applications.[15-17]

Patient monitoring

One of the major advantages of digital platform technologies is that they allow for patients' symptoms to be monitored continuously and remotely, outside of outpatient or inpatient settings.[9] Mobile phone applications and other wearable technologies, that patients can have on them at all times, can make use of remote sensors to monitor markers of disease, acting as sources of continuous real-time data for healthcare providers. There are numerous advantages to such technology[9]:

- Symptoms can be monitored continuously, with in-built alarms to detect severity and alert healthcare providers should intervention be necessary, allowing for rapid response
- These devices can be combined with others that act as preventative tools, by delivering therapy or suggesting behavioral modifications
- Tracking and analysis of data gathered may reveal new patterns that predict disease severity or progression, such as demographic or geographic predilections

Examples of mobile applications on the market, which allow for physiological monitoring through sensors built into the mobile platforms, include AliveCor's© electrocardiogram, Kinsa's Smart Thermometer©, and Sanofi's iBGStar© glucose monitor.[9] Wireless wrist monitors that monitor blood pressure using motion sensor technology are available. These are able to directly sync to smartphone applications, thereby acting not just as data-collection tools, but also as tools for intervention, with the applications able to show users the changes in their blood pressures and suggest appropriate therapies.[18] Wearable defibrillators for postmyocardial infarction patients are currently undergoing development.[19] A recent review of studies on digital technologies used in remote monitoring found that most studies were carried out on older adult populations, with small sample sizes and limited follow-up, indicating that there is still room for large-

scale trials of these technologies. However, although there is substantial diversity in health-related outcomes among the studies, they predominantly reported positive findings.[20]

Digital phenotyping

Traditional phenotyping involves the measurement of physiological markers of disease to determine disease severity. Examples include blood glucose levels to measure the severity of diabetes or serum troponin levels to measure myocardial damage postinfarction. The use of digital platforms makes novel, previously nonmeasurable data available to healthcare providers. This new data, when coupled with existing markers, act as novel digital markers of disease severity. A collection of these markers therefore allows for the creation of a "digital phenotype" for patients, a set of digitally measured markers that act as determinants of disease progression, and aid in the remote monitoring mentioned earlier.[9] An early example of this would be the use of internet search data to monitor outbreaks of communicable diseases such as salmonella and flu.[21] More recently, research has shown that digital cognitive tests can act as neural correlates for Alzheimer's disease progression.[22] Pfizer and Akili Interactive Labs are companies that are now combining traditional biomarkers of neural imaging with digital markers obtained through videogame measurements, to develop a prodromal profile for Alzheimer's disease.[9,23] Increasingly, mobile phones have in-built sensors that track activity levels and Global Positioning Satellite-based tracking sensors that track changes in location. Changes in activity levels and locations can be used as markers for physical and mental health. For example, frequency, length, and content of text messages or participation in social media can be used as a marker for mood states, and the timing of mobile phone activity can be used to monitor the severity of insomnia.[24] The use of these technologies in psychiatric medicine will be detailed in a later section.

Disease management

Although in theory the most beneficial form of medical management, primary prevention, is difficult, in practice it is usually based on behavioral modifications (exceptions being vaccines and prophylactic medications such as antibiotics and statins), and hence requires clinical observation and assessment of at-risk individuals. However, with continuous real-time monitoring of patients made possible by digital platform technologies, behavioral modification is poised to become a much more effective tool in primary prevention.[9,25,26] By allowing for constant communication between healthcare providers and patients, these technologies can improve adherence to primary preventative interventions and also allow for closer and more consistent follow-up. For example, a remote wireless sensor attached to bronchodilator inhalers has been developed by Propeller Health. It delivers real-time data on timing and locations of inhaler usage in patients with asthma or chronic obstructive pulmonary disease, allowing healthcare providers to study trends in these patients' exacerbations and usage, making it easier to identify potential triggers and suggest behavioral modifications to avoid these.[27,28] This technology has been shown to reduce inhaler use and improve control of disease. Another example includes Akili Interactive Labs' NeuroRacer video game, custom designed to monitor cognitive function in patients with Alzheimer's disease.[23] The assessment of multitasking abilities in the game platform acts as a digital correlate to cognitive decline, exemplifying the "digital phenotype" concept mentioned earlier. Furthermore, the game allows for interventions such as training these multitasking abilities, which has been shown to improve electroencephalographic markers of cognitive function, sustained attention, and working memory.[23]

Patient empowerment

Digital platforms allow patients to be more involved in their own healthcare.[9] Patients can monitor their own symptoms and submit reports on their experiences associated with conditions and treatments, allowing for the evaluation of these conditions and treatments by healthcare providers in a clinically relevant manner. Through the use of communication tools and platforms, such as social media, patients can share this information with other individuals who may be having similar symptoms or are at a similar stage of disease progression. Companies, such as PatientsLikeMe (Cambridge, MA, USA), Alliance Health's (Salt Lake City, UT, USA) social health communities, and 23andMe's (Mountain View, CA, USA) CureTogether.com are making use of this concept to bring together communities of engaged patients, who act as sources of clinical data on drugs and other interventions.[9,29] For example, the PatientsLikeMe website was used to evaluate the effectiveness of lithium carbonate treatment on patients with Amyotropic Lateral Sclerosis (ALS), with similar results to later randomized control trials.[30]

Thus, it is evident that there are numerous benefits to using internet and technology-based platforms in medical management. Table 11.1 summarizes these benefits[9]:

TABLE 11.1
Benefits of Technological Platforms in Medical Interventions.

Benefit	Description	Example
Patient education	Information on medical conditions is now more easily available and accessible to patients	m.CARAT ©provides information to patients with asthma and allergic rhinitis
Patient monitoring and early detection of symptoms	Mobile platforms/wearable technologies can be used to monitor patients' symptoms outside of the clinic or hospital settings. This technology will lead to early detection of symptoms and secondary prevention of diseases.	Wireless wrist blood pressure monitors
Digital phenotyping	Wearable technologies can be used to obtain new forms of objective data to assist in monitoring and management of conditions	Akili interactive labs' NeuroRacer© game acts as a correlate for cognitive impairment in Alzheimer's
Disease management	Mobile platforms can be used to deliver nonpharmacological interventions to patients outside the clinic or hospital settings	Propeller Health's remote wireless sensor attached to bronchodilators to suggests behavioral modifications to avoid potential triggers for asthma attacks
Patient empowerment	Patients have easier access to clinician expertise and are empowered to use it in self-monitoring and reporting of symptoms	PatientsLikeMe website helps to evaluate ALS patients' experience with lithium carbonate

INTERNET AND TECHNOLOGY-BASED INTERVENTIONS IN PSYCHIATRY

The psychiatric profession is one that could greatly benefit from the use of digital platform technologies. Psychiatrists are willing to embrace the use of smartphone applications in patient monitoring and management, and are even getting involved in the development of these applications.[31,32]

The Advantages of Digital Platforms in Psychiatry

Many of the benefits of these technologies mentioned above, such as remote monitoring and management, are very relevant and applicable to the field of psychiatry as well.

Remote patient monitoring in psychiatry

Psychiatric patients are unique in that they are primarily assessed through subjective self-reports and accounts that are made by patients to clinicians. Although clinicians can glean some information on the patients' wellbeing through observation in the clinical setting, this is done in isolation and is not as useful as personal reports that patients can provide, which account for the longer time period in between consults. For example, patients with bipolar disorder are evaluated using tools such as the Mood Disorders Questionnaire and the Clinical Monitoring Form, both of which requires active patients' input to answer specific questions about their mood.[33-36] Digital platforms would allow for such tools to be made available to patients at all times via a mobile phone application or the internet, thus allowing patients to continuously submit reports on their mood status to healthcare providers, who would then be able to monitor and evaluate them on a consistent basis. For example, the MONitoring, treAtment, and pRediCtion of bipolAr disorder episodes (MONARCA) trial evaluated a custom-designed smartphone application that allowed for patient self-monitoring and reporting of mood symptoms. The trial found that self-reports on the application correlated well with existing mood rating scales, indicating its potential for use as a remote-monitoring tool.[37] A similar application, to allow for passive collection of data by remote monitoring of patients with schizophrenia, has also been developed and trialed with positive results.[38]

Disease management and care delivery

One of the greatest challenges in psychiatry is non-pharmacological management, which is usually done in the form of psychological therapies and behavioral modifications. Psychiatric patients are very likely to miss outpatient appointments, therefore stalling management and treatment of their conditions.[39] Thus, if behavioral modifications and psychological therapies could be delivered to patients via their mobile phones or the internet, it would overcome the problem of missed clinic appointments and therefore allow for consistent management of patients. Smartphone applications have been conceptualized that help carers of patients with dementia in the management of these patients.[40,41] Similarly, applications that suggest behavioral modifications, such as warning compulsive gamblers when they are in the vicinity of gambling dens or warning alcoholics when their blood alcohol levels are too high, have also been conceptualised.[42,43]

Digital phenotyping

A major challenge in managing psychiatric patients is the lack of objective markers with which to assess disease progression. As mentioned previously, psychiatric assessment is based predominantly on clinic-based interviews and observations along with subjective accounts of patients' experiences. Diagnostic and assessment tools tend to take the form of questionnaires for patients to answer.[33-36] The disadvantage of this is evident with patients who are poor historians, either due to an inability to accurately recount their experiences, or because they want to influence the clinician's assessment by providing false information. Having objective markers of disease severity would allow clinicians to have continuous real-time data independent of that provided by the patients themselves with which to assess their mental states. Smartphones have been developed with in-built sensors to help pick up data from patients that can assist in overcoming this hurdle. For example, the application mentioned earlier, MONARCA, along with another similar application, the Social Information Monitoring for Patients with Bipolar Affective Disorder (SIMBA) application, makes use of in-built sensors in phones to track objective markers of physical and social activity in patients with bipolar disorder.[37,44,45] The applications track the number of calls and text messages sent and received by the user, along with speech durations during calls, as markers of social activity, and cell tower movement and GPS-tracked distance traveled as markers of physical activity. Thus, these new data sets can act as new digital phenotypic markers of disease severity for clinicians. In summary, the psychiatric profession can truly benefit from the addition of digital platform-based technologies, both in monitoring and management of patients, as summarized in Table 11.2:

DIGITAL TECHNOLOGIES IN THE ASSESSMENT AND MANAGEMENT OF MDD

A 2008 paper identified the key challenges in managing MDD[46]:

- Varied presentation causing difficulty in diagnosis
- Difficulties in identifying target groups for screening
- Poor treatment adherence
- Maximizing the impact of cognitive behavioral therapy (CBT)

TABLE 11.2
Technological Solutions to Challenges in Psychiatry.

Aspect of Treatment	Current Challenges	Technological Solutions
Remote management	High rate of patients missing clinic appointments	Applications can deliver psychological and behavior modification therapies remotely to patients
Remote monitoring	Clinicians are only able to assess patients during appointments, thereby only getting a snapshot of patients' conditions and otherwise relying on their subjective recounts to fill in gaps	Self-monitoring applications allow patients to track their own conditions more regularly, while information is sent to clinicians in real time
Assessing disease progression	Inability of patients to recount true experiences and potential of falsifying information	Sensors from mobile phones/wearable technologies can record objective data from patients

Another major impediment to treatment is access to adequate care. Many patients are unable or reluctant to access and participate in treatment due to barriers such as high costs, personal stigma, waiting lists, and a dearth of trained professionals to meet the rising burden.[47,48] The use of internet-based and other technologies can potentially help to address these difficulties.

Screening and Diagnosis of MDD

Depression is generally screened for and diagnosed via clinical interviews and questionnaires, which judge the likelihood of depression by ranking the severity of patients' symptoms. Examples of such questionnaires include the Patient Health Questionnaire 9 (PHQ-9), Beck Depression Inventory (BDI), and Hamilton Depression Rating Scale (HDRS).[49,50] Questionnaires need to be filled out before patients can be seen by clinicians, and the potential lack of patient adherence, in addition to difficulty in distribution and analysis, means that they are usually given to patients in clinic, before appointments, or mailed to them. The use of digital platforms can assist in improving patient access to these tools as well as the return of data collected from them to healthcare providers. It has been established that questionnaire data can be collected without compromising psychometric characteristics.[51–53] Administering questionnaires over the internet or via mobile phone applications can have numerous advantages[54]:

- Improved adherence as patients can access them without having to come to clinic
- The risk of missing items can be reduced
- Red flags can be automatically raised and acted upon
- Summary scores can be automatically generated
- Algorithms can be developed to help therapists monitor progress and actively intervene if necessary
- Costs of scoring and posting questionnaires can be reduced

"Depression Monitor©" is a free smartphone application that contains the PHQ-9. Users submit their demographics and baseline data before proceeding to complete the questionnaire, the results of which are saved onto the device history. Those with high depression score are advised by the application to take their results to their healthcare professional for further assessment. They are also provided with an explanation of their results, along with links to relevant websites form information on depression. The application also has an in-built weekly notification to remind users to complete the PHQ-9 questionnaire after download, and their results are automatically synchronized to the research database. Participants are also unable to submit the questionnaire without completing all the questions, to circumvent the problem of missing data.[55] A cross-sectional study of the application found that there was an overall response rate of 73.9% by those who downloaded it. Among those not previously diagnosed with depression, 82.5% and 66.8% were at high risk of depression using PHQ-9 thresholds of 11 and 15, respectively. Among them, 36.0% and 34.8%, respectively, responded "nearly every day" to the PHQ-9 suicidal ideation statement Item 9.[55] A more recent study has found that applications based on the PHQ-9 questionnaire produce estimates that correlate strongly with traditionally administered PHQ-9 scores ($r = 0.84$, 95% CI 0.55–0.95).[56] This study shows that smartphone applications have the potential to be effective screening tools for depression in the community. By prompting users with high scores to actively seek help, they could also help in earlier identification, diagnosis, and hence management of patients with depression.

A similar study was conducted on an internet-based screening tool for depression. The Centers for Epidemiological Studies Depression scale was adapted as an online screening test on the Intelihealth health information portal. Participants received feedback based on their probability of having depression upon completing the questionnaire. Those who scored in the moderate range were instructed to either retake the test later or seek advice from a health professional, while those who scored above 22 were earmarked as having a high likelihood of clinical depression and were advised to seek treatment. They were then presented with a postscreening questionnaire with questions on past treatment, attitudes regarding depression and treatment preferences, acting as a starting point for treatment discussions. Finally, these participants were advised to take a printed summary of their assessment for professional review.[57] The study found that 58% of respondents had a high probability of depression, consistent with previous public health screenings. Of those identified with depression, many had never received treatment, indicating that current nontechnological methods of screening may not be effective in identifying patients with depression requiring treatment. One of the reasons for this may be that routine screening does not reach all demographics. This internet-based tool was found to be more effective in identifying younger people with depression than previous screening programmes.[57,58]

Thus, digital platform technologies, by making depression screening tools more accessible to the public, have the potential to improve the identification and diagnosis of patients with depression, allowing them to be identified and started on treatment earlier by first, delivering real-time data from these screening tools to healthcare providers, and second, prompting users to actively seek out health from mental health professionals. Thus, it is imperative that more large-scale trials are carried to assess the efficacies of these applications and programs in improving rates of diagnosis.

Monitoring of MDD
Continuous real-time data
After patients have been identified and diagnosed with depression, it is important for them to be routinely monitored and followed up closely for a multitude of reasons:

- These patients are likely to miss routine clinic appointments, making follow-up difficult.[59]
- There is a high risk of recurrence of MDD in patients who are on treatment.[60]
- These patients have high suicide risk (MDD is one of the five major risk factors for suicide).[61–63]

Thus, the ability of digital platforms to provide a means for continuous real-time monitoring of patients with MDD, outside of the clinic setting, could prove to be extremely beneficial in reducing the risk of recurrence and suicide. By allowing users to be monitored for mood changes continuously, these technologies ensure that patients are under the constant care of clinicians, regardless of clinic appointments. Internet programs and mobile phone applications can be developed with in-built algorithms that can calculate the risks of suicide and recurrence, acting as early warning systems to flag up at-risk individuals to healthcare providers. These technologies can also provide means of objectively monitoring patients, as opposed to relying purely on patient-filled questionnaires and subjective daily accounts. This is an example of ecological momentary assessment, which permits psychiatric patients to report their symptoms immediately after occurrence.

Numerous mobile phone applications that track mood symptoms in patients have been trialed. The MONARCA application, mentioned earlier, is an example of such.[37,44] MONARCA specifically assesses objective (speech, social activity, physical activity, alcohol) and subjective (mood, irritability, sleep) symptoms of mood disorders. These symptoms are then run through scoring algorithms to provide clinicians, who receive this data in real time, with an objective means of assessing risk of mood deterioration. The application also tracks early warning signs, such as sudden changes in patients' behaviors, as potential red flags. Recently, a trial of 17 patients with bipolar disorder found that self-reported mood scores on MONARCA correlated significantly with HDRS scores; there was a 0.51-point decrease in the self-rated mood on the mood scale ($P < .0001$) for every 10 point increase on the HDRS. Similarly, there was a 10-point increase in HDRS corresponding to a 4.8 times decrease in patients changing between cell towers ($P = .020$). Thus, the MONARCA application is able to effectively track changes in mood through both objective and subjective measures.[37,44] The self-monitoring and psychoeducation in bipolar patients with a smart-phone application (SIMPLe) project, similar to MONARCA, was carried out to validate a smartphone application designed to monitor mood symptoms.[64] The application directs users to answer five daily questions on mood, energy, sleep time, irritability, and medication adherence, comparing answers week-to-week to identify relevant mood changes. Users with mood changes that determine them to be at risk of mood disorders are then directed to a more thorough questionnaire based on DSM-5 criteria. They are then given tailored psychoeducational advice based on their performance in this questionnaire. Users are also assessed for risk of substance abuse and suicide, with an immediate notification is sent to mental health teams should suicide be a concern. The application also suggests to the user to call emergency services to seek help. A web-based

interface is being developed to assist mental health teams in real-time monitoring of patients.[64] The SIMPLe application thus not only allows for patients to monitor their mood symptoms regularly, but also has in-built systems to notify professionals of red-flag symptoms, so that they can intervene and help the patients when necessary. Other mood-tracking applications, such as the T2 Mood Tracker and Mobile Mood Diary, work on a similar basis of allowing users to record their mood symptoms daily and tracking the changes over time in real time.[65,66]

Moving further on from just tracking mood symptoms, applications have also been the developed that can predict users' mood states based on previous trends. The Mobilyze! application has been designed as a context-aware system that functions in three phases, with the application sending data from the user to a "learner" who then analyses and uses the data to execute the application's predictive function, as shown in Fig. 11.1[67]:

The application works in conjunction with a website, which not only allows users to visualize their uploaded data, but also have access to psychoeducation and online "coaches" who can view their results and suggest necessary interventions. The application is also able to carry out "ecological momentary interventions" by tracking situations in which the user's mood can deteriorate and sending messages to the user suggesting

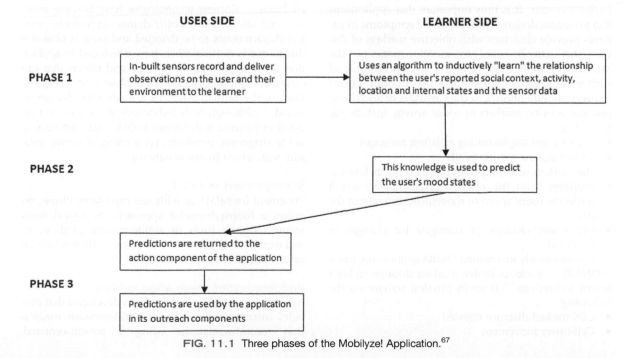

FIG. 11.1 Three phases of the Mobilyze! Application.[67]

interventions during these situations. Eight adults with MDD were trialed for 8 weeks using the Mobilyze! application. The study had numerous promising results:
- Mean location classification accuracy of 60.3% (95% CI 43.2–77.2)
- Decrease in depressive symptoms on the PHQ-9 ($t_{13} = 7.02$, beta$_{week} = -0.82$, $P < .001$)
- Decrease in depressive symptoms on the Quick Inventory of Depressive Symptomatology—clinician rating ($t_{13} = 8.22$, beta$_{week} = -0.81$, $P < .001$)
- Decrease in anxiety symptoms on the Generalized Anxiety Disorder 7-item scale ($t_{13} = 4.59$, beta$_{week} = -0.71$, $P < .001$)
- Reduction in participant meeting MDD diagnostic criteria ($Z = 2.15$, b$_{week} = -0.65$, $P = .03$)

A major challenge in managing MDD is the inability to predict and avoid risk factors for mood deterioration. Mobilyze! provides hope that mobile phone applications can help in overcoming this hurdle by predicting stressors for patients and intervening promptly and accordingly.[67]

Objective markers of disease
As mentioned earlier, patients with MDD can be poor historians or at worst, can attempt to mislead clinicians so as to avoid intervention. With regards to mood tracking technologies, patients may attempt to use these applications to portray their mood in a more positive light, thereby limiting the usefulness of data from subjective accounts. It is thus important that applications and programs designed to track mood symptoms in patients provide clinicians with objective markers of disease that can be used to monitor patients. The MONARCA application is, again, a good example of such technology.[37,44] MONARCA uses in-built sensors in users' mobile phones to track markers of social and physical activity. Markers of social activity include the following:
- No. of outgoing/incoming calls/text messages
- Speech duration during calls

The markers used for physical activity are as follows:
- Readings from the phone's accelerometer, which tracks the users' speed of movement throughout the day
- Cell tower changes (a surrogate for changes in location)

The previously mentioned SIMBA application, like a MONARCA, tracks objective markers through in-built sensor technology.[68] It tracks physical activity via the following:
- GPS-tracked distance traveled
- Cell-tower movement

- Accelerometer readings

It tracks social activity via the following:
- Number and duration of outgoing calls from the phone
- Number of outgoing text messages

Thus, these applications are able to deliver real-time objective, measurable data to clinicians that were previously not available in routine clinic-based monitoring. Additional trials on smartphone sensor technologies have shown that these have been able to achieve mood recognition accuracies of 76% and mood state change detection precision and recall of more than 97%.[68] Building on this, new wearable technologies, based on the same concept of incorporating built-in sensors, are being developed to assist in the monitoring of patients with mood disorders. For example, making use of known correlations between mood disorders and dysfunctions involving the autonomic nervous system (ANS), the personalized monitoring systems for care in mental health European project developed a sensorized t-shirt that records changes in the ANS as markers of mood change.[69] Similarly, "smart-watches" with sensor technologies that can continuously record physiological markers such as heart rate, skin conductance, and blood pressure are being developed to work in conjunction with mobile phone applications that track subjective changes in mood. These devices can then record data that are then processed through an algorithm to deliver an objective indicator of users' mood states to clinicians.[70] Current technologies have become more nuanced, allowing for subtler changes in patients' physical characteristics to be detected and used as objective disease markers. Researchers have developed an application for laptops, mobile phones, and tablets that can carry out computerized speech analysis to detect deviations in the human voice, as a marker for changes in mood.[71] Although such technology has yet to be validated in patients with known MDD, it has potential to aid in diagnosis, providing yet another objective measure with which to assess patients.

Management of MDD
Treatment for MDD, as with any psychiatric illness, requires a biopsychosocial approach. Biological treatments take the form of antidepressant medications and treatment of comorbid diseases, while psychological treatment is done via CBT.[72]

Antidepressant medication guidance
A smartphone application has been developed that provides instant, evidence-based antidepressant medication recommendations using a patient-centered,

symptom-based approach.[73] This application was trialed among family medicine residents and attending physicians to ascertain if it could assist them in deciding on antidepressant treatment for their patients. The physicians were assessed via questionnaires on their confidence with regards to three aspects:

- Managing outpatient adults with MDD
- Starting antidepressants for newly diagnosed MDD
- Choosing antidepressants based on patient factors

The study found that using the application led to an increase in confidence scores in these three categories at 6 and 12 weeks after commencing use (baseline vs. 6 weeks [P-value] vs. 12 weeks [P-value]):

- Managing outpatient adults with MDD (4.214 vs. 4.444 [$P = .607$] vs. 5.364 [$P = .048$])
- Starting antidepressants for newly diagnosed MDD (4.286 vs. 4.778 [$P = .297$] vs. 5.636 [$P = .018$])
- Choosing antidepressants based on patient factors (3.642 vs. 4.889 [$P = .034$] vs. 5.273 [$P = .010$])

Thus, although only confidence in choosing antidepressants based on patient factors increased significantly over 6 weeks, confidence in all three categories rose significantly over 12 weeks, indicating that longer access to the application led to greater improvements. In addition, the average scores on the antidepressant knowledge, assessed via quizzes, improved over the study period, though not significantly ($P = .205$). The improvement in knowledge can be attributed to the ability of smartphone applications to be automatically updated as soon as new information is released. They can therefore help to keep clinicians, who otherwise may be too busy to read medical journals regularly, up to date with the latest treatment guidelines. Thus, it is evident that such applications can assist in the treatment of MDD, by improving the knowledge and confidence of clinicians.[73]

Internet-CBT

Experts suggest that internet-based delivery of psychological treatments, such as CBT, can be as effective as face-to-face treatments, leading to sustained improvements. They can also improve access to these treatments and are likely to be more cost-effective than traditionally delivered treatments.[74] The process of delivering such "digital treatment" involves adapting standard face-to-face protocols into computerized self-help material, either as a self-help program or alongside live psychological treatment with a therapist, which is delivered over a specific time period. Treatments thus become automated and location independent.[75] Internet-CBT has delivered promising results in trials for a range of mental health conditions, including depression.[74,76]

A meta-analysis comparing internet-based guided self-help tools for depression with control groups found an effect size of $d = 0.56$ (95% CI 0.41−0.71; $Z = 7.48$, $P < .001$), a finding supported by another meta-analysis that included only studies on MDD.[77,78] These effect sizes correspond to those for face-to-face psychotherapy.[79] Further studies have found no significant differences in effect sizes between internet-based guided self-help and face-to-face therapies for depression.[80,81]

Deprexis is an interactive, web-based program that consists of 10 content modules representing different psychotherapeutic approaches. An integrative treatment tool draws from numerous psychological treatment concepts including, but not restricted to, CBT and psychoeducation.[82] Two studies have evaluated the efficacy of Deprexis in managing MDD. In the first study, participants were randomized either to the program with regular treatment, or to regular treatment alone, for 9 weeks. Participants were scored on the BDI at pre- and posttreatment. The study found that at 9 weeks, those who used Deprexis had significantly lower BDI scores (Deprexis 19.87 vs. Control 27.15; $t_{214} = 4.14$, $P < .001$, $d = 0.64$) and improved social functioning. Participants in the immediate access group also experienced a reduction in depressive symptoms and recovered more often.[82] In the second study, participants were given 3 months of access to either Deprexis or usual treatment, and then scored on the PHQ-9. Again, treatment with Deprexis was associated with significant reductions in PHQ-9 scores (Deprexis 10.08 vs. Control 13.64; $d = 0.57$).[83] However, for both trials, the differences became nonsignificant at 6-month follow-up, as the control groups were started on Deprexis after the initial trial periods, indicating that even delayed treatment with the program can have catch-up effects.[82,83] Another internet-CBT website is MoodGYM, designed to manage depression in adolescents.[84] It consists of a set of five cognitive behavioral training modules, a personal workbook containing 29 exercises, an interactive game, and an evaluation form. Compared to controls, MoodGYM significantly reduced Center for Epidemiologic Studies depression scores by 4.5 (95% CI 1.8−7.3, $P < .05$) and dysfunctional thinking scores on the Automatic Thoughts Questionnaire by 8.4 (95% CI 3.2−13.6, $P < .05$). The program also improved medical and CBT literacy.[84] Another internet-CBT program, the Sadness Program, also resulted in significant reductions in depression scores on the HDRS for patients with MDD, and was found to be equally effective when delivered via a smartphone application.[85,86] Currently, online and live therapies are being combined into "Blended therapy" to optimize the beneficial effects of both by allowing therapists to guide patients' use of internet-CBT.[87] Therapists can help to determine the suitability of different treatments by making diagnoses, and assist clinicians in individualizing the program for specific patients. A mixture of online and live therapy may also help to improve adherence.[54] In general, internet programs have been shown to be effective in delivering CBT and may be of greater benefit when combined with live therapy, which is gaining acceptance among mental health stakeholders.[75]

LIMITATIONS

There are a few limitations to using digital platform-based interventions. Practical issues such as limited access to smartphones or internet connectivity issues can affect the accessibility of these platforms.[88] More importantly, there is the issue of patient confidentiality and data security.[89] A recent review found that clinicians and patients are using mobile technologies before providers are able to guarantee security and privacy. Furthermore, they tend to be unaware of the privacy and security aspects of their smartphones. The review raises concerns that new healthcare applications are not able to ensure the privacy and safety of patients' health information.[90] Some patients, such as those who are suicidal or in crises, may not be suitable for internet-CBT, and the lack of personal contact can have drawbacks such as poor adherence to or understanding of therapy.[88] Lastly, there is a lack of regulatory bodies monitoring and ensuring the quality of smartphone apps.

CONCLUSION

In summary, there are numerous internet and other technology-based interventions that can assist in the screening, diagnosis, monitoring, and management of MDD. Many of these have been demonstrated to produce significant improvements in patients, and mental health professionals are showing an increased willingness to integrate these platforms into their management programs. However, there are limitations that should be addressed before such interventions are legislated for public use.

REFERENCES

1. Lim GY, Tam WW, Lu Y, Ho CS, Zhang MW, Ho RC. Prevalence of depression in the community from 30 countries between 1994 and 2014. *Sci Rep*. February 12, 2018;8(1): 2861. https://doi.org/10.1038/s41598-018-21243-x.

2. Tofighi B, Abrantes A, Stein MD. The role of technology-based interventions for substance use disorders in primary care: a review of the literature. *Med Clin*. July 2018;102(4):715−731. https://doi.org/10.1016/j.mcna.2018.02.011.

3. Gordon MS, Carswell SB, Schadegg M, et al. Avatar-assisted therapy: a proof-of-concept pilot study of a novel technology-based interventionto treat substance use disorders. *Am J Drug Alcohol Abuse*. September 2017;43(5):518−524. https://doi.org/10.1080/00952990.2017.1280816.

4. Gell NM, Grover KW, Humble M, Sexton M, Dittus K. Efficacy, feasibility, and acceptability of a novel technology-based intervention to support physical activity in cancer survivors. *Support Care Canc*. April 2017; 25(4):1291−1300. https://doi.org/10.1007/s00520-016-3523-5.

5. Senn TE, Braksmajer A, Coury-Doniger P, Urban MA. Carey MP Mobile technology use and desired technology-based intervention characteristics among HIV+ Black men who have sex with men. *AIDS Care*. April 2017;29(4):423−427. https://doi.org/10.1080/0950121.2016.1220479.

6. Number of Internet Users. *Internet Live Stats*; 2016. Available from: http://www.internetlivestats.com/internet-users/.

7. Mobile and tablet internet usage exceeds desktop for first time worldwide. [Online] StatCounter Global Stats. Available from: http://gs.statcounter.com/press/mobile-and-tablet-internet-usage-exceeds-desktop-for-first-time-worldwide [Accessed: 4th August 2017].

8. Topol EJ, Steinhubl SR, Torkamani A. Digital medical tools and sensors. *JAMA*. 2015;313(4):353−354. Available from: http://jamanetwork.com/journals/jama/article-abstract/2091997?linkid=11957339.

9. Elenko E, Underwood L, Zohar D. Defining digital medicine. *Nat Biotechnol*. 2015;33(5):456−461. Available from: http://www.nature.com/nbt/journal/v33/n5/full/nbt.3222.html.

10. Boulos MNK, Brewer AC, Karimkhani C, Buller DB, Dellavalle RP. Mobile medical and health apps: state of the art, concerns, regulatory control and certification. *Online J Public Health Inform*. 2014;5(3):229. https://doi.org/10.5210/ojphi.v5i3.4814.

11. Bauer AM, Thielke SM, Katon W, Unützer J, Areán P. Aligning health information technologies with effective service delivery models to improve chronic disease care. *Prev Med*. 2014;0:167−172. https://doi.org/10.1016/j.ypmed.2014.06.017.

12. Diaz JA, Griffith RA, Ng JJ, Reinert SE, Friedmann PD, Moulton AW. Patients' use of the internet for medical information. *J Gen Intern Med*. 2002;17(3):180−185. https://doi.org/10.1046/j.1525-1497.2002.10603.x.

13. Shepperd S, Charnock D, Gann B. Helping patients access high quality health information. *BMJ*. 1999; 319(7212):764−766. https://doi.org/10.1136/bmj.319.7212.764.

14. Burnay E, Cruz-Correia R, Jacinto T, Sousa AS, Fonseca J. Challenges of a mobile application for asthma and allergic

rhinitis patient enablement-interface and synchronization. *Telemed J E Health.* 2013;19(1):13−18. https://doi.org/10.1089/tmj.2012.0020.

15. Winker MA, Flanagin A, Chi-Lum B, et al. Guidelines for medical and health information sites on the internet: principles governing AMA web sites. *J Am Med Assoc.* 2000;283(12):1600−1606. https://doi.org/10.1001/jama.283.12.1600.

16. Lewis TL. A systematic self-certification model for mobile medical apps. *J Med Internet Res.* 2013;15(4):e89. https://doi.org/10.2196/jmir.2446.

17. Stoyanov SR, Hides L, Kavanagh DJ, Zelenko O, Tjondronegoro D, Mani M. Mobile app rating scale: a new tool for assessing the quality of health mobile apps. *JMIR mHealth and uHealth.* 2015;3(1). https://doi.org/10.2196/mhealth.3422.

18. An HS, Bubak M, Dinkel DM, Slivka D, Lee JM. Validity of the iHealth-BP7 and Withings-BP800 Self Measurement Blood Pressure Monitor. Available from: http://digitalcommons.unomaha.edu/pahppresentations/20/?utm_source=digitalcommons.unomaha.edu%2Fpahpp resentations%2F20&utm_medium=PDF&utm_campaign=PDFCoverPages [Accessed: 5th August 2017].

19. Adler A, Halkin A, Viskin S. Wearable cardioverter-defibrillators. *Circulation.* 2013;127(7):854−860. Available from: http://circ.ahajournals.org/content/127/7/854.short.

20. Vegesna A, Tran M, Angelaccio M, Arcona S. Remote patient monitoring via non-invasive digital technologies: a systematic review. *Telemed J e Health.* 2017;23(1):3−17. https://doi.org/10.1089/tmj.2016.0051.

21. Brownstein JS, Freifeld CC, Madoff LC. Digital disease detection–harnessing the Web for public health surveillance. *N Engl J Med.* 2009;360(21):2153−2155. https://doi.org/10.1056/NEJMp0900702, 2157.

22. Lim YY, Maruff P, Pietrzak RH, et al. Aβ and cognitive change: examining the preclinical and prodromal stages of Alzheimer's disease. *Alzheimer's Dementia.* 2014;10(6):743−751.e1. https://doi.org/10.1016/j.jalz.2013.11.005.

23. Anguera JA, Boccanfuso J, Rintoul JL, et al. Video game training enhances cognitive control in older adults. *Nature.* 2013;501(7465):97−101. https://doi.org/10.1038/nature12486.

24. Jain SH, Powers BW, Hawkins JB, Brownstein JS. The digital phenotype. *Nat Biotechnol.* 2015;33(5):462−463. https://doi.org/10.1038/nbt.3223.

25. Avery L, Flynn D, Wersch A van, Sniehotta FF, Trenell MI. Changing physical activity behavior in type 2 diabetes: a systematic review and meta-analysis of behavioral interventions. *Diabetes Care.* 2012;35(12):2681−2689. https://doi.org/10.2337/dc11-2452.

26. Lin JS, O'Connor E, Evans CV, Senger CA, Rowland MG, Groom HC. Behavioral counseling to promote a healthy lifestyle in persons with cardiovascular risk factors: a systematic review for the U.S. Preventive services task force. *Ann Intern Med.* 2014;161(8):568. https://doi.org/10.7326/M14-0130.

27. Sickle DV, Magzamen S, Truelove S, Morrison T. Remote monitoring of inhaled bronchodilator use and weekly feedback about asthma management: an open-group, short-term pilot study of the impact on asthma control. *PLoS One.* 2013;8(2):e55335. https://doi.org/10.1371/journal.pone.0055335.

28. Merchant RK, Inamdar R, Quade RC. Effectiveness of population health management using the propeller health asthma platform: a randomized clinical trial. *J Allergy Clin Immunol: In Pract.* 2016;4(3):455−463. https://doi.org/10.1016/j.jaip.2015.11.022.

29. Hafen E, Kossmann D, Brand A. Health data cooperatives - citizen empowerment. *Methods Inf Med.* 2014;53(2):82−86. https://doi.org/10.3414/ME13-02-0051.

30. Wicks P, Vaughan TE, Massagli MP, Heywood J. Accelerated clinical discovery using self-reported patient data collected online and a patient-matching algorithm. *Nat Biotechnol.* 2011;29(5):411−414. https://doi.org/10.1038/nbt.1837.

31. Zhang MWB, Ho RCM. Enabling psychiatrists to explore the full potential of E-health. *Front Psychiatry.* 2015;6. https://doi.org/10.3389/fpsyt.2015.00177.

32. Zhang MW, Tsang T, Cheow E, Ho CS, Yeong NB, Ho RC. Enabling psychiatrists to be mobile phone app developers: insights into app development methodologies. *JMIR mHealth and uHealth.* 2014;2(4). https://doi.org/10.2196/mhealth.3425.

33. Baldassano CF. Assessment tools for screening and monitoring bipolar disorder. *Bipolar Disord.* 2005;7:8−15. https://doi.org/10.1111/j.1399-5618.2005.00189.x.

34. Hirschfeld RMA, Williams JBW, Spitzer RL, et al. Development and validation of a screening instrument for bipolar spectrum disorder: the mood disorder questionnaire. *Am J Psychiatry.* 2000;157(11):1873−1875. https://doi.org/10.1176/appi.ajp.157.11.1873.

35. Hirschfeld RMA, Holzer C, Calabrese JR, et al. Validity of the mood disorder questionnaire: a general population study. *Am J Psychiatry.* 2003;160(1):178−180. https://doi.org/10.1176/appi.ajp.160.1.178.

36. Sachs GS, Guille C, McMurrich SL. A clinical monitoring form for mood disorders. *Bipolar Disord.* 2002;4(5):323−327. https://doi.org/10.1034/j.1399-5618.2002.01195.x.

37. Bardram JE, Frost M, Szántó K, Faurholt-Jepsen M, Vinberg M, Kessing LV. Designing mobile health technology for bipolar disorder: a field trial of the monarca system. In: *Proceedings of the SIGCHI Conference on Human Factors in Computing Systems.* New York, NY, USA: ACM; 2013:2627−2636. https://doi.org/10.1145/2470654.2481364.

38. Palmier-Claus JE, Ainsworth J, Machin M, et al. The feasibility and validity of ambulatory self-report of psychotic symptoms using a smartphone software application. *BMC Psychiatry.* 2012;12:172. https://doi.org/10.1186/1471-244X-12-172.

39. Lim LE, Poo KP, Lein T, Chew SK. Why patients fail to attend psychiatric outpatient follow-up-A pilot study.

Singap Med J. 1995;36:403–405. Available from: http://smj.sma.org.sg/3604/3604a12.pdf.

40. Zhang MWB, Chan S, Wynne O, et al. Conceptualization of an evidence-based smartphone innovation for caregivers and persons living with dementia. *Technol Health Care.* 2016;24(5):769–773. https://doi.org/10.3233/THC-161165.

41. Zhang MWB, Ho RCM. Personalized reminiscence therapy M-health application for patients living with dementia: innovating using open source code repository. *Technol Health Care.* 2017;25(1):153–156. https://doi.org/10.3233/THC-161253.

42. Zhang MWB, Ho RCM. Tapping onto the potential of smartphone applications for psycho-education and early intervention in addictions. *Front Psychiatry.* 2016;7. https://doi.org/10.3389/fpsyt.2016.00040.

43. Zhang MWB, Ward J, Ying JJB, Pan F, Ho RCM. The alcohol tracker application: an initial evaluation of user preferences. *BMJ Innovations.* 2015. https://doi.org/10.1136/bmjinnov-2015-000087.

44. Faurholt-Jepsen M, Vinberg M, Christensen EM, Frost M, Bardram J, Kessing LV. Daily electronic self-monitoring of subjective and objective symptoms in bipolar disorder—the MONARCA trial protocol (MONitoring, treAtment and pRediCtion of bipolAr disorder episodes): a randomised controlled single-blind trial. *BMJ Open.* 2013;3(7):e003353. https://doi.org/10.1136/bmjopen-2013-003353.

45. Beiwinkel T, Kindermann S, Maier A, et al. Using smartphones to monitor bipolar disorder symptoms: a pilot study. *JMIR Mental Health.* 2016;3(1). https://doi.org/10.2196/mental.4560.

46. Lester H, Howe A. Depression in primary care: three key challenges. *Postgrad Med.* 2008;84(996):545–548. https://doi.org/10.1136/pgmj.2008.068387.

47. Cuijpers P. Bibliotherapy in unipolar depression: a meta-analysis. *J Behav Ther Exp Psychiatry.* 1997;28(2):139–147.

48. Greenberg DB. Barriers to the treatment of depression in cancer patients. *J Natl Cancer Inst Monogr.* 2004;(32):127–135. https://doi.org/10.1093/jncimonographs/lgh019.

49. Kroenke K, Spitzer RL, Williams JBW. The PHQ-9. *J Gen Intern Med.* 2001;16(9):606–613. https://doi.org/10.1046/j.1525-1497.2001.016009606.x.

50. Aben I, Verhey F, Lousberg R, Lodder J, Honig A. Validity of the Beck depression inventory, hospital anxiety and depression scale, SCL-90, and Hamilton depression rating scale as screening instruments for depression in stroke patients. *Psychosomatics.* 2002;43(5):386–393. https://doi.org/10.1176/appi.psy.43.5.386.

51. Hedman E, Ljótsson B, Rück C, et al. Internet administration of self-report measures commonly used in research on social anxiety disorder: a psychometric evaluation. *Comput Hum Behav.* 2010;26(4):736–740. https://doi.org/10.1016/j.chb.2010.01.010.

52. Coles ME, Cook LM, Blake TR. Assessing obsessive compulsive symptoms and cognitions on the internet:

evidence for the comparability of paper and Internet administration. *Behav Res Ther.* 2007;45(9):2232–2240. https://doi.org/10.1016/j.brat.2006.12.009.

53. Carlbring P, Brunt S, Bohman S, et al. Internet vs. paper and pencil administration of questionnaires commonly used in panic/agoraphobia research. *Comput Hum Behav.* 2007;23(3):1421–1434. https://doi.org/10.1016/j.chb.2005.05.002.

54. Andersson G, Titov N. Advantages and limitations of Internet-based interventions for common mental disorders. *World Psychiatr.* 2014;13(1):4–11. https://doi.org/10.1002/wps.20083.

55. BinDhim NF, Shaman AM, Trevena L, Basyouni MH, Pont LG, Alhawassi TM. Depression screening via a smartphone app: cross-country user characteristics and feasibility. *J Am Med Inform Assoc.* 2015;22(1):29–34. https://doi.org/10.1136/amiajnl-2014-002840.

56. Torous J, Staples P, Shanahan M, et al. Utilizing a personal smartphone custom app to assess the patient health questionnaire-9 (PHQ-9) depressive symptoms in patients with major depressive disorder. *JMIR Mental Health.* 2015;2(1). https://doi.org/10.2196/mental.3889.

57. Houston TK, Cooper LA, Vu HT, Kahn J, Toser J, Ford DE. Screening the public for depression through the internet. *Psychiatr Serv.* 2001;52(3):362–367. https://doi.org/10.1176/appi.ps.52.3.362.

58. Magruder K, Norquist G, Feil Al E. Who comes to a voluntary depression screening program? *Year Bk Psychiatr Appl Ment Health.* 1997;1997(7):253–254.

59. Curran GM, Kirchner JE, Worley M, Rookey C, Booth BM. Depressive symptomatology and early attrition from intensive outpatient substance use treatment. *J Behav Health Serv Res.* 2002;29(2):138–143.

60. Burcusa SL, Iacono WG. Risk for recurrence in depression. *Clin Psychol Rev.* 2007;27(8):959–985. https://doi.org/10.1016/j.cpr.2007.02.005.

61. Cheng ATA, Chen THH, Chen C-C, Jenkins R. Psychosocial and psychiatric risk factors for suicide: case—control psychological autopsy study. *Br J Psychiatry.* 2000;177(4):360–365. https://doi.org/10.1192/bjp.177.4.360.

62. Blair-West GW, Cantor CH, Mellsop GW, Eyeson-Annan ML. Lifetime suicide risk in major depression: sex and age determinants. *J Affect Disord.* 1999;55(2–3):171–178.

63. Holma KM, Melartin TK, Haukka J, Holma IAK, Sokero TP, Isometsä ET. Incidence and predictors of suicide attempts in DSM-IV major depressive disorder: a five-year prospective study. *Am J Psychiatry.* 2010;167(7):801–808. https://doi.org/10.1176/appi.ajp.2010.09050627.

64. Hidalgo-Mazzei D, Mateu A, Reinares M, et al. Self-monitoring and psychoeducation in bipolar patients with a smart-phone application (SIMPLe) project: design, development and studies protocols. *BMC Psychiatry.* 2015;15:52. https://doi.org/10.1186/s12888-015-0437-6.

65. Bush NE, Ouellette G, Kinn J. Utility of the T2 mood tracker mobile application among army warrior transition

unit service members. *Mil Med.* 2014. https://doi.org/10.7205/MILMED-D-14-00271.

66. Matthews M, Doherty G. In the mood: engaging teenagers in psychotherapy using mobile phones. In: *Proceedings of the SIGCHI Conference on Human Factors in Computing Systems.* New York, NY, USA: ACM; 2011:2947–2956. https://doi.org/10.1145/1978942.1979379.

67. Burns MN, Begale M, Duffecy J, et al. Harnessing context sensing to develop a mobile intervention for depression. *J Med Internet Res.* 2011;13(3). https://doi.org/10.2196/jmir.1838.

68. Grünerbl A, Muaremi A, Osmani V, et al. Smartphone-based recognition of states and state changes in bipolar disorder patients. *IEEE J Biomed Health Inform.* 2015;19(1):140–148. http://ieeexplore.ieee.org/abstract/document/6866115/?reload=true.

69. Valenza G, Gentili C, Lanatà A, Scilingo EP. Mood recognition in bipolar patients through the PSYCHE platform: preliminary evaluations and perspectives. *Artif Intell Med.* 2013;57(1):49–58. http://www.sciencedirect.com/science/article/pii/S0933365712001492.

70. Hänsel K, Alomainy A, Haddadi H. Large scale mood and stress self-assessments on a smartwatch. In: *Proceedings of the 2016 ACM International Joint Conference on Pervasive and Ubiquitous Computing: Adjunct.* New York, NY, USA: ACM; 2016:1180–1184. https://doi.org/10.1145/2968219.2968305.

71. Braun S, Annovazzi C, Botella C, et al. Assessing chronic stress, coping skills, and mood disorders through speech analysis: a self-assessment 'voice app' for laptops, tablets, and smartphones. *Psychopathology.* 2016;49(6):406–419. https://doi.org/10.1159/000450959.

72. Schotte CKW, Van Den Bossche B, De Doncker D, Claes S, Cosyns P. A biopsychosocial model as a guide for psychoeducation and treatment of depression. *Depress Anxiety.* 2006;23(5):312–324. https://doi.org/10.1002/da.20177.

73. Man C, Nguyen C, Lin S. Effectiveness of a smartphone app for guiding antidepressant drug selection. *Fam Med.* 2014;46(8):626–630. http://www.stfm.org/FamilyMedicine/Vol46Issue8/Man626.

74. Andersson G. Internet-delivered psychological treatments. *Annu Rev Clin Psychol.* 2016;12(1):157–179. https://doi.org/10.1146/annurev-clinpsy-021815-093006.

75. Topooco N, Riper H, Araya R, et al. Attitudes towards digital treatment for depression: a European stakeholder survey. *Internet Interv.* 2017;8:1–9. https://doi.org/10.1016/j.invent.2017.01.001.

76. Cuijpers P, Riper H, Andersson G. Internet-based treatment of depression. *Curr Opin Psychol.* 2015;4:131–135. https://doi.org/10.1016/j.copsyc.2014.12.026.

77. Richards D, Richardson T. Computer-based psychological treatments for depression: a systematic review and meta-analysis. *Clin Psychol Rev.* 2012;32(4):329–342. https://doi.org/10.1016/j.cpr.2012.02.004.

78. Andrews G, Cuijpers P, Craske MG, McEvoy P, Titov N. Computer therapy for the anxiety and depressive disorders is effective, acceptable and practical health care: a meta-analysis. *PLoS One.* 2010;5(10):e13196. http://journals.plos.org/plosone/article?id=10.1371/journal.pone.0013196.

79. Cuijpers P, Riper H. Internet interventions for depressive disorders: an overview. *Rev Psicopatol Psicol Clínica.* 2014;19(3):209–216. https://doi.org/10.5944/rppc.vol.19.num.3.2014.13902.

80. Cuijpers P, Donker T, Straten A van, Li J, Andersson G. Is guided self-help as effective as face-to-face psychotherapy for depression and anxiety disorders? A systematic review and meta-analysis of comparative outcome studies. *Psychol Med.* 2010;40(12):1943–1957. https://doi.org/10.1017/S0033291710000772.

81. Andersson G, Cuijpers P, Carlbring P, Riper H, Hedman E. Guided Internet-based vs. face-to-face cognitive behavior therapy for psychiatric and somatic disorders: a systematic review and meta-analysis. *World Psychiatr.* 2014;13(3):288–295. http://onlinelibrary.wiley.com/doi/10.1002/wps.20151/full.

82. Meyer B, Berger T, Caspar F, Beevers CG, Andersson G, Weiss M. Effectiveness of a novel integrative online treatment for depression (Deprexis): randomized controlled trial. *J Med Internet Res.* 2009;11(2). https://doi.org/10.2196/jmir.1151.

83. Meyer B, Bierbrodt J, Schröder J, et al. Effects of an Internet intervention (Deprexis) on severe depression symptoms: randomized controlled trial. *Internet Interv.* 2015;2(1):48–59. https://doi.org/10.1016/j.invent.2014.12.003.

84. Christensen H, Griffiths KM, Korten A. Web-based cognitive behavior therapy: analysis of site usage and changes in depression and anxiety scores. *J Med Internet Res.* 2002;4(1). https://doi.org/10.2196/jmir.4.1.e3.

85. Rosso IM, Killgore WDS, Olson EA, et al. Internet-based cognitive behavior therapy for major depressive disorder: a randomized controlled trial. *Depress Anxiety.* 2017;34(3):236–245. https://doi.org/10.1002/da.22590.

86. Watts S, Mackenzie A, Thomas C, et al. CBT for depression: a pilot RCT comparing mobile phone vs. computer. *BMC Psychiatry.* 2013;13(1):49. https://doi.org/10.1186/1471-244X-13-49.

87. Wentzel J, van der Vaart R, Bohlmeijer ET, van Gemert-Pijnen JEWC. Mixing online and face-to-face therapy: how to benefit from blended care in mental health care. *JMIR Mental Health.* 2016;3(1). https://doi.org/10.2196/mental.4534.

88. Andersson G. Using the Internet to provide cognitive behaviour therapy. *Behav Res Ther.* 2009;47(3):175–180. Available from: http://www.sciencedirect.com/science/article/pii/S0005796709000291.

89. Yuen EK, Goetter EM, Herbert JD, Forman EM. Challenges and opportunities in internet-mediated telemental health.

Prof Psychol Res Pract. 2012;43(1):1. Available from: http://psycnet.apa.org/record/2011-24864-001.

90. Martínez-Pérez B, Torre-Díez I de la, López-Coronado M. Privacy and security in mobile health apps: a review and recommendations. *J Med Syst.* 2015;39(1):181. https://doi.org/10.1007/s10916-014-0181-3.

FURTHER READING

1. Simmonds M, Lomas J, Llewellyn A, et al. *Vortioxetine for Treating Major Depressive Disorder: A Single Technology Appraisal.* CRD/CHE Technology Assessment Group; 2015. Available from: https://www.nice.org.uk/guidance/ta367/documents/major-depressive-disorder-vortioxetine-id583-final-scope2.

CHAPTER 12

Dysregulation of the Glutamatergic System in Major Depressive Disorder

TIMOTHY M. COOPER, MD • DAN V. IOSIFESCU, MD, MSC

The monoamine hypothesis, which posits that depression results from deficiencies in levels of synaptic monoamine neurotransmitters, has been the dominant neurochemical theory in major depressive disorder (MDD) research for decades. Although the monoamine hypothesis has had a significant impact on our understanding of the neurobiology of depression and guided the search for many of our current pharmacological interventions, it has become apparent that there are limitations to this approach. First, monoaminergic antidepressants have modest efficacy. In the large Sequenced Treatment Alternatives to Relieve Depression (STAR*D) study, fewer than one-third of patients achieved remission after an initial course of selective serotonin reuptake inhibitor (SSRI) pharmacotherapy, and more than one-third did not improve even after four consecutive antidepressant trials.[1] Second, the timeframe of monoaminergic antidepressants' clinical activity is discordant with their pharmacological effects. Patients improve gradually over weeks to months, though synaptic levels of monoamines increase shortly after antidepressant administration. Third, depletion of monoamines does not universally lead to severe depression, suggesting that monoamine abnormalities do not provide a sufficient explanation for the underlying neurobiology of MDD. It has become clear that traditional antidepressants acting at the level of the synapse have downstream effects that are thought to mediate the delayed clinical response. Research efforts have focused increasingly on the role of synaptic plasticity and functional connectivity in the pathogenesis and treatment of depression.[2,3]

Glutamate is the principal excitatory neurotransmitter in vertebrates and is distributed widely throughout the human brain.[4] Glutamate is synthesized from glutamine in the presynaptic neuron and then packaged by vesicular glutamate transporters for release into the synaptic cleft. Once released, glutamate may interact with three classes of postsynaptic ionotropic receptors, N-methyl-D-aspartate receptors (NMDARs), α-amino-3-hydroxy-6-methyl-4-isoxazolepropionic acid receptors (AMPARs), and kainate receptors, in addition to metabotropic glutamate receptors (mGluRs), which are present both pre- and postsynaptically. Binding of glutamate to NMDA and AMPA receptors causes depolarization of the postsynaptic membrane and downstream activation of brain-derived neurotrophic factor, the mTOR signaling pathway, and transcription factors, ultimately resulting in modifications in synaptic plasticity. Glial cells also play a major role in glutamatergic neurotransmission by taking up synaptic glutamate through excitatory amino acid transporters (EAATs). Once inside the glial cell, glutamate may then be converted to glutamine and transported back to the presynaptic neuron for further use in the messaging cycle.[2]

Glutamatergic neurotransmission is a key modulator of neuronal plasticity and functional connectivity, processes that are disrupted in MDD.[5,6] It is perhaps unsurprising, then, that a growing body of research in humans has demonstrated abnormalities in glutamate signaling in MDD, which we review here.

STUDIES OF CIRCULATING GLUTAMATE LEVELS

Early studies analyzed levels of glutamate and glutamine in serum and plasma. Kim and colleagues reported increased serum glutamate (but not glutamine) levels in 64 depressed inpatients compared to controls, but this increase was seen only in those receiving antidepressants.[7] Similarly, no initial differences in levels of serum glutamate or glutamine were reported in 35 unmedicated inpatients with MDD compared to controls, though elevations in both glutamate and glutamine emerged after 5 weeks of antidepressant treatment.[8] In contrast, several studies of plasma glutamate and

Major Depressive Disorder. https://doi.org/10.1016/B978-0-323-58131-8.00012-4

glutamine levels have reported baseline differences between controls and unmedicated depressed subjects. Three small studies reported increased plasma glutamate (but not glutamine) in MDD subjects compared to controls,[9-11] whereas another reported both plasma glutamate and glutamine elevations in depression, with a direct correlation between plasma glutamate levels and depression severity as assessed by Hamilton Depression Rating Scale scores.[12] Although the significance of these reports is debatable given the lack of an established correlation between levels of glutamate in the circulation and in specific brain areas, these early studies have the merit of raising the question of glutamatergic abnormalities in MDD.

DIRECT MEASUREMENTS OF BRAIN GLUTAMATE LEVELS

There are few studies that directly measure brain glutamate levels. In the CSF, increased levels of glutamine[13] were reported in a small group of unmedicated depressed subjects. Another study[14] that included both unipolar and bipolar subjects showed decreased levels of glutamate in the CSF of unmedicated depressed patients. Brain tissue studies are also limited. No difference was reported in tissue levels of glutamate and glutamine within the superior frontal gyrus in a sample of 21 medicated MDD inpatients undergoing psychosurgery compared to nondepressed neurosurgical controls.[15] However, a brain bank study found decreased levels of frontal cortex glutamate (but not glutamine) in 15 MDD and 15 bipolar patients compared to controls.[16] Taken together, these metabolic studies show a mixed picture of changes in glutamate (and less frequently glutamine) levels in the blood, CSF, and brain tissue. Interestingly, some of these changes were reported during treatment with antidepressants, which may reflect downstream activation of glutamatergic signaling by these agents.

GENETIC STUDIES

Genetic studies are suggestive of abnormalities in glutamatergic signaling in mood disorders. A gene analysis of 26 male suicide victims showed global glutamatergic abnormalities.[17] A meta-analysis of genome-wide association studies in MDD found significant alterations in genes involved in glutamatergic synaptic neurotransmission.[18] Choudary and colleagues conducted a genetic microarray study of nine brain bank samples of patients with MDD, examining the anterior cingulate cortex (ACC) and dorsolateral prefrontal cortex (DLPFC).[19] Both of these areas showed downregulation of

glutamate transporters (SLC1A2 and SLC1A3) and glutamine synthetase. AMP1 and GluR-KA2 were upregulated in the ACC, whereas AMP3, GluR5, and GluR-KA2 were upregulated in the DLPFC. Genetic studies have also demonstrated abnormalities in glutamate receptors in the prefrontal cortex (PFC)[20,21] and locus coeruleus.[22]

GLUTAMATE RECEPTOR AND STRUCTURAL PROTEIN ABNORMALITIES

Various abnormalities have been detected in **NMDA receptor** binding and composition in MDD. Decreased NMDAR binding was described in brain bank studies in the frontal cortex (BA 10) of 22 suicide victims[23] and in the superior temporal cortex (BA 22) of 15 MDD subjects.[24] In MDD, decreased levels of the NR2A and NR2B subunits of the NMDAR were described in the PFC,[25] while decreased NR2A and NR1 were reported in the DLPFC.[26] Karolewicz et al. showed decreased expression of NR2C in the locus coeruleus[27] and increased expression of NR2A in the amygdala[28] of MDD subjects. Beneyto and colleagues reported decreased expression of NR2A and NR2B in the perirhinal cortex and increased NMDAR binding (but intact NMDAR subunit composition) in the hippocampus.[29] Others have reported no change in NR1 levels in the hippocampus or orbitofrontal cortex (OFC) in MDD.[30] Using in situ hybridization of the DLPFC in brain bank samples from 15 MDD subjects, significant decreases were reported in **AMPA receptor** subunits GluR2 and GluR3, but not in subunits GluR1 or GluR4, or in other signaling proteins NSF, PICK1, stargazin, and syntenin.[31] Independent studies described decreased levels of GluR1, GluR3, and GluR5 in the perirhinal cortex in MDD,[29] but no changes in NMDARs, AMPARs, or kainate receptors in the striatum.[32]

In addition to receptor abnormalities, changes in levels of **structural proteins involved in glutamatergic signaling** have been observed in MDD. In a brain bank study[33] including 15 MDD subjects, significantly decreased levels of striatal SAP-102 were detected by in situ hybridization in MDD compared to controls (though there were no differences for striatal PSD-93, PSD-95, or NF-L). These proteins have been found to be crucial in normal NMDAR membrane trafficking and signaling.[34] Another brain bank study including 15 patients with MDD reported decreased striatal levels of the glutamate transporter EAAT4 (though EAAT1, EAAT2, and EAAT3 were not significantly altered).[35] Glutamate transporters are involved in the critical step of removing excess glutamate from the synapse, and their dysfunction may be related to glutamate excitotoxicity.[36] Others have found decreased levels of EAAT1 in the OFC of MDD subjects (although levels of EAAT2 and glutamine synthase were not significantly altered).[37] No changes in levels of PSD-95, NF-L, or SAP-102 were reported in the DLPFC,[26] and no changes in levels of PSD-95 were reported in the hippocampus or OFC.[30] By contrast, PSD-95 levels were elevated in the amygdala and decreased in the PFC.[25,28]

The receptor and protein studies reviewed earlier tend to be relatively small and differ in the methods and brain areas studied. Their results are sometimes contradictory. Although none of the findings has been replicated at this time, in aggregate these studies are suggestive of significant abnormalities in the glutamate receptors and associated structural proteins in mood disorders.

IMAGING STUDIES

Imaging studies, primarily those using proton magnetic resonance spectroscopy (^{1}H-MRS), have provided in vivo evidence of abnormalities of the glutamatergic system in MDD. Measuring glutamate with ^{1}H-MRS is technically challenging, although robust methods have been validated.[38] ^{1}H-MRS studies have several limitations: (a) most used methods that were not able to separate glutamate and glutamine, instead reporting the combined glutamate + glutamine peak (Glx), (b) the MRS voxels were relatively large and collected signals from multiple brain areas and CSF, poorly matching the anatomical boundaries of the brain areas investigated, and (c) the glutamate levels measured were a combination of intra- and extracellular levels. Despite these limitations, ^{1}H-MRS remains one of the best tools to investigate the brain glutamate system in vivo. Earlier studies of Glx in MDD (before 2006) have been summarized in a meta-analysis by Yildiz-Yesiloglu and Ankerst.[39]

Several ^{1}H-MRS studies focusing on Glx changes in the **ACC**, a region with key roles in mediating emotion and cognition, have led to mixed results. Some reported decreased ACC levels of Glx in MDD compared to controls.[40] Decreased Glx levels in the ACC were reported in MDD subjects treated with antidepressants[41] and in unmedicated MDD patients.[42,43] Notably, this abnormality normalized in treatment responders after treatment with electroconvulsive therapy (ECT)[44] or SSRIs.[43] In contrast, a study that separated glutamate and glutamine signals did not find significant decreases in ACC levels of glutamate, though it did find a significant decrease in glutamine levels among a subset of highly anhedonic MDD patients.[45] Negative and even contradictory findings in glutamatergic alterations in

the ACC have been reported by several other investigators. Some reported no changes in ACC levels of Glx[46,47] or in levels of pure glutamate or glutamine.[48] Others found increased glutamate levels in the midcingulate cortex (which comprises the posterior portion of the ACC)[49] and increased levels of Glx, glutamate, and glutamine in the ACC of MDD patients.[50]

Other parts of the limbic system that have been investigated include the **hippocampus**, where depression has well-established deleterious effects. Decreased levels of Glx were reported in the left amygdala/anterior hippocampus significant only in MDD patients as opposed to combined unipolar and bipolar depressed patients.[51] Interestingly, Glx increased in the pooled analysis of 13 unipolar and 15 bipolar depressed patients following ECT treatment. Others also found a pattern of decreased hippocampal Glx and pure glutamine in patients with MDD, though these findings did not resolve after 8 weeks of treatment with antidepressants.[52] Decreased hippocampal Glx was demonstrated in treatment-resistant and recurrent-remitted depressed patients relative to controls.[53] In contrast, other studies either failed to show changes in Glx in the left hippocampus[54] or had discordant findings in the left and right hippocampus (no change in Glx in the right hippocampus but elevated in the left).[55] Following treatment with ECT, Glx levels were found to decrease in the left hippocampus.[55]

The **prefrontal cortex (PFC)** has been another region of active investigation in depression research. The majority of ^{1}H-MRS studies suggest a decrease in glutamatergic signaling in the PFC. Decreased Glx levels have been reported in the DLPFC in unmedicated MDD patients,[56] in both the dorsal and ventral aspects of the PFC,[57] and in the medial PFC.[42,58] Glx levels in the ventromedial PFC were reduced in remitted-recurrent and chronic depressed patients compared to controls and first-episode MDD subjects.[59] Moreover, Glx abnormalities in the DLPFC normalized after a course of ECT.[56] In contrast, other studies demonstrated no changes in Glx or pure glutamate levels in the DLFPC of MDD patients.[43,49,60] In one study, elevated baseline DLPFC glutamate predicted treatment response to antidepressant pharmacotherapy.[49]

Several other regions that have been imaged for glutamatergic abnormalities include the **insula and occipital cortex**. In a study of 33 depressed patients (29 of whom had MDD), glutamate (but not glutamine) levels were increased in the occipital cortex.[61] Consistent with this, a more recent study using carbon-13 nuclear magnetic resonance spectroscopy (^{13}C-NMR) noted decreased oxidative mitochondrial energy production of glutamatergic neurons in the occipital cortex (OCC).[62] However, others did not report abnormal Glx levels[46] or changes in glutamate and glutamine levels in the OCC.[48] Few studies described Glx abnormalities in other brain areas, such as the putamen,[48] or the anterior insula, where a significant inverse relationship between Glx and HDRS scores was reported.[63]

Although a number of ^{1}H-MRS imaging studies have suggested several trends for abnormalities in glutamate-related neurometabolite levels in different regions of the brain implicated in MDD, the current findings are often contradictory and difficult to interpret. However, taken together, the preponderance of existing research on the glutamatergic system has demonstrated abnormalities in MDD in a variety of contexts, from early studies of peripheral levels of neurotransmitters to genetic, protein, and imaging studies. Furthermore, research is needed to better characterize these changes, particularly given promising advances in imaging that may allow for more precise examination of glutamatergic pathways as well as the development of novel glutamatergic antidepressants.

REFERENCES

1. Sinyor M, Schaffer A, Levitt A. The sequenced treatment alternatives to relieve depression (STAR*D) trial: a review. *Can J Psychiatr.* 2010;55(3):126–135. https://doi.org/10.1177/070674371005500303. PubMed PMID: 20370962.
2. Murrough JW, Abdallah CG, Mathew SJ. Targeting glutamate signalling in depression: progress and prospects. Epub 2017/03/18 *Nat Rev Drug Discov.* 2017;16(7): 472–486. https://doi.org/10.1038/nrd.2017.16. PubMed PMID: 28303025.
3. Sanacora G, Zarate CA, Krystal JH, Manji HK. Targeting the glutamatergic system to develop novel, improved therapeutics for mood disorders. Epub 2008/04/22 *Nat Rev Drug Discov.* 2008;7(5):426–437. https://doi.org/10.1038/nrd2462. PubMed PMID: 18425072; PMCID: PMC2715836.
4. Meldrum BS. Glutamate as a neurotransmitter in the brain: review of physiology and pathology. *J Nutr.* 2000;130(4S Suppl):1007S–1015S. PubMed PMID: 10736372.
5. Marsden WN. Synaptic plasticity in depression: molecular, cellular and functional correlates. Epub 2012/12/27 *Prog Neuro-Psychopharmacol Biol Psychiatry.* 2013;43:168–184. https://doi.org/10.1016/j.pnpbp.2012.12.012. PubMed PMID: 23268191.
6. Duman RS, Aghajanian GK, Sanacora G, Krystal JH. Synaptic plasticity and depression: new insights from stress and rapid-acting antidepressants. Epub 2016/03/05 *Nat Med.* 2016;22(3):238–249. https://doi.org/10.1038/nm.4050. PubMed PMID: 26937618; PMCID:PMC5405628.
7. Kim JS, Schmid-Burgk W, Claus D, Kornhuber HH. Increased serum glutamate in depressed patients. *Arch Psychiatr Nervenkr.* 1982;232(4):299–304. PubMed PMID: 6133511.
8. Maes M, Verkerk R, Vandoolaeghe E, Lin A, Scharpe S. Serum levels of excitatory amino acids, serine, glycine, histidine, threonine, taurine, alanine and arginine in treatment-resistant depression: modulation by treatment with antidepressants and prediction of clinical responsivity. *Acta Psychiatr Scand.* 1998;97(4):302–308. PubMed PMID:9570492.
9. Altamura CA, Mauri MC, Ferrara A, Moro AR, D'Andrea G, Zamberlan F. Plasma and platelet excitatory amino acids in psychiatric disorders. *Am J Psychiatry.* 1993;150(11): 1731–1733. https://doi.org/10.1176/ajp.150.11.1731. PubMed PMID:8214185.
10. Altamura C, Maes M, Dai J, Meltzer HY. Plasma concentrations of excitatory amino acids, serine, glycine, taurine and histidine in major depression. *Eur Neuropsychopharmacol.* 1995;5(Suppl):71–75. PubMed PMID:8775762.
11. Mauri MC, Ferrara A, Boscati L, et al. Plasma and platelet amino acid concentrations in patients affected by major depression and under fluvoxamine treatment. *Neuropsychobiology.* 1998;37(3):124–129. PubMed PMID:9597668.
12. Mitani H, Shirayama Y, Yamada T, Maeda K, Ashby Jr CR, Kawahara R. Correlation between plasma levels of glutamate, alanine and serine with severity of depression. *Prog Neuro-Psychopharmacol Biol Psychiatry.* 2006;30(6): 1155–1158. https://doi.org/10.1016/j.pnpbp.2006.03.036. PubMed PMID: 16707201.
13. Levine J, Panchalingam K, Rapoport A, Gershon S, McClure RJ, Pettegrew JW. Increased cerebrospinal fluid glutamine levels in depressed patients. *Biol Psychiatry.* 2000;47(7):586–593. PubMed PMID: 10745050.
14. Frye MA, Tsai GE, Huggins T, Coyle JT, Post RM. Low cerebrospinal fluid glutamate and glycine in refractory affective disorder. *Biol Psychiatry.* 2007;61(2):162–166. https://doi.org/10.1016/j.biopsych.2006.01.024. PubMed PMID: 16735030.
15. Francis PT, Poynton A, Lowe SL, et al. Brain amino acid concentrations and Ca2+-dependent release in intractable depression assessed antemortem. *Brain Res.* 1989;494(2): 315–324. PubMed PMID:2570624.
16. Hashimoto K, Sawa A, Iyo M. Increased levels of glutamate in brains from patients with mood disorders. *Biol Psychiatry.* 2007;62(11):1310–1316. https://doi.org/10.1016/j.biopsych.2007.03.017. PubMed PMID: 17574216.
17. Sequeira A, Mamdani F, Ernst C, et al. Global brain gene expression analysis links glutamatergic and GABAergic alterations to suicide and major depression. *PLoS One.* 2009;4(8):e6585. https://doi.org/10.1371/journal.pone.0006585. PubMed PMID: 19668376; PMCID:PMC2719799.
18. Lee PH, Perlis RH, Jung JY, et al. Multi-locus genome-wide association analysis supports the role of glutamatergic synaptic transmission in the etiology of major depressive disorder. *Transl Psychiatry.* 2012;2:e184. https://doi.org/

10.1038/tp.2012.95. PubMed PMID: 23149448; PMCID: PMC3565768.

19. Choudary PV, Molnar M, Evans SJ, et al. Altered cortical glutamatergic and GABAergic signal transmission with glial involvement in depression. *Proc Natl Acad Sci U S A.* 2005;102(43):15653—15658. https://doi.org/10.1073/pnas.0507901102. PubMed PMID: 16230605; PMCID: PMC1257393.

20. Gray AL, Hyde TM, Deep-Soboslay A, Kleinman JE, Sodhi MS. Sex differences in glutamate receptor gene expression in major depression and suicide. *Mol Psychiatr.* 2015;20(9):1139. https://doi.org/10.1038/mp.2015.114. PubMed PMID: 26216299.

21. Deschwanden A, Karolewicz B, Feyissa AM, et al. Reduced metabotropic glutamate receptor 5 density in major depression determined by [(11)C]ABP688 PET and post-mortem study. *Am J Psychiatry.* 2011;168(7):727—734. https://doi.org/10.1176/appi.ajp.2011.09111607. PubMed PMID: 21498461; PMCID:PMC3129412.

22. Chandley MJ, Szebeni A, Szebeni K, et al. Elevated gene expression of glutamate receptors in noradrenergic neurons from the locus coeruleus in major depression. *Int J Neuropsychopharmacol.* 2014;17(10):1569—1578. https://doi.org/10.1017/S1461145714000662. PubMed PMID: 24925192.

23. Nowak G, Ordway GA, Paul IA. Alterations in the N-methyl-D-aspartate (NMDA) receptor complex in the frontal cortex of suicide victims. *Brain Res.* 1995; 675(1—2):157—164. PubMed PMID:7796124.

24. Nudmamud-Thanoi S, Reynolds GP. The NR1 subunit of the glutamate/NMDA receptor in the superior temporal cortex in schizophrenia and affective disorders. *Neurosci Lett.* 2004;372(1—2):173—177. https://doi.org/10.1016/j.neulet.2004.09.035. PubMed PMID: 15531111.

25. Feyissa AM, Chandran A, Stockmeier CA, Karolewicz B. Reduced levels of NR2A and NR2B subunits of NMDA receptor and PSD-95 in the prefrontal cortex in major depression. *Prog Neuro-Psychopharmacol Biol Psychiatry.* 2009;33(1):70—75. https://doi.org/10.1016/j.pnpbp.2008.10.005. PubMed PMID: 18992785; PMCID: PMC2655629.

26. Beneyto M, Meador-Woodruff JH. Lamina-specific abnormalities of NMDA receptor-associated postsynaptic protein transcripts in the prefrontal cortex in schizophrenia and bipolar disorder. *Neuropsychopharmacology.* 2008;33(9):2175—2186. https://doi.org/10.1038/sj.npp.1301604. PubMed PMID: 18033238.

27. Karolewicz B, Stockmeier CA, Ordway GA. Elevated levels of the NR2C subunit of the NMDA receptor in the locus coeruleus in depression. *Neuropsychopharmacology.* 2005;30(8):1557—1567. https://doi.org/10.1038/sj.npp.1300781. PubMed PMID: 15920498; PMCID:PMC2921564.

28. Karolewicz B, Szebeni K, Gilmore T, Maciag D, Stockmeier CA, Ordway GA. Elevated levels of NR2A and PSD-95 in the lateral amygdala in depression. *Int J Neuropsychopharmacol.* 2009;12(2):143—153. https://doi.org/

10.1017/S1461145708008985. PubMed PMID: 18570704; PMCID:PMC2645479.

29. Beneyto M, Kristiansen LV, Oni-Orisan A, McCullumsmith RE, Meador-Woodruff JH. Abnormal glutamate receptor expression in the medial temporal lobe in schizophrenia and mood disorders. *Neuropsychopharmacology.* 2007;32(9):1888—1902. https://doi.org/10.1038/sj.npp.1301312. PubMed PMID: 17299517.

30. Toro C, Deakin JF. NMDA receptor subunit NRI and post-synaptic protein PSD-95 in hippocampus and orbitofrontal cortex in schizophrenia and mood disorder. *Schizophr Res.* 2005;80(2—3):323—330. https://doi.org/10.1016/j.schres.2005.07.003. PubMed PMID: 16140506.

31. Beneyto M, Meador-Woodruff JH. Lamina-specific abnormalities of AMPA receptor trafficking and signaling molecule transcripts in the prefrontal cortex in schizophrenia. *Synapse.* 2006;60(8):585—598. https://doi.org/10.1002/syn.20329. PubMed PMID: 16983646.

32. Meador-Woodruff JH, Hogg Jr AJ, Smith RE. Striatal ionotropic glutamate receptor expression in schizophrenia, bipolar disorder, and major depressive disorder. *Brain Res Bull.* 2001;55(5):631—640. PubMed PMID: 11576760.

33. Kristiansen LV, Meador-Woodruff JH. Abnormal striatal expression of transcripts encoding NMDA interacting PSD proteins in schizophrenia, bipolar disorder and major depression. *Schizophr Res.* 2005;78(1):87—93. https://doi.org/10.1016/j.schres.2005.06.012. PubMed PMID: 16023328.

34. Perez-Otano I, Ehlers MD. Learning from NMDA receptor trafficking: clues to the development and maturation of glutamatergic synapses. *Neurosignals.* 2004;13(4):175—189. https://doi.org/10.1159/000077524. PubMed PMID: 15148446.

35. McCullumsmith RE, Meador-Woodruff JH. Striatal excitatory amino acid transporter transcript expression in schizophrenia, bipolar disorder, and major depressive disorder. *Neuropsychopharmacology.* 2002;26(3):368—375. https://doi.org/10.1016/S0893-133X(01)00370-0. PubMed PMID: 11850151.

36. O'Shea RD. Roles and regulation of glutamate transporters in the central nervous system. *Clin Exp Pharmacol Physiol.* 2002;29(11):1018—1023. Epub 2002/10/09. PubMed PMID: 12366395.

37. Miguel-Hidalgo JJ, Waltzer R, Whittom AA, Austin MC, Rajkowska G, Stockmeier CA. Glial and glutamatergic markers in depression, alcoholism, and their comorbidity. *J Affect Disord.* 2010;127(1—3):230—240. https://doi.org/10.1016/j.jad.2010.06.003. PubMed PMID: 20580095; PMCID:PMC2975814.

38. Henry ME, Lauriat TL, Shanahan M, Renshaw PF, Jensen JE. Accuracy and stability of measuring GABA, glutamate, and glutamine by proton magnetic resonance spectroscopy: a phantom study at 4 Tesla. Epub 2010/12/07 *J Magn Reson.* 2011;208(2):210—218. https://doi.org/10.1016/j.jmr.2010.11.003. PubMed PMID: 21130670; PMCID:PMC4641575.

39. Yildiz-Yesiloglu A, Ankerst DP. Review of 1H magnetic resonance spectroscopy findings in major depressive disorder: a meta-analysis. Epub 2006/06/30 *Psychiatr Res.* 2006;147(1):1–25. https://doi.org/10.1016/j.pscychresns.2005.12.004. PubMed PMID: 16806850.

40. Auer DP, Putz B, Kraft E, Lipinski B, Schill J, Holsboer F. Reduced glutamate in the anterior cingulate cortex in depression: an in vivo proton magnetic resonance spectroscopy study. *Biol Psychiatry.* 2000;47(4):305–313. PubMed PMID: 10686265.

41. Jarnum H, Eskildsen SF, Steffensen EG, et al. Longitudinal MRI study of cortical thickness, perfusion, and metabolite levels in major depressive disorder. *Acta Psychiatr Scand.* 2011;124(6):435–446. https://doi.org/10.1111/j.1600-0447.2011.01766.x. PubMed PMID: 21923809.

42. Li H, Xu H, Zhang Y, et al. Differential neurometabolite alterations in brains of medication-free individuals with bipolar disorder and those with unipolar depression: a two-dimensional proton magnetic resonance spectroscopy study. *Bipolar Disord.* 2016;18(7):583–590. https://doi.org/10.1111/bdi.12445. PubMed PMID: 27870506.

43. Chen LP, Dai HY, Dai ZZ, Xu CT, Wu RH. Anterior cingulate cortex and cerebellar hemisphere neurometabolite changes in depression treatment: a 1H magnetic resonance spectroscopy study. *Psychiatr Clin Neurosci.* 2014;68(5):357–364. https://doi.org/10.1111/pcn.12138. PubMed PMID: 24393367.

44. Pfleiderer B, Michael N, Erfurth A, et al. Effective electroconvulsive therapy reverses glutamate/glutamine deficit in the left anterior cingulum of unipolar depressed patients. *Psychiatr Res.* 2003;122(3):185–192. PubMed PMID: 12694892.

45. Walter M, Henning A, Grimm S, et al. The relationship between aberrant neuronal activation in the pregenual anterior cingulate, altered glutamatergic metabolism, and anhedonia in major depression. *Arch Gen Psychiatr.* 2009;66(5):478–486. https://doi.org/10.1001/archgenpsychiatry.2009.39. PubMed PMID: 19414707.

46. Price RB, Shungu DC, Mao X, et al. Amino acid neurotransmitters assessed by proton magnetic resonance spectroscopy: relationship to treatment resistance in major depressive disorder. *Biol Psychiatry.* 2009;65(9):792–800. https://doi.org/10.1016/j.biopsych.2008.10.025. PubMed PMID: 19058788; PMCID:PMC2934870.

47. Li M, Metzger CD, Li W, et al. Dissociation of glutamate and cortical thickness is restricted to regions subserving trait but not state markers in major depressive disorder. *J Affect Disord.* 2014;169:91–100. https://doi.org/10.1016/j.jad.2014.08.001. PubMed PMID: 25173431.

48. Godlewska BR, Masaki C, Sharpley AL, Cowen PJ, Emir UE. Brain glutamate in medication-free depressed patients: a proton MRS study at 7 Tesla. *Psychol Med.* 2017:1–7. https://doi.org/10.1017/S0033291717003373. PubMed PMID: 29224573.

49. Grimm S, Luborzewski A, Schubert F, et al. Region-specific glutamate changes in patients with unipolar depression. *J Psychiatr Res.* 2012;46(8):1059–1065. https://doi.org/10.1016/j.jpsychires.2012.04.018. PubMed PMID: 22595871.

50. Abdallah CG, Hannestad J, Mason GF, et al. Metabotropic glutamate receptor 5 and glutamate involvement in major depressive disorder: a multimodal imaging study. *Biol Psychiatry Cogn Neurosci Neuroimaging.* 2017;2(5):449–456. https://doi.org/10.1016/j.bpsc.2017.03.019. PubMed PMID: 28993818; PMCID:PMC5630181.

51. Michael N, Erfurth A, Ohrmann P, Arolt V, Heindel W, Pfleiderer B. Neurotrophic effects of electroconvulsive therapy: a proton magnetic resonance study of the left amygdalar region in patients with treatment-resistant depression. *Neuropsychopharmacology.* 2003;28(4):720–725. https://doi.org/10.1038/sj.npp.1300085. PubMed PMID: 12655317.

52. Block W, Traber F, von Widdern O, et al. Proton MR spectroscopy of the hippocampus at 3 T in patients with unipolar major depressive disorder: correlates and predictors of treatment response. *Int J Neuropsychopharmacol.* 2009;12(3):415–422. https://doi.org/10.1017/S1461145708009516. PubMed PMID: 18845018.

53. de Diego-Adelino J, Portella MJ, Gomez-Anson B, et al. Hippocampal abnormalities of glutamate/glutamine, N-acetylaspartate and choline in patients with depression are related to past illness burden. *J Psychiatry Neurosci.* 2013;38(2):107–116. https://doi.org/10.1503/jpn.110185. PubMed PMID: 23425950; PMCID:PMC3581591.

54. Milne A, MacQueen GM, Yucel K, Soreni N, Hall GB. Hippocampal metabolic abnormalities at first onset and with recurrent episodes of a major depressive disorder: a proton magnetic resonance spectroscopy study. *Neuroimage.* 2009;47(1):36–41. https://doi.org/10.1016/j.neuroimage.2009.03.031. PubMed PMID: 19324095.

55. Njau S, Joshi SH, Espinoza R, et al. Neurochemical correlates of rapid treatment response to electroconvulsive therapy in patients with major depression. *J Psychiatry Neurosci.* 2017;42(1):6–16. https://doi.org/10.1503/jpn.150177. PubMed PMID: 27327561; PMCID: PMC5373714.

56. Michael N, Erfurth A, Ohrmann P, Arolt V, Heindel W, Pfleiderer B. Metabolic changes within the left dorsolateral prefrontal cortex occurring with electroconvulsive therapy in patients with treatment resistant unipolar depression. *Psychol Med.* 2003;33(7):1277–1284. PubMed PMID: 14580081.

57. Hasler G, van der Veen JW, Tumonis T, Meyers N, Shen J, Drevets WC. Reduced prefrontal glutamate/glutamine and gamma-aminobutyric acid levels in major depression determined using proton magnetic resonance spectroscopy. *Arch Gen Psychiatr.* 2007;64(2):193–200. https://doi.org/10.1001/archpsyc.64.2.193. PubMed PMID: 17283286.

58. Tan HZ, Li H, Liu CF, et al. Main effects of diagnoses, brain regions, and their interaction effects for cerebral metabolites in bipolar and unipolar depressive disorders. *Sci Rep.* 2016;6:37343. https://doi.org/10.1038/srep37343. PubMed PMID: 27869127; PMCID:PMC5116758.

59. Portella MJ, de Diego-Adelino J, Gomez-Anson B, et al. Ventromedial prefrontal spectroscopic abnormalities over the course of depression: a comparison among first episode, remitted recurrent and chronic patients. *J Psychiatr Res.* 2011;45(4):427—434. https://doi.org/10.1016/j.jpsychires. 2010.08.010. PubMed PMID: 20875647.

60. Nery FG, Stanley JA, Chen HH, et al. Normal metabolite levels in the left dorsolateral prefrontal cortex of unmedicated major depressive disorder patients: a single voxel (1) H spectroscopy study. *Psychiatr Res.* 2009;174(3): 177—183. https://doi.org/10.1016/j.pscychresns.2009. 05.003. PubMed PMID: 19910168.

61. Sanacora G, Gueorguieva R, Epperson CN, et al. Subtype-specific alterations of gamma-aminobutyric acid and glutamate in patients with major depression. *Arch Gen Psychiatr.* 2004;61(7):705—713. https://doi.org/10.1001/ archpsyc.61.7.705. PubMed PMID: 15237082.

62. Abdallah CG, Jiang L, De Feyter HM, et al. Glutamate metabolism in major depressive disorder. Epub 2014/07/31 *Am J Psychiatry.* 2014;171(12):1320—1327. https://doi.org/ 10.1176/appi.ajp.2014.14010067. PubMed PMID: 25073688; PMCID:PMC4472484.

63. Demenescu LR, Colic L, Li M, et al. A spectroscopic approach toward depression diagnosis: local metabolism meets functional connectivity. *Eur Arch Psychiatry Clin Neurosci.* 2017;267(2):95—105. https://doi.org/10.1007/ s00406-016-0726-1. PubMed PMID: 27561792.

CHAPTER 13

Glutamate Modulators in Major Depressive Disorder

TIMOTHY M. COOPER, MD • DAN V. IOSIFESCU, MD, MSC

As we discussed previously, the current pharmacologic methods of treating major depressive disorder (MDD) are limited by modest efficacy and delayed clinical response, leading investigators to search for novel antidepressants operating through different mechanisms of action. Several agents with direct modulatory effects on glutamate receptors and/or neurotransmission have demonstrated compelling evidence in treating MDD, making this an active area of pharmaceutical research.

The first demonstration of the antidepressant action of glutamatergic agents dates back to 1959, when D-cycloserine was reported to be effective in treatment of depression in patients receiving it for tuberculosis.[1] There has been a renewed interest in modulators of the glutamatergic system, starting with studies in the 1990s demonstrating efficacy in animal models of depression.[2] Perhaps the most promising of these agents is ketamine. Ketamine is a selective N-methyl-D-aspartate (NMDA) receptor antagonist, where it binds close to the channel pore and prevents depolarization of the postsynaptic membrane.

HOW DOES KETAMINE'S MECHANISM OF ACTION SUPPORT THE HYPOTHESIS OF GLUTAMATE DYSREGULATION IN DEPRESSION?

Although the mechanism by which ketamine produces antidepressant effects remains incompletely understood, significant advances in this area have been made in the last decade. Studies of the cellular signaling mechanisms underlying the synaptic actions of ketamine demonstrate that the ketamine-mediated blockade of NMDA receptors at rest results in a relative increase in activation of intrasynaptic α-amino-3-hydroxy-5-methyl-4-isoxazolepropionic acid (AMPA) receptors, the net effect of which is increased glutamatergic neurotransmission and a cascade of secondary messengers with neurotrophic and neuroplastic functions, and activation of pathways that increase the synthesis of synaptic proteins.

For example, NMDA blockade by ketamine deactivates eukaryotic elongation factor 2 (eEF2) kinase, resulting in reduced eEF2 phosphorylation and desuppression of translation of brain-derived neurotrophic factor (BDNF), thereby increasing BDNF expression in pyramidal neurons.[3] BDNF plays a key role in mediating antidepressant efficacy to classical antidepressants.[4] That ketamine effects are mediated by BDNF is supported by findings that the antidepressant actions of ketamine are blocked in conditional BDNF knockout mice,[3] and in knockout mice with the BDNF Val66Met allele, which blocks the processing and activity-dependent release of BDNF.[5]

Increased synthesis of synaptic proteins also occurs via regulation of mammalian target of rapamycin complex 1 (mTORC1), in addition to eEF2 kinase. Ketamine rapidly increases the phosphorylation of mTOR and downstream signaling proteins that stimulate synaptic protein synthesis. In contrast, the behavioral actions of ketamine are blocked by rapamycin, a selective inhibitor of mTORC1.[6]

The net effect of these increases in neuroplastic factors and synaptic proteins is rapid increases in the number and function of dendritic spines, which tend to decrease after chronic stress exposure and increase in conditions associated with resilience to such stress.[7] A single dose of ketamine rapidly increases the number and function of dendritic spines in layer V pyramidal neurons in the medial prefrontal cortex (mPFC), and rapidly reverses the synaptic deficits of these neurons caused by 3 weeks of chronic stress exposure.[6,8] Increased levels of synaptic proteins, such as the glutamate AMPA receptor GluA1, were observed 1–4 hours after ketamine administration, consistent with the onset of the therapeutic actions of ketamine.[9] These studies

Major Depressive Disorder. https://doi.org/10.1016/B978-0-323-58131-8.00013-6

demonstrate that ketamine rapidly increases synaptic function in the mPFC, and that this corrects or reverses the synaptic changes associated with chronic stress and depression.[6,8] Ketamine has also been speculated to decrease excitotoxic effects of excessive glutamate by inhibiting extrasynaptic NMDA receptors.[10]

CLINICAL EFFECTS OF KETAMINE

Ketamine is widely used as an anesthetic, particularly in children and in patients with severe injuries due to its relatively favorable safety profile. Administration of ketamine is associated with transient psychotic symptoms of dissociation, hallucinations, and disorientation, as well as transient elevations in blood pressure. Less frequently, genitourinary complications including cystitis have been described and appear to be associated with repeated administration.

The first reports of ketamine's efficacy in the treatment of depression were small, saline-controlled studies with a crossover design. Berman and colleagues (2000) reported that in nine unmedicated depressed subjects (8 MDD, 1 bipolar, current episode depressed) a single administration of intravenous (IV) ketamine 0.5 mg/kg was associated with rapid, robust antidepressant effects compared to saline.[11] Separation in depression scores between the study arms emerged at 6 hours with sustained response through day 3. By contrast, the acute psychotogenic effects of ketamine generally resolved within several hours of infusion. Zarate et al. subsequently reported that in 20 treatment-resistant MDD (TRD) subjects, a single dose of IV ketamine 0.5 mg/kg was associated with a 71% rate of clinical response[1] at 24 hours, with 35% of subjects maintaining response for 1 week. Another study of 27 depressed inpatients receiving 0.54 mg/kg IV ketamine within 30 minutes found significant antidepressant response[2] compared to saline sustained for 1 week.[12]

Early studies of ketamine as an antidepressant were limited by small sample sizes, use of saline as a control, and crossover study design. Murrough and colleagues attempted to address these shortcomings in a larger RCT (73 TRD subjects) with straight randomization and using midazolam as an active control to improve blinding.[13] They reported that the ketamine group had greater improvement in the Montgomery–Åsberg Depression Rating Scale (MADRS) score than the

midazolam group (64% vs. 28% response[3]) 24 hours after treatment. The differences between treatment groups remained statistically significant at day 3 but were no longer significant at day 7. Transient dissociative side effects and blood pressure elevations were greater in subjects receiving ketamine, highlighting the importance of raters at primary outcome blind to infusion side effects, as was done in this study. Overall, midazolam offered superior blinding to saline placebo.

Although previous studies tested ketamine as monotherapy, superior results were also reported for ketamine as an adjuvant to antidepressants. In a study of 30 severely depressed subjects receiving escitalopram, a single IV ketamine (vs. saline) administration was associated with 92.3% versus 57.1% response[4] and 76.9% versus 14.3% remission[5] at 4 weeks.[14] However, data regarding ketamine augmentation of ECT are mixed. Some studies have reported faster initial improvement in subjects receiving ketamine compared to other anesthetics, but these separations were notably transient and did not separate from ECT controls on subsequent evaluations.[15–17] Other studies have reported no advantage for ketamine in ECT.[18,19]

Several studies have also demonstrated rapid, sustained antisuicidal action in depressed patients receiving ketamine,[20–23] raising interest in applications in emergency psychiatric settings.

Given the limitations of IV administration, several investigators have examined alternative routes of ketamine administration in depression. An initial study reported antidepressant efficacy of intranasal ketamine (50 mg), although improvement in depression scores was sustained for only 2 days.[24] A recent large study randomized 67 TRD subjects to 2 weeks of twice weekly intranasal esketamine (the S enantiomer of ketamine) followed by open treatment.[25] All three esketamine doses (28 mg, 56 mg, or 84 mg) were superior to placebo, with a significant ascending dose-response relationship ($p < .001$). Improvement in depressive symptoms appeared to be sustained for more than 2 months despite reduced dosing frequency in the open-label phase.

Others have shown that oral ketamine is well tolerated,[26] as is subcutaneous administration,[27] but these routes of administration are associated with significant variability in the rates of absorption.

---

[1]Defined as 50% or greater reduction in Hamilton Rating Scale for Depression (HRSD) score from baseline.
[2]Defined as 50% or greater reduction in Montgomery–Åsberg Depression Rating Scale (MADRS) score from baseline.

[3]Defined as 50% or greater reduction in MADRS score from baseline.
[4]Defined as 50% or greater reduction in MADRS score from baseline.
[5]Defined as MADRS score of 10 or lower.

Most studies on ketamine in MDD have examined the effects of a single administration of the drug. The effects of repeated administration are less well established. A randomized, placebo-controlled study of repeated IV ketamine treatment twice to thrice weekly showed superiority compared to placebo for up to 4 weeks.[28] Interestingly, subjects receiving twice versus thrice weekly dosing showed similar improvement. Ongoing treatment with ketamine also raises concerns about the potential for development of glutamatergic neurotoxicity. Although several studies support ketamine as a safe, well-tolerated, and sustainable ongoing treatment for depression,[29–34] further research is needed to better characterize ketamine's long-term safety and efficacy in the treatment of depression.

Newport and colleagues conducted a meta-analysis reporting that in studies of primarily MDD patients (though some bipolar depressed patients were included), ketamine was about 10 times as likely to induce response and about 14.5 times as likely to induce remission at 24 hours after administration compared to controls as assessed by Hamilton Rating Scale for Depression (HRSD) or MADRS scores.[35] A separate meta-analysis of eight randomized, controlled studies of ketamine treatment in depressed subjects (including bipolar patients) was conducted by McGirr and colleagues and showed robust antidepressant effects.[36] Similar findings were reported in a Cochrane Review by Caddy and colleagues.[37]

Taken together, these studies make the case for ketamine as a rapid-acting, effective treatment for MDD. Its efficacy in suicidal and treatment-resistant subjects is clinically significant. However, there are important limitations to the current literature on ketamine including relatively smaller study samples, concerns about the integrity of the study blinding, and an incomplete understanding of ketamine's long-term safety.

Ketamine is a racemate consisting of the R-ketamine enantiomer (arketamine) and the S-ketamine enantiomer (esketamine). Esketamine has a higher affinity for the NMDA receptor than arketamine and has been investigated as an IV and intranasal (IN) antidepressant. In a study of 30 subjects with treatment-resistant MDD, administration of IV esketamine resulted in rapid, robust improvement in depression scores that did not appear to differ by dose (0.2 mg/kg vs. 0.4 mg/kg).[38] As described earlier, a phase 2 study of IN ketamine in outpatients with treatment-resistant MDD showed good efficacy with an ascending dose-response relationship (28 mg, 56 mg, 84 mg).[25] In some preclinical studies, however, arketamine is associated with longer lasting antidepressant-like effects and with greater neuroplasticity changes than esketamine.[39,40] It is not yet clear if either of the two enantiomers is superior to racemic ketamine.

BEYOND KETAMINE: OTHER GLUTAMATERGIC MODULATORS AS NOVEL ANTIDEPRESSANTS

Several other glutamatergic agents have been studied in humans as putative novel antidepressants. D-cycloserine's antidepressant properties were first observed in the 1950s when it was used as an antibiotic in the treatment of tuberculosis.[1] D-cycloserine is a partial agonist at the NMDA receptor glycine binding site where it acts as a functional NMDAR agonist at doses up to 250 mg/day and as an NMDAR antagonist at doses greater than 500 mg/day.[41,42] In the modern era, a study of 26 treatment-resistant MDD subjects receiving 6 weeks of high-dose (1000 mg/d) D-cycloserine demonstrated a 54% response rate as assessed by HRSD score.[43] As expected, an earlier study examining use of lower dose D-cycloserine (250 mg/d) as an adjuvant agent in treatment-resistant MDD subjects did not demonstrate antidepressant efficacy.[44]

GLYX-13 (rapastinel) is an amidated tetrapeptide (Thr-Pro-Pro-Thr-NH_2) currently in phase 2 testing for treatment of depression. GLYX-13 acts as a functional partial agonist (mixed antagonist/agonist) of the allosteric glycine site of the NMDA receptor. In a study of 116 subjects with MDD who had failed treatment with at least one standard (monoamine) antidepressant, a single dose of GLYX-13 was reported to rapidly reduce depressive symptoms with sustained effect for an average of 7 days.[45]

CERC-301 (MK-0657 or Rislenemdaz) is an NMDA NR2B subunit antagonist. A small crossover pilot study in which five subjects with treatment-resistant MDD received oral CERC-301 showed improvement in depression scores on the HRSD and Beck Depression Inventory, though the primary study outcome of MADRS score did not demonstrate significant effects.[46] Investigation of another NMDA NR2B antagonist, CP-101,606, suggested that it may have antidepressant effects,[47] but its development was discontinued after it was found to cause abnormalities of cardiac conduction.

Nitrous oxide (N_2O), commonly used as an inhalational anesthetic, acts as an NMDA receptor antagonist. In a proof-of-concept trial of 20 subjects with TRD, inhalational nitrous oxide (50% N_2O/50% O_2) showed rapid and robust antidepressant effect compared to placebo and had relatively good tolerability.[48]

Dextromethorphan (DXM), commonly used as an over-the-counter antitussive, acts as an antagonist at the NMDA receptor when administered at higher doses. Combination with quinidine serves to delay DXM metabolism and prolong its effects on the NMDAR. There is ongoing investigation into the potential role of DXM-containing compounds in the treatment of depression, for example, Nuedexta (DXM/quinidine), which is FDA-approved for treatment of pseudobulbar affect, and AVP-786 (deuterated DXM/quinidine). An initial pilot study of DXM/quinidine in 20 TRD subjects suggested potential antidepressant effect.[49] Another ongoing study is evaluating the combination of DXM with bupropion (NCT02741791).

It is less clear that agents active at metabotropic glutamate receptors can have antidepressant effects. Basimglurant is a negative allosteric modulator of the postsynaptic metabotropic glutamate subtype 5 (mGluR5) receptor. In a phase 2 study of 333 subjects with MDD with inadequate response to an SSRI or SNRI, oral basimglurant was administered at 0.5 or 1.5 mg daily in addition to ongoing antidepressant treatment. Outcomes for those receiving 0.5 mg daily administration were not found to differ significantly from placebo, though patient-rated measures improved with 1.5 mg daily administration.[50]

The recent advances in psychiatric drug development raise many possibilities (and many questions) about the future of antidepressants, which have traditionally targeted abnormalities of monoamine neurotransmission. Data from molecular, genetic, and imaging studies demonstrate abnormalities of the glutamatergic system in subjects with MDD. Ketamine acts as a glutamate receptor antagonist, initial studies of which have demonstrated rapid, robust antidepressant effects and a relatively favorable safety profile. Ketamine's efficacy in the treatment of depression adds support to the hypothesis of glutamatergic abnormalities and has paved the way for the development of other novel glutamatergic agents. Although more research is needed to further characterize the benefits and drawbacks of glutamatergic modulators, these agents may signal a new era of pharmacotherapy in the treatment of depression, particularly for patients who have failed to respond to traditional antidepressants or emergently require rapid clinical improvement.

REFERENCES

1. Crane GE. Cyloserine as an antidepressant agent. *Am J Psychiatry*. 1959;115(11):1025–1026. https://doi.org/10.1176/ajp.115.11.1025. Epub 1959/05/01. PubMed PMID: 13637281.

2. Trullas R, Skolnick P. Functional antagonists at the NMDA receptor complex exhibit antidepressant actions. *Eur J Pharmacol*. 1990;185(1):1–10. Epub 1990/08/21. Pub Med PMID: 2171955.

3. Autry AE, Adachi M, Nosyreva E, et al. NMDA receptor blockade at rest triggers rapid behavioural antidepressant responses. *Nature*. 2011;475(7354):91–95. https://doi.org/10.1038/nature10130. Epub 2011/06/17. PubMed PMID: 21677641; PMCID: PMC3172695.

4. Monteggia LM, Barrot M, Powell CM, et al. Essential role of brain-derived neurotrophic factor in adult hippocampal function. *Proc Natl Acad Sci U S A*. 2004;101(29):10827–10832. https://doi.org/10.1073/pnas.0402141101. Epub 2004/07/14. PubMed PMID: 15249684; PMCID: PMC490019.

5. Liu RJ, Lee FS, Li XY, Bambico F, Duman RS, Aghajanian GK. Brain-derived neurotrophic factor Val66Met allele impairs basal and ketamine-stimulated synaptogenesis in prefrontal cortex. *Biol Psychiatry*. 2012;71(11):996–1005. https://doi.org/10.1016/j.biopsych.2011.09.030. Epub 2011/11/01. PubMed PMID: 22036038; PMCID: PMC3290730.

6. Li N, Lee B, Liu RJ, et al. mTOR-Dependent synapse formation underlies the rapid antidepressant effects of NMDA antagonists. *Science*. 2010;329(5994):959–964. https://doi.org/10.1126/science.1190287. Epub 2010/08/21. PubMed PMID: 20724638; PMCID: PMC3116441.

7. McEwen BS, Eiland L, Hunter RG, Miller MM. Stress and anxiety: structural plasticity and epigenetic regulation as a consequence of stress. *Neuropharmacology*. 2012;62(1):3–12. https://doi.org/10.1016/j.neuropharm.2011.07.014. Epub 2011/08/03. PubMed PMID: 21807003; PMCID: PMC3196296.

8. Li N, Liu RJ, Dwyer JM, et al. Glutamate N-methyl-D-aspartate receptor antagonists rapidly reverse behavioral and synaptic deficits caused by chronic stress exposure. *Biol Psychiatry*. 2011;69(8):754–761. https://doi.org/10.1016/j.biopsych.2010.12.015. Epub 2011/02/05. PubMed PMID: 21292242; PMCID: PMC3068225.

9. Zhang K, Yamaki VN, Wei Z, Zheng Y, Cai X. Differential regulation of GluA1 expression by ketamine and memantine. *Behav Brain Res*. 2017;316:152–159. https://doi.org/10.1016/j.bbr.2016.09.002. Epub 2016/09/08. PubMed PMID: 27599619.

10. Murrough JW, Abdallah CG, Mathew SJ. Targeting glutamate signalling in depression: progress and prospects. *Nat Rev Drug Discov*. 2017;16(7):472–486. https://doi.org/10.1038/nrd.2017.16. Epub 2017/03/18. PubMed PMID: 28303025.

11. Berman RM, Cappiello A, Anand A, et al. Antidepressant effects of ketamine in depressed patients. *Biol Psychiatry*. 2000;47(4):351–354. PubMed PMID: 10686270.

12. Sos P, Klirova M, Novak T, Kohutova B, Horacek J, Palenicek T. Relationship of ketamine's antidepressant and psychotomimetic effects in unipolar depression. *Neuroendocrinol Lett*. 2013;34(4):287–293. PubMed PMID: 23803871.

13. Murrough JW, Iosifescu DV, Chang LC, et al. Antidepressant efficacy of ketamine in treatment-resistant major depression: a two-site randomized controlled trial. *Am J Psychiatry*. 2013;170(10):1134−1142. https://doi.org/10.1176/appi.ajp.2013.13030392. PubMed PMID: 23982301; PMCID: PMC3992936.

14. Hu YD, Xiang YT, Fang JX, et al. Single i.v. ketamine augmentation of newly initiated escitalopram for major depression: results from a randomized, placebo-controlled 4-week study. *Psychol Med*. 2016;46(3):623−635. https://doi.org/10.1017/S00332917150021 59. PubMed PMID: 26478208.

15. Wang X, Chen Y, Zhou X, Liu F, Zhang T, Zhang C. Effects of propofol and ketamine as combined anesthesia for electroconvulsive therapy in patients with depressive disorder. *J ECT*. 2012;28(2):128−132. https://doi.org/10.1097/YCT.0b013e31824d1d02. Epub 2012/05/25. PubMed PMID: 22622291.

16. Yoosefi A, Sepehri AS, Kargar M, et al. Comparing effects of ketamine and thiopental administration during electroconvulsive therapy in patients with major depressive disorder: a randomized, double-blind study. *J ECT*. 2014;30(1):15−21. https://doi.org/10.1097/YCT.0b013e3182a4b4c6. Epub 2013/10/05. PubMed PMID: 24091902.

17. Okamoto N, Nakai T, Sakamoto K, Nagafusa Y, Higuchi T, Nishikawa T. Rapid antidepressant effect of ketamine anesthesia during electroconvulsive therapy of treatment-resistant depression: comparing ketamine and propofol anesthesia. *J ECT*. 2010;26(3):223−227. https://doi.org/10.1097/YCT.0b013e3181c3b0aa. Epub 2009/11/26. PubMed PMID: 19935085.

18. Jarventausta K, Chrapek W, Kampman O, et al. Effects of S-ketamine as an anesthetic adjuvant to propofol on treatment response to electroconvulsive therapy in treatment-resistant depression: a randomized pilot study. *J ECT*. 2013;29(3):158−161. https://doi.org/10.1097/YCT.0b013e318283b7e9. Epub 2013/03/12. PubMed PMID: 23475029.

19. Abdallah CG, Fasula M, Kelmendi B, Sanacora G, Ostroff R. Rapid antidepressant effect of ketamine in the electroconvulsive therapy setting. *J ECT*. 2012;28(3):157−161. https://doi.org/10.1097/YCT.0b013e31824f8 296. Epub 2012/08/01. PubMed PMID: 22847373; PMCID: PMC3426617.

20. Price RB, Nock MK, Charney DS, Mathew SJ. Effects of intravenous ketamine on explicit and implicit measures of suicidality in treatment-resistant depression. *Biol Psychiatry*. 2009;66(5):522−526. https://doi.org/10.1016/j.biopsych.2009.04.029. Epub 2009/06/24. PubMed PMID: 19545857; PMCID: PMC2935847.

21. Price RB, Iosifescu DV, Murrough JW, et al. Effects of ketamine on explicit and implicit suicidal cognition: a randomized controlled trial in treatment-resistant depression. *Depress Anxiety*. 2014;31(4):335−343. https://doi.org/10.1002/da.22253. Epub 2014/03/29. PubMed PMID: 24668760; PMCID: PMC4112410.

22. Ballard ED, Ionescu DF, Vande Voort JL, et al. Improvement in suicidal ideation after ketamine infusion: relationship to reductions in depression and anxiety. *J Psychiatr Res*. 2014;58:161−166. https://doi.org/10.jpsychires.2014.07.027. Epub 2014/08/30. PubMed PMID: 25169854; PMCID: PMC4163501.

23. Murrough JW, Soleimani L, DeWilde KE, et al. Ketamine for rapid reduction of suicidal ideation: a randomized controlled trial. *Psychol Med*. 2015;45(16):3571−3580. https://doi.org/10.1017/S0033291715001506. Epub 2015/08/13. PubMed PMID: 26266877.

24. Lapidus KA, Levitch CF, Perez AM, et al. A randomized controlled trial of intranasal ketamine in major depressive disorder. *Biol Psychiatry*. 2014;76(12):970−976. https://doi.org/10.1016/j.biopsych.2014.03.026. PubMed PMID: 24821196; PMCID: PMC4185009.

25. Daly EJ, Singh JB, Fedgchin M, et al. Efficacy and safety of intranasal esketamine adjunctive to oral antidepressant therapy in treatment-resistant depression: a randomized clinical trial. *JAMA Psychiatry*. 2018;75(2):139−148. https://doi.org/10.1001/jamapsychiatry.2017.3739. Epub 2017/12/29. PubMed PMID: 29282469.

26. Schoevers RA, Chaves TV, Balukova SM, Rot MA, Kortekaas R. Oral ketamine for the treatment of pain and treatment-resistant depression. *Br J Psychiatry*. 2016;208(2):108−113. https://doi.org/10.1192/bjp.bp.115.165498. Epub 2016/02/03. PubMed PMID: 26834167.

27. Loo CK, Galvez V, O'Keefe E, et al. Placebo-controlled pilot trial testing dose titration and intravenous, intramuscular and subcutaneous routes for ketamine in depression. *Acta Psychiatr Scand*. 2016;134(1):48−56. https://doi.org/10.1111/acps.12572. Epub 2016/03/31. PubMed PMID: 27028832.

28. Singh JB, Fedgchin M, Daly EJ, et al. A double-blind, randomized, placebo-controlled, dose-frequency study of intravenous ketamine in patients with treatment-resistant depression. *Am J Psychiatry*. 2016;173(8):816−826. https://doi.org/10.1176/appi.ajp.2016.16010037. PubMed PMID: 27056608.

29. aan het Rot M, Collins KA, Murrough JW, et al. Safety and efficacy of repeated-dose intravenous ketamine for treatment-resistant depression. *Biol Psychiatry*. 2010;67(2):139−145. https://doi.org/10.1016/j.biopsych.2009.08.038. Epub 2009/11/10. PubMed PMID: 19897179.

30. Murrough JW, Perez AM, Pillemer S, et al. Rapid and longer-term antidepressant effects of repeated ketamine infusions in treatment-resistant major depression. *Biol Psychiatry*. 2013;74(4):250−256. https://doi.org/10.1016/j.biopsych.2012.06.022. Epub 2012/07/31. PubMed PMID: 22840761; PMCID: PMC3725185.

31. Shiroma PR, Johns B, Kuskowski M, et al. Augmentation of response and remission to serial intravenous subanesthetic ketamine in treatment resistant depression. *J Affect Disord*. 2014;155:123−129. https://doi.org/10.1016/j.jad.2013.10.036. Epub 2013/11/26. PubMed PMID: 24268616.

32. Rasmussen KG, Lineberry TW, Galardy CW, et al. Serial infusions of low-dose ketamine for major depression. *J Psychopharmacol*. 2013;27(5):444−450. https://doi.org/10.1177/0269881113478283. Epub 2013/02/23. PubMed PMID: 23428794.

33. Segmiller F, Ruther T, Linhardt A, et al. Repeated S-ketamine infusions in therapy resistant depression: a case series. *J Clin Pharmacol*. 2013;53(9):996–998. https://doi.org/10.1002/jcph.122. Epub 2013/07/31. PubMed PMID: 23893490.

34. Cusin C, Ionescu DF, Pavone KJ, et al. Ketamine augmentation for outpatients with treatment-resistant depression: preliminary evidence for two-step intravenous dose escalation. *Aust N Z J Psychiatr*. 2017;51(1):55–64. https://doi.org/10.1177/0004867416631828. Epub 2016/02/20. PubMed PMID: 26893373.

35. Newport DJ, Carpenter LL, McDonald WM, Potash JB, Tohen M, Nemeroff CB, Biomarkers APACoRTFoN, treatments. Ketamine and other NMDA antagonists: early clinical trials and possible mechanisms in depression. *Am J Psychiatry*. 2015;172(10):950–966. https://doi.org/10.1176/appi.ajp.2015.15040465. Epub 2015/10/02. PubMed PMID: 26423481.

36. McGirr A, Berlim MT, Bond DJ, Fleck MP, Yatham LN, Lam RW. A systematic review and meta-analysis of randomized, double-blind, placebo-controlled trials of ketamine in the rapid treatment of major depressive episodes. *Psychol Med*. 2015;45(4):693–704. https://doi.org/10.1017/S0033291714001603. Epub 2014/07/11. PubMed PMID: 25010396.

37. Caddy C, Amit BH, McCloud TL, et al. Ketamine and other glutamate receptor modulators for depression in adults. *Cochrane Database Syst Rev*. 2015;9:CD011612. https://doi.org/10.1002/14651858.CD011612.pub2. Epub 2015/09/24. PubMed PMID: 26395901.

38. Singh JB, Fedgchin M, Daly E, et al. Intravenous esketamine in adult treatment-resistant depression: a double-blind, double-randomization, placebo-controlled study. *Biol Psychiatry*. 2016;80(6):424–431. https://doi.org/10.1016/j.biopsych.2015.10.018. Epub 2015/12/29. PubMed PMID: 26707087.

39. Fukumoto K, Toki H, Iijima M, et al. Antidepressant potential of (R)-Ketamine in rodent models: comparison with (S)-Ketamine. *J Pharmacol Exp Ther*. 2017;361(1):9–16. https://doi.org/10.1124/jpet.116.239228. Epub 2017/01/25. PubMed PMID: 28115553.

40. Yang C, Shirayama Y, Zhang JC, et al. A rapid-onset and sustained antidepressant without psychotomimetic side effects. *Transl Psychiatry*. 2015;5:e632. https://doi.org/10.1038/tp.2015.136. Epub 2015/09/04. PubMed PMID: 26327690; PMCID: PMC5068814.

41. Hood WF, Compton RP, Monahan JB. D-cycloserine: a ligand for the N-methyl-D-aspartate coupled glycine receptor has partial agonist characteristics. *Neurosci Lett*. 1989;98(1):91–95. Epub 1989/03/13. PubMed PMID: 2540460.

42. Emmett MR, Mick SJ, Cler JA, Rao TS, Iyengar S, Wood PL. Actions of D-cycloserine at the N-methyl-D-aspartate-associated glycine receptor site in vivo. *Neuropharmacology*. 1991;30(11):1167–1171. Epub 1991/11/01. PubMed PMID: 1663594.

43. Heresco-Levy U, Gelfin G, Bloch B, et al. A randomized add-on trial of high-dose D-cycloserine for treatment-resistant depression. *Int J Neuropsychopharmacol*. 2013; 16(3):501–506. https://doi.org/10.1017/S146115712000910. Epub 2012/11/24. PubMed PMID: 23174090.

44. Heresco-Levy U, Javitt DC, Gelfin Y, et al. Controlled trial of D-cycloserine adjuvant therapy for treatment-resistant major depressive disorder. *J Affect Disord*. 2006;93(1–3): 239–243. https://doi.org/10.1016/j.jad.2006.03.004. Epub 2006/05/09. PubMed PMID: 16677714.

45. Preskorn S, Macaluso M, Mehra DO, et al. Randomized proof of concept trial of GLYX-13, an N-methyl-D-aspartate receptor glycine site partial agonist, in major depressive disorder nonresponsive to a previous antidepressant agent. *J Psychiatr Pract*. 2015;21(2):140–149. https://doi.org/10.1097/01.pra.0000462606.17725.93. Epub 2015/03/19. PubMed PMID: 25782764.

46. Ibrahim L, Diaz Granados N, Jolkovsky L, et al. A randomized, placebo-controlled, crossover pilot trial of the oral selective NR2B antagonist MK-0657 in patients with treatment-resistant major depressive disorder. *J Clin Psychopharmacol*. 2012;32(4):551–557. https://doi.org/10.1097/JCP.0b013e31825d70d6. Epub 2012/06/23. PubMed PMID: 22722512; PMCID: PMC3438886.

47. Preskorn SH, Baker B, Kolluri S, Menniti FS, Krams M, Landen JW. An innovative design to establish proof of concept of the antidepressant effects of the NR2B subunit selective N-methyl-D-aspartate antagonist, CP-101,606, in patients with treatment-refractory major depressive disorder. *J Clin Psychopharmacol*. 2008;28(6):631–637. https://doi.org/10.1097/JCP.0b013e31818a6cea. Epub 2008/11/18. PubMed PMID: 19011431.

48. Nagele P, Duma A, Kopec M, et al. Nitrous oxide for treatment-resistant major depression: a proof-of-concept trial. *Biol Psychiatry*. 2015;78(1):10–18. https://doi.org/10.1016/j.biopsych.2014.11.016. Epub 2015/01/13. PubMed PMID: 25577164.

49. Murrough JW, Wade E, Sayed S, et al. Dextromethorphan/quinidine pharmacotherapy in patients with treatment resistant depression: a proof of concept clinical trial. *J Affect Disord*. 2017;218:277–283. https://doi.org/10.1016/j.jad.2017.04.072. Epub 2017/05/10. PubMed PMID: 28478356.

50. Quiroz JA, Tamburri P, Deptula D, et al. Efficacy and safety of basimglurant as adjunctive therapy for major depression: a randomized clinical trial. *JAMA Psychiatry*. 2016;73(7):675–684. https://doi.org/10.1001/jamapsychiatry2016.0838. Epub 2016/06/16. PubMed PMID: 27304433.

CHAPTER 14

Depression in Children and Adolescents

JUSTIN N. CHEE, PHD(C), MSC, HONBSC • KAREN WANG, MD, MED, FRCP(C) •
AMY CHEUNG, MD, MSC, FRCP(C)

DEPRESSION IN CHILDREN AND ADOLESCENTS

Case Vignette

Macy is a 16-year-old female who was identified as gifted since she was 10 years old. She has previously done very well in school, maintaining high marks in all her subject areas. However, over the past year, she began isolating herself in her room and spending most mornings fighting with her mother, as she does not want to go to school. She recently ended a relationship with her boyfriend and spent most nights crying herself to sleep, thinking of all the horrible things she said to him.

Her parents became concerned as she began to articulate feeling very hopeless and not wanting to live anymore. They sought assistance from a mental health professional who diagnosed her with major depressive disorder. She was prescribed one of the selective serotonin reuptake inhibitors, and over the course of the subsequent 3 months, continued to report a moderately low mood and difficulties with appetite and motivation.

Her psychiatrist referred her for cognitive behavioral therapy, and she met with a therapist once a week for 12 weeks. Together, they were able to identify some of the problematic thoughts that she continued to hold on to regarding her previous relationship, including self-criticism and an excessive need for reassurance and approval.

With the support of her therapist, Macy slowly began to build up a new social network and also developed steps to improve her eating and activity levels. Macy also received school accommodations to enable her more time to complete assignments. By the end of the 6 months of treatment, Macy was able to complete her school year feeling better and was even contemplating obtaining a summer job.

Children and adolescents with depression often present with a diverse range of symptoms that can be easily recognized by the untrained eye. For a skilled clinician, however, being able to distinguish these indicators from ordinary characteristics may lead to a formal diagnosis, with appropriate clinical criteria and instruments to facilitate the process. Common presentations of depression may include: low or persistently sad mood; decreased interest or pleasure in almost all activities; increased irritability, agitation, or worry; boredom; decreased energy and goal-directed activities; weight loss or weight gain; difficulty with sleep; withdrawn or isolative behavior; poor concentration and memory; somatic complaints (e.g., headaches, stomach aches); feelings of worthlessness; self-harming behavior; suicidal thinking or gestures; and an impairment with respect to social relationships, school work, and family life. Subsyndromal symptoms may also impact functioning and contribute to the development of other mental health disorders. Nevertheless, in spite of the many signs of depression, major depression continues to be both underidentified and undertreated in primary care settings. This is counterintuitive, given that awareness of depressive disorders and their impact on those affected appears to be increasing, particularly in developed countries.

The prevalence and onset of depression have been examined in several research studies so far. According to this literature, lifetime prevalence rates of depressive disorders are estimated to be between 15% and 20%.[1,2] Although depressive disorders are commonly observed in children, they are typically more prevalent among adolescents. A meta-analysis of 26 studies, for example, revealed that the prevalence of depressive disorders was 2.8% for children under age 13, but 5.6% for patients between 13 and 18 years old.[3] Furthermore, according to retrospective studies of adults with depression, its onset was reported to have first occurred between mid-to-late adolescence and young adulthood. Approximately 25% of adults with major depression or persistent depressive disorder, in particular, disclosed

Major Depressive Disorder. https://doi.org/10.1016/B978-0-323-58131-8.00014-8

that the onset of symptoms occurred before young adulthood. In fact, the early expression of core features of depression also appeared to increase the likelihood of these individuals meeting the criteria for major depressive disorder in later years. As a result, depression has been recognized as one of the most common mental illnesses affecting children and adolescents, and it has significant long-term sequelae (e.g., suicide) that these young people are forced to confront as they progress into adulthood.

Another factor that has to be taken into consideration when examining the onset of depression, and how it manifests in children and adolescents, is sex-related differences. Before the onset of puberty, there is an equal prevalence of depression among boys and girls. However, once puberty begins, girls are shown to be at a higher risk of developing depression than their male counterparts. Several theories have been postulated to explain this gender imbalance, including the hypothesis that girls are more likely to experience negative events in life and exhibit more cognitive vulnerability, such as a negative ruminative style and negative cognitions.[4-6] Furthermore, in comparison to girls, boys with depression are far more likely to exhibit a sad mood, fatigue, and problems with concentration.[7] Therefore, the sex of the child or adolescent must be considered when diagnosing and treating him or her for depression.

In addition, the median duration of an episode of depression as well as its rate of relapse is important to consider when assessing or treating patients with this disorder. Research indicates that, in clinical samples, the median duration of an episode among children or adolescents is 7−9 months. In addition, the relapse rate was found to be considerable (i.e., at approximately 60%), particularly among those who present with an early onset of depression. This is especially troubling, given that depressed patients exhibit higher rates of impaired functioning, substance abuse, suicide attempts, and psychiatric hospitalizations.[8] The likelihood of relapse is further increased by the presence of co-occurring anxiety disorders.[9] As a result, these findings suggest that establishing treatment plans that sufficiently span a depressive episode and providing early treatment for this disorder in younger patients may have positive long-term consequences.

In this chapter, we examine the assessment and diagnosis of depressive disorders, as well as best practices for their treatment approaches and the initial and ongoing management techniques employed by clinicians. This overview is a culmination of both existing literature and expert opinion on these topics, and we provide additional resources for those interested to explore with respect to issues that fall outside the scope of this book.

Assessment and Diagnosis

The assessment and diagnosis of depression in children and adolescents most commonly involves conducting a comprehensive interview, which may additionally involve using or supplementing it with validated instruments, clinical diagnostic criteria, physical examinations, laboratory evaluations, and an analysis of co-occurring psychiatric diagnoses. In the first place, the interview process will often necessitate participation by, not only the patient, but also his or her parents or primary caregivers. As well, engaging third parties, such as schools, external agencies (e.g., child protection agencies), and previous health care professionals or therapists, will be necessary to obtain collateral information. During the interview itself, obtaining key information from the patient directly can be augmented by establishing a solid rapport with the child or adolescent. Toward that goal, it is often beneficial to validate and normalize their concerns, which goes a long way to allay those concerns.

In addition, the interview provides a means by which the clinician can assess the patient for changes to mood, sleep, energy, appetite, focus/concentration, daily functioning, academic functioning, social relationships, and suicidality, all of which are important factors in arriving at an appropriate diagnosis of major depression. In obtaining the patient's mental health history, details regarding the onset of the depressive episode and possible precipitants for depression should be examined carefully. There may be particular temperamental or personality features (e.g., borderline personality traits), medical comorbidities (e.g., diabetes, epilepsy) and intellectual or learning challenges that increase the likelihood for depressive episodes. Ongoing school difficulties, bullying, trauma, substance use, and interpersonal conflict may also perpetuate depressive symptoms and perpetuate a loss of functioning. Understanding protective factors, such as parental warmth/understanding, low levels of environmental stress, and access to supportive relationships, would also help to guide decisions regarding treatment and improve prognosis.

There are several tools available to clinicians seeking to assess and diagnose depression among children and adolescents. First, a validated instrument should always be utilized during the initial assessment period as well as regularly throughout treatment to facilitate the screening, evaluation, and monitoring of depressive symptoms. Examples of such instruments, which have high specificity and sensitivity, include the Beck Depression Inventory (BDI I or BDI I—II) and the Patient Health Questionnaire modified for Adolescents (PHQ-A). Furthermore, diagnosing depression in children and adolescents should be based primarily on the DSM-5 criteria[10] for major depressive disorder. Lastly, the screening process may also include a physical examination and appropriate laboratory investigations. Although arriving at a diagnosis using these tools alone is not recommended, they still serve as an important complement to the clinical interview.

The last important consideration we will examine in the assessment and diagnosis of depressive disorders is the impact of comorbid conditions. As depression often co-occurs with other psychiatric diagnoses, it would be important to screen for those other disorders as well. Of particular concern are anxiety, eating disorders, substance use, learning disorders, and behavioral disorders (e.g., oppositional defiant disorder). In light of this, it is not surprising that children and adolescents may meet the criteria for a number of different depressive disorders, including major depression, persistent depressive disorder (formerly known as dysthymia), and adjustment disorder with depressed mood. In fact, a portion of adolescents who present with major depression are later discovered to have had bipolar disorder. Therefore, a careful assessment of the patient's periods of elevated mood, grandiosity, decreased need for sleep, heightened distractibility, and increased risky behavior would need to be ascertained.

Initial Management
Clinicians are first tasked with providing the initial management of depression to a patient once he or she has been identified as presenting with depressive symptoms. There are several components to initial management including active monitoring, psychoeducation, safety planning, and referral for peer support.

Active monitoring
The individualized treatment regimen that is developed for a patient varies depending on the suspected severity of depression under observation, as does the utilization of active monitoring in the process. For example, in cases where a child or adolescent presents with mild depressive symptoms without any complicating factor (e.g., trauma, family history, comorbid illnesses or previous history of mood disorders, etc.), clinicians may consider a period of active monitoring without initiating treatment. In other cases, when the severity of depression being monitored is higher, research from

randomized controlled trials revealed that brief psychosocial interventions, including symptom monitoring, psychoeducation, and supportive therapy, can result in the resolution of symptoms.[11] We will now examine a couple of these interventions, which have been proven to be effective: psychoeducation and peer support.

Psychoeducation
Psychoeducation is critical to patients and their families in order for them to better understand mental illness. As many children and adolescents struggle with depressive symptoms for weeks, months, or even years before being identified, providing them with information about the chronic and recurrent nature of their illness and the benefit of treatment is imperative. It improves adherence with the treatment course and reduces the risk of relapse or recurrence.

Critical components of psychoeducation include (1) peer support for patients and caregivers and (2) safety planning. A recent systematic review of randomized controlled trials, conducted by Bevan Jones et al.[12] identified 15 psychoeducational interventions (PI) and found that they can play a role in preventing and managing adolescent depression as a first-line or adjunct therapy. Examples of types of PI interventions include Family PI (e.g., focusing on parental depression, psychosocial stress, etc.); Simple Low-Intensity PI (e.g., focusing on lifestyle psychoeducation on such topics as physical activity, sleep and substance use, etc.); and Computerized/Online PI (e.g., games with cognitive behavioral therapy content, modules on problem solving, conflict resolution, etc.). Although the evidence base on the effectiveness of these interventions is limited, they have been demonstrating promising results. Positive effects on a wide range of mental health and wellbeing outcomes have been observed (e.g., reduced depressive symptoms, psychosocial stress, etc.). Furthermore, Dardas et al.[13] completed a systematic review examining the role of parental involvement in the effectiveness of depression interventions among adolescents. They identified 16 randomized controlled trials on the topic and found that health outcomes appeared dependent on the nature of how the parents were involved in interventions. Specifically, the more effective interventions were those that facilitated interactions between adolescents and their parents and in which the parents played an integral role.

Patients and their families need to know about the common signs and symptoms of depression, the impact of depression on functioning, and the need to adjust to the "sick role." Symptoms such as mood reactivity, where a patient with depression can appear bright when he/she is in a social setting, can cause confusion for doctors and caregivers alike, need to be discussed. Patients and families may also not understand how normal activities, such as school attendance or involvement of sporting activities, can be impacted by the symptoms of depression (e.g., distractibility and loss of energy). A discussion about the common endorsement of hopelessness and thoughts of death is also critical, as patients may not have shared these with their caregivers. This will naturally lead to a discussion about suicide prevention and safety planning (see side box below). Furthermore, those who are struggling with academics will need support from the clinician on obtaining accommodations for school work. Table 14.1 outlines common accommodations that can be helpful to children and adolescents with depression.

Side Box: Suicidality and Safety Planning

Thoughts of death and suicide are common among teenagers, and especially common among teenagers with depression. Although few will follow through with these thoughts, clinicians must still be vigilant about the risk of suicide in patients. Although patients are being treated for depression, clinicians have to develop **safety plans** with patients and their caregivers. Caregivers should safety proof the home environment, including securing or removing lethal means, such as firearms, knives, ropes/cables/belts, and medications. Clinicians, along with patients and caregivers, should also develop a **crisis plan**. This will include a list of individuals who patients can contact if they are feeling upset or suicidal, for example: family members, friends, or other adults, such as coaches or teachers. As an alternative, some children and adolescents may choose to contact crisis centers or helplines. A final option would be for them to go directly to the emergency room of the nearest hospital. Suicide contracts, which have been previously popular in clinical practice, have been shown to be ineffective in preventing suicide.

Peer support

Peer support is another important intervention that is commonly used in the initial management of depression for children and adolescents. It is important to recognize that the journey to recovery can be difficult for both patients and their caregivers. As a result, children or adolescents struggling with depression may benefit from the support of peers with lived experience as they recover from their illness. Similarly, caregivers may also benefit from peer support. Many advocacy organizations in Canada, the United States, and Australia, as well as healthcare institutions, now provide peer support to patients and caregivers. This is reflective of the vital role that peer support plays in the initial management of depression.

Treatment

The next stage in the clinical management of depression is the treatment phase. Effective treatments for child and adolescent depression include psychotherapy and medication, both of which we will examine in subsequent sections.

Psychotherapy

The efficacy of psychotherapy for the treatment of depression in children and adolescents has been effectively demonstrated in numerous studies as well as in high-quality quantitative and qualitative syntheses of the literature (i.e., meta-analyses and narrative reviews respectively). For childhood depression, cognitive behavioral therapy or CBT has been demonstrated to be effective. For depression in adolescents, both CBT and interpersonal therapy for adolescents (IPT-A) are well-supported evidence-based treatments.

Interpersonal therapy for adolescents. IPT-A is a time-limited therapy that has strong empirical support. It is based on the premise that the current depressive symptoms are affected by interpersonal relationships and vice versa. Consequently, to improve a patient's mood, the therapy targets improvements in interpersonal relationships. Key components of IPT-A include identifying a focus for therapy (e.g., grief, interpersonal conflicts, major life transitions, etc.), enhancing interpersonal problem-solving skills, and modifying communication patterns.

Although initially developed for the treatment of depression in adult populations, Mufson and colleagues successfully adapted this approach for use in adolescents.[14] In their seminal study, a randomized controlled trial was conducted in which 48 adolescents between 12 and 18 years old were randomly assigned to treatment groups for major depressive disorder (DSM–III–R) involving 12 weeks of either IPT-A or standard clinical monitoring. Greater reductions in depressive symptoms and improvements to overall social functioning were observed in those who received treatment with IPT-A. The approach has since been demonstrated to be effective when delivered in both individual and group. Positive outcomes have also been demonstrated compared to treatment as usual in a more recent clinical trial in which IPT-A was administered in a real-world setting (e.g., school-based mental health clinics[15]).

Cognitive behavioral therapy. CBT is an evidence-based treatment for depression in children and

TABLE 14.1
Classroom and Examination Accommodations.

My Illness or Medication Causes Problems With:		Possible Accommodations[29]
CLASSROOM ACCOMMODATIONS		
Concentration, keeping focused, processing information, organizing my thoughts, dealing with social situations	*Peer note-taker/Lecture notes from the professor* *Taping the lecture*	A formal arrangement where someone in the class takes notes for you. You still have to attend class, but it may help to reduce your anxiety and allow you to participate more in class. This can supplement your own note-taking and reduce the pressure of having to capture all the information. If you use a digital recorder, the software will allow you to download the lecture to your computer for easy access. You will need to get the permission of your teacher before taping.
	Preferential seating	You can arrange to sit in the front of the classroom and away from windows to help to reduce audio and visual distractions.
	Note-taking technology	Laptops, personal digital assistants (PDAs) with folding keyboards or small word-processing keyboards such as *AlphaSmart* (www.alphasmart.com/products/as3000_overview.html) or *Dana* (www.alphasmart.com/products/dana_overview.html) are an option if you find taking notes using a keyboard easier than handwriting.
Anxiety/low stress tolerance	*Reduced course load—but still remain registered as full-time student* *More frequent breaks*	You can arrange to step out of class when you need to move around to relieve stress, anxiety or restlessness.
	Exempt from group work *Exempt from presentations—option to present to professor alone*	
Missing or not participating in class	*Not graded for participation*	
EXAMINATION ACCOMMODATIONS		
Concentration, keeping focused, processing information, dealing with social situations	*Preferential seating*	You can arrange to sit in the front of the exam room and away from windows to help reduce audio and visual distractions.
Anxiety	*Quiet location or separate room for exam*	It may be possible to write an exam in a separate room with only a few students on your own in a supervised area.
	Supervised breaks during exam	You can arrange to step out of the exam when you need to move around to relieve stress, anxiety, or restlessness.
	Changes to scheduled exam dates	Arrangements can be made to write tests on different dates if you have several taking place in close succession.
Fatigue, concentration	*Extended times for exams*	You may be able to arrange for additional time to complete your exam.
	Exam broken into segments with rest breaks	This reduces the effects of fatigue and allows you to focus on one section at a time.
	Changes to scheduled exam times	Exams can be scheduled for times when you work best, for example, afternoon rather than morning.
	Exam counting for a smaller portion of your grade	

adolescents. CBT is time limited and focuses on thoughts, behaviors, and feelings and how these components interact and influence each other. In CBT, the therapist facilitates improvements to overall functioning and reductions in symptom severity (e.g., reduced hopelessness) with different strategies including behavioral activation (i.e., encouraging an increase in pleasurable activities), cognitive restructuring (i.e., reducing negative or maladaptive thoughts or beliefs), and enhancing assertiveness and problem-solving skills.

The efficacy of CBT has been established in a substantial body of the literature.[16] For example, a clinical trial was conducted using 107 patients between 13 and 18 years old with major depressive disorder (DSM—III—R) who were randomized to treatment groups involving 12—16 sessions of (1) individual CBT ($N = 37$), (2) systemic behavior family therapy (SBFT; $N = 35$), another intervention used effectively in families, and (3) nondirective supportive treatment (NST; $N = 35$), which was designed to serve as the control (e.g., the therapists refrained from giving advice).[17] The efficacy of CBT was found to be superior relative to SBFT and NST, among the 78 participants who completed the study. Specifically, those who were treated with CBT exhibited a lower rate of major depressive disorder at the end of treatment, relative to the group treated with NST, as well as a more rapid treatment response and a higher rate of remission than both the SBFT and NST treatment groups. All participants had decreased suicidality and increased functioning at the end of the study.

More recently, CBT has also been demonstrated as effective when administered as a computerized intervention (i.e., cCBT). Computer-based online therapies for children and adolescents with depression and anxiety were recently reviewed.[18] In that analysis, four cCBT-based interventional programs (i.e., *MoodGYM*, *Think Feel Do*, *The Journey*, and *SPARX*) were identified to have specifically targeted depression in children and adolescents. The effectiveness of these programs was evaluated in seven randomized controlled trials, providing evidence that such programs can improve depressive symptoms (i.e., 6/7 studies showed either a positive effect on reducing depressive symptoms or on preventing depression, relative to waitlist, placebo, active, or treatment-as-usual control groups). For example, a randomized controlled trial was performed in which 32 adolescents between 13 and 18 years old were randomly assigned to a 5-week cCBT intervention called SPARX or to a waitlist control group. Those in the SPARX group were found to exhibit significant reductions in depressive symptoms and a greater likelihood of being in remission.[19]

Medication

Despite concerns about potential adverse effects, there is still strong empirical evidence supporting the treatment of adolescent depression from both clinical trial data as well as quantitative and qualitative syntheses of the literature. Bridge and colleagues[20] demonstrated that treatment with antidepressants is beneficial for six times as many teenagers as it harms. That being said, using an individualized approach for selecting the specific treatment regimen would be prudent and should involve discussing the benefits and risks of different pharmacotherapies with adolescent patients and their caregivers.

Tricyclic antidepressants or TCAs were among the first generation of antidepressant medications that were prescribed for the treatment of depression in children and adolescents. However, clinical trials demonstrated no benefit of treating children and adolescents with this class of medications. Tricyclic antidepressants were also linked to significant cardiac side effects in patients.

Selective serotonin reuptake inhibitors (SSRIs) are among the second generation of antidepressants used to treat child and adolescent depression. Prescription rates for these medications have been on the rise over the past 2 decades. In fact, the use of this class of antidepressant may have outpaced the evidence base that supports their efficacy for use in young age groups in the 1990s and early 2000s. A recent literature review identified 27 peer-reviewed studies on this topic,[21] including randomized controlled trials on the effectiveness of (1) numerous SSRIs relative to placebo interventions (e.g., fluoxetine, paroxetine, citalopram, etc.) and (2) switching prescriptions from SSRIs to a serotonin norepinephrine reuptake inhibitor (SNRI) called venlafaxine. According to the literature review, the overall outlook on the use of SSRIs for the treatment of child and adolescent depression is positive. The clinical trials to-date, taken as a whole, reveal significant differences between children and adolescents on SSRIs for depression versus those taking placebo interventions; specifically, reporting that between 47% and 69% of patients respond to antidepressants compared to only 33%—57% for those on placebo. The findings at the level of the individual study, on the contrary, are less encouraging. In particular, the strength of the treatment effect appears to vary depending on the specific antidepressant that is studied. For example, at least three trials involving paroxetine have demonstrated negative effects for its influence on the primary outcome measures. Studies on three other SSRIs (i.e., citalopram, escitalopram, and sertraline) have revealed that these particular agents are associated with some improvements in several important outcome measures, but not in all.[20] Of all the agents in the SSRI class of antidepressants, fluoxetine has received the most consistent, high-quality empirical support for its efficacy in treating depression in children and adolescents. Consequently, it is often the first-line treatment, with other SSRIs chosen as a second or third option if the depression appears to be resistant to first-line combination treatment. Table 14.2 summarizes the response rates, dosing, as well as both adverse reactions and effects for common SSRIs.

Adverse effects (e.g., headaches, gastrointestinal upset, etc.) have been found to occur in most children and adolescents who are being treated with antidepressants. Duloxetine, venlafaxine, and paroxetine were the least tolerable in that respect.[21] It is also imperative to draw attention to the controversy that exists in the literature surrounding the treatment of adolescent depression with antidepressant medication given its association with emergent suicidality in children and adolescents. This controversy was addressed in a clinical trial involving 88 medication-free adolescent outpatients between 13 and 18 years old who were receiving treatment for major depressive disorder (DSM–III–R) with 12–16 weeks of psychotherapy only. The adolescents were reported to have no current suicidality at baseline and they were administered one of three forms of psychotherapy: CBT, systemic behavioral family therapy, or nondirective supportive therapy. At the end of treatment, psychotherapy was found to produce rates of new-onset or worsening suicidality that were similar to adolescents being treated with antidepressant medication.[22] The results suggest that having self-reported suicidal thoughts at intake was a significant predictor of emergent suicidality during treatment and intake suicidality should be assessed using self-report as opposed to interview-rated measures.

Regardless of which SSRI is selected for treatment, routine monitoring by clinicians is essential to determine whether there is clinical improvement with treatment, identify the emergence of adverse side effects, and revise the treatment plan accordingly. Clinical practice guidelines dictate that standardized measures and/or forms should be used to document clinical encounters.

Combination therapy. A landmark study, the Treatment for Adolescents with Depression Study (TADS), was a nationally funded randomized controlled trial in which 439 patients between 12 and 17 years old with major depressive disorder (DSM-IV) were assigned randomly to 12 weeks of (1) CBT alone, (2) antidepressant medication alone (i.e., 10–40 mg/d fluoxetine),

(3) a combination of CBT and antidepressant medication, and (4) a placebo (i.e., the equivalent of 10–40 mg/d).[23] The combination therapy (i.e., both CBT and fluoxetine) proved to be superior than the interventions involving either CBT or antidepressant medication alone, as it resulted in higher rates of response and remission, as well as better functioning among study patients. In fact, when treatment with antidepressants was initiated first or in combination with therapy, a more rapid initial response could be observed. The results suggested that, for adolescents with mild-to-moderate depression and no complicating factors (e.g., psychosis or comorbidities), either CBT or antidepressant medication alone can be attempted as an initial treatment. Combination therapy could then be initiated if the patient does not respond to the monotherapeutic approach. On the contrary, for child or adolescent outpatients who have been diagnosed with major depressive disorder, emerging evidence suggests that clinicians should begin combination therapy without delay.

Combination therapy can also play a role in the treatment of depressive episodes that are difficult to treat, as was established by the Treatment of SSRI-Resistant Depression in Adolescents (TORDIA) trial.[24] In that pivotal study, 334 adolescents between 12 and 18 years old who had treatment-resistant major depressive disorder and did not respond to one full regimen of an SSRI were randomly assigned to one of four interventions for a 12-week period: (1) being switched to another SSRI, i.e., paroxetine (Paxil), citalopram (Celexa), or fluoxetine (Prozac); (2) being switched to a different SSRI plus CBT; (3) being switched to venlafaxine (Effexor), an SNRI that some research has shown to be more effective at managing treatment-resistant depression; or (4) being switched to venlafaxine plus CBT. The key finding was that higher response rates were observed in patients who had CBT added to their treatment regimen and had their medication changed to a second SSRI or the SNRI (55%) compared to those who changed their medication alone (41%; $P = .009$). There were no significant differences in the response rate observed between those who were switched to another SSRI or to the SNRI. The three SSRIs tested were also equally effective at eliciting improvements. However, more adverse effects were observed in those treated with the SNRI (i.e., venlafaxine), including the emergence of skin infections and cardiovascular side effects. Therefore, clinicians should first consider switching patients to another SSRI instead.

The treatment of patients who present with both psychotic and depressive symptoms require combination

TABLE 14.2
Selective Serotonin Reuptake Inhibitors: Response Rates, Dosing, and Adverse Reactions/Effects.

Medication	RESPONSE RATES[a, 21]			DOSING[21]				COMMON ADVERSE REACTIONS/EFFECTS[21]					
	Drug (%)	Placebo (%)	Significance (P)	Starting Dose (mg/od)	Effective Dose (mg)	Maximum Dose (mg)	Contraindicated Medications	Headaches	GI Upset	Insomnia	Drowsiness	Agitation	Anxiety
Citalopram	47–51	45–53	NS	10	20	60		⊕	⊕	⊕			⊕
Fluoxetine	52–61	35–37	<0.001–0.03	10	20	60		⊕	⊕	⊕		⊕	
Fluvoxamine		NA[b]		50	150	300	MAOIs	⊕	⊕		⊕		
Paroxetine	65–69	46–57	<0.005–NS	10	20	60		⊕	⊕	⊕		⊕	⊕
Sertraline	63	53	0.05	25	100	200		⊕	⊕	⊕			
Escitalopram	63	52	NS	10	10	20		⊕	⊕	⊕			

⊕, applicable adverse effect; *GI*, gastrointestinal; *MAOIs*, monoamine oxidase inhibitors (a first-generation antidepressant medication); *NA*, not available; *NS*, not significant.

[a] Response rates in randomized controlled trials of antidepressants based on clinical global impression (CGI).

[b] No high-quality studies on the efficacy of treating adolescent depression, but successful for other disorders (e.g., obsessive-compulsive disorder).

treatment. These individuals are commonly prescribed antipsychotics along with antidepressant medications until the psychotic symptoms resolve. Atypical antipsychotics (e.g., risperidone, olanzapine, and quetiapine) are often the first-line treatment. However, there is a paucity of research in this area and therefore, guidance around dosing and medication selection are based on extrapolation from other patient populations, including adults as well as children or adolescents with primary psychotic disorders and/or bipolar disorder. Pappadopulos and colleagues[25] established a collection of 14 evidence- and consensus-based recommendations for treating children and adolescents with serious psychiatric disorders and externalizing behaviors to serve as a guide until more research is conducted on this topic. A comprehensive review of the literature on this topic is presented in the study by Pappadopulos et al.[25] and readers interested in learning more about the use of atypical antipsychotics in children and adolescents are directed to that resource.

In summary, if a child or adolescent fails to respond from initial treatment with an antidepressant, it is recommended that psychotherapy be initiated. Conversely, if a child or adolescent fails to respond to psychotherapy initially, an antidepressant should be considered as adjunct treatment. If combination treatment is initiated as first-line, and response is not established within 12 weeks, clinicians should reassess the child or adolescent to confirm the diagnosis of depression and the occurrence of comorbid illness(es) that might have attenuated treatment benefit. For example, a patient might not respond to depression treatment because their depressive symptoms were secondary to bipolar disorder. Depressive symptoms might also be unresponsive to treatment because of an unrecognized comorbid disorder(s). For example, a patient might have depression and an undiagnosed substance misuse disorder. In cases of undiagnosed comorbid illness(es), clinicians should reconsider the treatment plan to include effective treatment for the comorbid condition(s).

Ongoing Management
Lastly, subsequent to the treatment phase of the clinical management of child and adolescent depression is the ongoing management of this disorder. This phase involves clinical follow-up and continued treatment, as needed. Several long-term studies on the use of antidepressants have been conducted in adolescents with depression. Emslie et al.[26] and Cheung et al.[27] have both examined the effectiveness of continued treatment of antidepressants after acute response (12 weeks). Both

studies demonstrated benefit in continued treatment beyond the first 12 weeks. Furthermore, one additional study (Cheung et al.)[28] examined the benefit of continued treatment after acute response (12 weeks) and continued treatment (24 weeks) and found a trend in support of continued treatment. This emerging evidence supports the clinical guidance from the American Academy of Child and Adolescent Psychiatry Practice Parameters regarding ongoing management.

Summary
Major depression appears to manifest in children and adolescents as a diverse range of symptoms, which if not dealt with, can have significant short and long-term repercussions on the lives of those affected as well as their families. The recent update to the Diagnostic and Statistical Manual of Mental Disorders (DSM-5) reflects the new knowledge that has been generated on this disorder in recent years and coincides with advances in treatment.[10] The assessment and diagnosis of major depression in children and adolescents includes conducting a comprehensive interview with the patient and caregivers as well as a physical examination and appropriate laboratory investigations, establishing rapport with the patient, utilizing validated instruments to assess depressive symptoms, and screening for co-occurring psychiatric disorders. Active monitoring, psychoeducation, safety planning, and referral for peer support are critical components in the initial management of the disorder. Established evidence-based treatments include psychotherapy (e.g., CBT and IPT-A), pharmacotherapy (SSRIs), or a combination of the two approaches. The treatment plan should be tailored for each patient and should involve finding the most suitable balance between the benefits and risks of the therapeutic approach in consultation with patients and their caregivers.

Although the diagnosis and management of depression in the pediatric population continue to bear a strong resemblance to approaches used in adults, clinicians should consider the influence of developmental issues associated with pediatric patients. Future research will undoubtedly lead to more targeted and effective diagnostic and therapeutic approaches for depression in children and adolescents.

REFERENCES
1. Birmaher B, Ryan ND, Williamson DE, Brent DA, Kaufman J. Childhood and adolescent depression: a review of the past 10 years. Part II. *J Am Acad Child Adolesc Psychiatry.* 1996;27:248–251.

2. Kessler R, Walters E. Epidemiology of DSM-III-R major depression and minor depression among adolescents and young adults in the National Comorbidity Survey. *Depress Anxiety*. 1998;7:3−14.

3. Jane Costello E, Erkanli A, Angold A. Is there an epidemic of child or adolescent depression? *J Child Psychol Psychiatry*. 2006;47:1263−1271.

4. Hankin BL, Abramson LY. Development of gender differences in depression: an elaborated cognitive vulnerability-transactional stress theory. *Psychol Bull*. 2001;127:773−796.

5. Hankin BL, Fraley R, Abela J. Daily depression and cognitions about stress: evidence for trait like depressogenic cognitive style and the prediction of depression symptoms trajectories in a prospective daily diary study. *J Personal Soc Psychol*. 2005;88:673−685.

6. Schwartz J, Keonig L. Response styles and negative affect among adolescents. *Cogn Ther Res*. 1996;20:13−36.

7. Gudmundsen G, Rhew I, McCauley E, Kim J, Vander Stoep A. Emergence of depressive symptoms from kindergarten to sixth grade. *J Clin Child Adolesc Psychol*. 2018;7:1−15.

8. Weissman MM, Wolk S, Goldstein RB, et al. Depressed adolescents grown up. *J Am Med Assoc*. 1999;281(18):1707−1713.

9. Curry J, Silva S, Rohde P, Ginsburg G, Kratochvil C, Simons A. Recovery and recurrence following treatment for adolescent major depression. *Arch Gen Psychiatr*. 2011;68:263−269.

10. American Psychiatric Association. *Diagnostic and Statistical Manual of Mental Disorders (DSM-5)*. 5th ed. American Psychiatric Association; 2014.

11. Goodyer I, Dubicka B, Wilkinson P, et al. Selective serotonin reuptake inhibitors (SSRIs) and routine specialist care with and without cognitive behaviour therapy in adolescents with major depression: randomised controlled trial. *BMJ*. 2007;335(7611):142.

12. Bevan Jones R, Thapar A, Stone Z, et al. Psychoeducational interventions in adolescent depression: a systematic review. *Patient Educ Counsel*. 2018;101(5):804−816.

13. Dardas LA, van de Water B, Simmons LA. Parental involvement in adolescent depression interventions: a systematic review of randomized clinical trials. *Int J Ment Health Nurs*. 2018;27:555−570.

14. Mufson L, Weissman MM, Moreau D, Garfinkel R. Efficacy of interpersonal psychotherapy for depressed adolescents. *Arch Gen Psychiatr*. 1999;56:573−579.

15. Mufson L, Dorta KP, Wickramaratne P, Nomura Y, Olfson M, Weissman MM. A randomized effectiveness trial of interpersonal psychotherapy for depressed adolescents. *Arch Gen Psychiatr*. 2004;61(6):577−584.

16. Compton SN, March JS, Brent D, Albano AM, Weersing VR, Curry J. Cognitive-behavioral psychotherapy for anxiety and depressive disorders in children and adolescents: an evidence-based medicine review. *J Am Acad Child Adolesc Psychiatry*. 2004;43(8):930−959.

17. Brent DA, Holder D, Kolko D, et al. A clinical psychotherapy trial for adolescent depression comparing cognitive, family, and supportive therapy. *Arch Gen Psychiatr*. 1997;54(9):877−885.

18. Stasiak K, Fleming T, Lucassen MFG, Shepherd MJ, Whittaker R, Merry SN. Computer-based and online therapy for depression and anxiety in children and adolescents. *J Child Adolesc Psychopharmacol*. 2016;26(3):235−245.

19. Fleming T, Dixon R, Frampton C, Merry S. A pragmatic randomized controlled trial of computerized CBT (SPARX) for symptoms of depression among adolescents excluded from mainstream education. *Behav Cognit Psychother*. 2011;40:529−541.

20. Bridge JA, Iyengar S, Salary CB, et al. Clinical response and risk for reported suicidal ideation and suicide attempts in pediatric antidepressant treatment: a meta-analysis of randomized controlled trials. *J Am Med Assoc*. 2007;297(15):1683−1696.

21. Cheung AH, Zuckerbrot RA, Jensen PS, Laraque D, Stein REK, GLAD-PC Steering Group. Guidelines for adolescent depression in primary care (GLAD-PC): part II. Treatment and ongoing management. *Pediatrics*. 2018;141(3). e20174082−18.

22. Bridge JA, Barbe RP, Birmaher B, Kolko DJ, Brent DA. Emergent suicidality in a clinical psychotherapy trial for adolescent depression. *Am J Psychiatry*. 2005;162(11):2173−2175.

23. March J, Silva S, Petrycki S, et al. Fluoxetine, cognitive-behavioral therapy, and their combination for adolescents with depression: treatment for adolescents with depression study (TADS) randomized controlled trial. *J Am Med Assoc*. 2004;292(7):807−820.

24. Brent DA. The treatment of SSRI-resistant depression in adolescents (TORDIA): in search of the best next step. *Depress Anxiety*. 2009;26(10):871−874.

25. Pappadopulos E, Macintyre II JC, Crismon ML, et al. Treatment recommendations for the use of antipsychotics for aggressive youth (TRAAY). Part II. *J Am Acad Child Adolesc Psychiatry*. 2003;42(2):145−161.

26. Emslie GJ, Heiligenstein JH, Hoog SL, et al. Fluoxetine treatment for prevention of relapse of depression in children and adolescents: a double-blind, placebo-controlled study. *J Am Acad Child Adolesc Psychiatry*. 2004;43(11):1397−1405.

27. Cheung A, Levitt A, Cheng M, et al. A pilot study of citalopram treatment in preventing relapse of depressive episode after acute treatment. *J Can Acad Child Adolesc Psychiatry*. 2016;25(1):11−16.

28. Cheung A, Kusumakar V, Kutcher S, et al. Maintenance study for adolescent depression. *J Child Adolesc Psychopharmacol*. 2008;18(4):389−394.

29. Huestis L. *Your Education-Your Future*. Canadian Mental Health Association; 2004.

Index

Note: Page numbers followed by "t" indicate tables and "f" indicate figures.